The **Integrated Case Management Manual**

*Assisting Complex Patients Regain
Physical and Mental Health*

Roger G. Kathol, MD, acquired extensive experience in the clinical integration of general medical and mental health services for complex patients as the director of a Complexity Intervention Unit (the new term for Medical Psychiatry Unit) at the University of Iowa Hospitals between 1986 and 1999. Thereafter, he assisted in the integration of physical and mental health care management as medical director at Blue Cross Blue Shield of Minnesota for several years. As president of Cartesian Solutions, Inc., he has consulted to numerous national and international organizations, hospitals and clinics, insurance companies, care management companies, employers, and government agencies wishing to coordinate medical and mental health care management services. In these positions, he has designed many integrated case management programs and trained case managers and practicing physicians from varied specialties in cross-disciplinary techniques so that they could coordinate care for patients with multimorbidity. Dr. Kathol has over 150 peer-reviewed publications related to the interaction of general medical and mental health disorders, and, with Suzanne Gatteau, has authored a book, *Healing Body and Mind: A Critical Issue for Health Care Reform,* (2007) which explains how to transition today's siloed care to integrated care through purchaser, health plan, provider, and patient partnerships.

Rebecca Perez, RN, BSN, CCM, has experienced firsthand the impact that segregation of physical and behavioral health has on the coordination of care, health service delivery, and patient outcomes during 15 years in acute care nursing and 15 in case management. As a result, Ms. Perez, a resident of St. Louis, Missouri, coauthored the depression chapter of the *Case Management Adherence Guidelines* (2006), has written numerous patient education articles on case management integration, and has presented nationally on and contributed to the development of integrated case management curricula. She currently serves on the national board of directors for the Case Management Society of America and has been active in her local chapter. Ms. Perez is president and owner of Carative Health Solutions, which provides direct care/case management services and consults to case management professionals on strategies to apply integrated case management principles in their programs. She has been involved in the creation of the integrated case management training curriculum at the Case Management Society of America since its inception and is currently an accredited trainer.

Janice S. Cohen, PhD, CPsych, is a clinical psychologist at the Children's Hospital of Eastern Ontario (CHEO), as well as clinical professor in the School of Psychology at the University of Ottawa. Throughout her career, Dr. Cohen's clinical and research activities have focused on children and youth who have complex medical and mental health issues. As clinical head of the Behavioural Neurosciences and Consultation Liaison Team at CHEO, she has championed integrative collaborative health care, most recently through her initiative to develop a multifaceted clinical decision-making tool, the Pediatric INTERMED Complexity Assessment Grid (PIM-CAG), to improve assessment and treatment planning for children and youth with complex health needs. Dr. Cohen is currently principal investigator of a funded research project at CHEO examining the psychometric properties of the PIM-CAG in children and youth with inflammatory bowel diseases. She is a recipient of an Expertise Mobilization Award from the Provincial Centre of Excellence for Child and Youth Mental Health at CHEO in support of her work on the development of the PIM-CAG. Dr. Cohen's other ongoing research projects include a multisite Canadian study investigating knowledge translation strategies in pediatric procedural pain. For over a decade, Dr. Cohen also served as the Director of Training in Psychology at CHEO and has received awards from national and international professional bodies for her contributions to training.

The Integrated Case Management Manual

Assisting Complex Patients Regain Physical and Mental Health

Roger G. Kathol, MD

Rebecca Perez, RN, BSN, CCM

Janice S. Cohen, PhD, CPsych

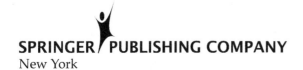
SPRINGER PUBLISHING COMPANY
New York

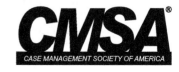
CASE MANAGEMENT SOCIETY OF AMERICA

Springer Publishing Company, LLC
11 West 42nd Street
New York, NY 10036
www.springerpub.com

Acquisitions Editor: Margaret Zuccarini
Production Editor: Gayle Lee
Cover Design: Armen Kojoyian
Composition: Emily Johnston at Apex CoVantage

ISBN: 978-0-8261-0633-9
E-book ISBN: 978-0-8261-0634-6

10 11 12 13 / 5 4 3 2 1

The authors and the publisher of this Work have made every effort to use sources believed to be reliable to provide information that is accurate and compatible with the standards generally accepted at the time of publication. Because medical science is continually advancing, our knowledge base continues to expand. Therefore, as new information becomes available, changes in procedures become necessary. We recommend that the reader always consult current research and specific institutional policies before performing any clinical procedure. The authors and publisher shall not be liable for any special, consequential, or exemplary damages resulting, in whole or in part, from the readers' use of, or reliance on, the information contained in this book. The publisher has no responsibility for the persistence or accuracy of URLs for external or third-party Internet Web sites referred to in this publication and does not guarantee that any content on such Web sites is, or will remain, accurate or appropriate.

Library of Congress Cataloging-in-Publication Data

Kathol, Roger G.
   The integrated case management manual : assisting complex patients regain physical and mental health / Roger G. Kathol, Rebecca Perez, Janice S. Cohen.
      p. ; cm.
   Includes bibliographical references and index.
   ISBN 978-0-8261-0633-9 (print) — ISBN 978-0-8261-0634-6 (e-book)   1. Hospitals—Case management services.   I. Perez, Rebecca.   II. Cohen, Janice S.   III. Title.
   [DNLM: 1. Case Management—organization & administration.   2. Comorbidity.   3. Continuity of Patient Care—organization & administration.   4. Delivery of Health Care, Integrated—organization & administration.   W 84.7 K195i   2010]
   RA975.5.C36K37 2010
   362.11068—dc22   2010017014

Printed in the United States of America by Bang Printing.

Contents

Appendices

Case Management Flowcharts

Triaging and Informed Consent Tools

INTERMED-Complexity Assessment Grids

Templates for Care Plan Development and Outcome Measurement

Abbreviations and Terminology

European INTERMED in English

Appendices Available on Springer Web Site (www.springerpub.com/kathol)

Foreword

In today's U.S. health care system, mental illness is either treated separately from physical disease (15%) or goes poorly or untreated (85%), leading to persistent physical and mental illness, disability, and high health care service use. At the same time there is increasing empirical evidence that integrated care—that is, combining physical and mental condition treatment—in multimorbid patients improves quality of life and medical outcomes while reducing total health care costs.

Case managers are a vital element in the health care delivery system. They work with patients and their family/caregivers in providing case management, care coordination, and resource management. Yet, in today's world, case managers coming from physical health backgrounds focus *solely* on assisting with physical disease, and those coming from mental health backgrounds focus *solely* on mental health care, with little or no coordination of the support services they provide. Patients find this type of care management frustrating and often voice their dissatisfaction with such a fragmented approach to their care needs. This fragmented approach may lead not only to patient dissatisfaction but also to medication errors, to patient safety concerns, to miscommunication, and to duplication of resource use.

Case managers need to learn and deploy a new set of skills in supporting multimorbid patients. It is essential to assess both medical and mental health issues in a single evaluation and to coordinate appropriate integrated health interventions and treatment planning to achieve effective strategies for safe care. Yet case managers need tools and resources for deploying an integrated health model (physical and mental health treatment) to the medically complex patient.

The Case Management Society of America (CMSA), a multidisciplinary organization committed to support-ing the development of case management professionals, is excited about the new approach to care outlined in this book. Case managers studying this manual will enhance their knowledge about physical and mental health conditions and will learn a new evaluation and assistance technology to help facilitate care for complex patients. The program is particularly appropriate for case managers who wish to augment their skill sets. Additionally, disease managers who are involved with the thorough assessment of medically complex patients will also find this program of value.

Case managers are part of a collaborative partnership in emerging models of care delivery within multidisciplinary health care teams. Being prepared and using an integrated case management approach will assist them in contributing to the research of improving efficiency, effectiveness, accountability, and positive outcomes in their clinical settings.

CMSA would like to acknowledge Dr. Roger Kathol for his commitment to case management and his efforts in developing a comprehensive educational resource for the professional development of integrated health case managers. Dr. Kathol, working with a collaborative team, has published this manual and has created an accompanying course that builds on CMSA's strategic initiative of education and research in acknowledging case managers as pioneers of health care change.

CMSA encourages you to enhance your ability to work with complex patients, learn how to apply new, evidence-based assessments, and push forward the change needed for improved quality and safe care for all patients.

Cheri Lattimer, RN, BSN
Executive Director, Case Management
Society of America

Preface

Having provided clinical services to patients at the interface of general medicine and psychiatry throughout our professional careers, we have been impressed with the degree to which health issues related to the mind and body interact. Yet each of us work in systems of care that rigorously separate and approach physical and mental conditions as if the mind and body have no connection. The purpose of this book, therefore, is to help case managers see that the assessment and treatment of mental health and general medical conditions are more similar than dissimilar. Segregation of care in these domains, and in other domains that create barriers to health, is counterproductive. Rather, assistance with return to health can be more effectively and efficiently accomplished when a unified approach is used.

This manual was written to apply this principle to the practice of case management, a discipline in which nurses and other health professionals assist patients/clients (hereafter referred to as patients) with health complexity in overcoming barriers to improvement. Case managers were chosen as the target audience for this manual because they primarily and routinely work with patients who have multiple, poorly controlled health conditions, a high percentage of which involve both general medical and mental health issues and/or social and health system challenges. Their patients are also the ones who use a high percentage of health resources. Thus, if improved support for their care can be achieved through the systematic application of complexity measurement and an integrated approach to breaking down complexity-based health barriers in multiple domains, we reason that case managers can become major contributors to better health at a lower total health-related cost as care delivery and payment reform measures are introduced.

We consider this manual to be an introduction to the next generation of case management: integrated case management. Unlike traditional case management, it guides case managers with either medical or mental health backgrounds as they develop skills that will allow them to connect and assist with health issues in the biological, psychological, social, and health system domains while maintaining a personal relationship with the patient. Patient handoffs are the exception and follow through on care manager assistance over time is the rule.

Integrated case management does this by linking health complexity assessments to integrated assistance techniques. Based on a color-coded level of complexity grid (see color tables), case managers prioritize associated barriers to improvement in various domains, build care plans, and assist patients as they stabilize or return to health. Core components in the integrated case management process include: a relationship and communication between complex patients and the case manager, a longitudinal outcomes orientation, the systematic assessment of complexity, the use of complexity item scores and their interactions to guide health improvement actions, and case manager accountability for health outcomes in all risks and needs domains. In essence, the integrated process transforms traditional case management into an approach that systematizes assessments, connects evaluation findings to multi-domain actions, and moves managed patients toward documentable improvement and graduation.

Case managers studying this manual will develop new and important cross-disciplinary skills, which will allow them to alter the health trajectory of some of the most needy patients in the health system.

Tools, which help them initiate programs and complete this task, can be found in the Appendices at the back of the manual. Additional support documents can be found on the Springer Publishing Web site (www.springerpub.com/kathol) and Case Management Society of America (CMSA) Web site. For those wishing to initiate integrated case management programs in their practice location and have completed training in integrated case management practices, Health Insurance Portability and Accountability Act (HIPAA) compliant software documentation support is available on the CMSA Web site or can be purchased for onsite installation from CMSA.

Roger G. Kathol, MD
Rebecca Perez, RN, BSN, CCM
Janice S. Cohen, PhD, CPsych

Acknowledgments

The following professionals deserve recognition for the ideas, insights, editorial comments, and general suggestions that they made to this completed work. Some contributed to formative development of the organization and content, as the original drafts were written (Rachel Happel, RN, and Byron Bair, MD), while others reviewed content shortly before the manual was sent to the publisher (Jessica Cox, RN, Frits Huyse, MD, PhD, Mary Kathol, MD, Corine Latour, RN, PhD, Dan Rome, MD, and Pat Stricker, RN, MEd). Some provided suggestions and edits for specific sections of the book (Peter Dehnel, MD, Jos Dobber, MSc, Corine Latour, RN, PhD, John Lyons, PhD, William Sheehan, MD, Read Sulik, MD, Steve Thurber, PhD, and Shirelle Washington, RN).

Others, many of whom are members of the INTERMED Foundation Board, contributed through discussions, by providing general insights about various topics included in the book (Peter de Jonge, PhD, Frits Huyse, MD, PhD, Corine Latour, RN, PhD, Elena Lobo, PhD, Joris Slaets, MD, PhD, Wolfgang Söllner, MD, and Frederick Stiefel, MD). Still others contributed ideas related to iterative changes made as field testing with case managers was performed during the two years prior to publication (Deborah Gutteridge, MS, Shirelle Washington, RN, and Cheri Lattimer, RN, BSN). The authors also wish to thank over 80 case managers who participated in developmental phases of integrated case management training for their valuable feedback about the manual and the training process. Without their input, this manual would not have been possible.

Finally, special appreciation goes to Mary Kathol, MD, who provided invaluable suggestions regarding the educational presentation and manual formatting.

Overview of the Development
of the INTERMED Method

The literature presents relevant arguments substantiating the effectiveness of the assessment and treatment of psychosocial comorbidities when they are integrated into the provision of general medical care. Based on this, in 1995, an international group, including Frits Huyse (the Netherlands), John Lyons (United States), Fritz Stiefel (Switzerland), Joris Slaets (the Netherlands), and Peter De Jonge (the Netherlands), supported by a European grant, began to synchronize their individual research and clinical strategies to develop an integrated approach toward the care of the complex medically ill. In 2008 Roger Kathol (United States), among others, joined the group. The outcome of this group's work is the INTERMED method: a practical, visualized approach to risk and needs management, including decision support and outcomes management. One goal of the INTERMED method is to operationalize the biopsychosocial model of disease and to fill the gap between general medical care and mental health care. Another goal is to improve the health care provider's awareness of patients' integrated health risks and needs through the systematic assessment represented in the Complexity Assessment Grids, which counteract these risks and deliver preventive and thereby cost-effective care. Three specialized versions of the Complexity Assessment Grid are currently in a process of validation; a *geriatric version,* a *U.S. case management adult version,* and a *U.S. case management pediatric version.*

The INTERMED method is supported by an Internet-based software in Europe (www.intermedfoundation.org). The current adult European version 6, which was developed based on empirical studies using previous versions, makes the method generic for application in epidemiologic studies, as well as in primary and secondary care.

THE PEDIATRIC INTERMED COMPLEXITY ASSESSMENT GRID (PIM-CAG)

In 2005 Frits Huyse, John Lyons, Lise Bisnaire (Children's Hospital of Eastern Ontario) and Janice Cohen (Children's Hospital of Eastern Ontario) began developing an adaptation of the INTERMED tool for use with children and youth. Other members of the development group included Roger Kathol (Cartesian Solutions, Inc.), Peter Dehnel (pediatrician in Minnesota), and Read Sulik (jointly boarded child psychiatrist and pediatrician from Minnesota), among others. In fall 2009 a pediatric version for case managers, which is complementary to the U.S. case management adult version (25 variables), was developed for inclusion in this manual. Janice Cohen, involved in the construction of the case management version, continues to conduct her research with the original version of the tool, which consists of 33 variables. In Lausanne, Switzerland, in November 2009, during a council meeting of the INTERMED Foundation, the 33-variable version was endorsed as the Pediatric INTERMED, version 1 (PIM v1). The 25-variable version is a specialized version of the PIM v1 for case managers.

Introduction

OBJECTIVES

- To give an overview of the manual
- To summarize the principles and value of integrated case management
- To explain the importance of studying the manual
- To describe the addition of integrated pediatric case management
- To indicate the level of proficiency at the completion of manual study
- To encourage international application of integrated case management principles and practice

Integrated case management is characterized by a health professional giving personal multidimensional assistance to targeted patients with health complexity as they learn how to regain stable health and function.

MANUAL OVERVIEW

This manual is an introductory text for integrated case management. It is intended to expand the skill set of practicing case managers, from nursing and other health professions. It has been written to address the training needs of case managers coming from either general medical or mental health sector backgrounds and should allow them to work with patients experiencing both physical and mental health barriers to improvement. It teaches them a new and systematic approach to the evaluation of and assistance for biological, psychological, social, and health system problems. These are four targeted domains that contribute to health complexity and lead to medical and mental health treatment resistance, persistent symptoms and illness complications, functional impairment, and high health care service use.

The manual can also serve as a companion textbook for advanced-level nursing and social work courses given at academic institutions worldwide. While it is an introductory text for integrated case management, this is an area of practice with sufficient complexity that those studying the manual should have a firm grasp of basic knowledge and skills in their specialty area, such as nursing (nurses), social services (social workers), medicine (physicians), rehabilitation (disability/workers' compensation counselors), and so forth; comfort with general medical *or* mental health care; and a willingness to learn the cross-disciplinary and health complexity content used in integrated case management.

Finally, the manual will serve as the source for knowledge-based material associated with the Case Management Society of America (CMSA) integrated case management certificate course. Those studying the manual for this course will be expected to attend local or Web-based seminars and pass tests related to each chapter prior to entry into a face-to-face onsite training experience.

INTEGRATED CASE MANAGEMENT

The integrated case management manual has been under development since 2006, albeit in pieces, and is based on 15 years of research from sources throughout the world. It is the composite work of many individuals and research groups that have had a vested interest in addressing the needs of patients heretofore orphaned because their illnesses fell at the interface of noncommunicating segments of the health system, the general medical and behavioral health sectors. Evidence accumulating now shows that a high percentage of the few patients with health complexity, which use the majority of health care resources, have concurrent physical and behavioral issues contributing to poor outcomes. With this knowledge, it has now been possible to garner support for the development of this manual and the training program associated with it.

A core component of integrated case management, grounded in a relationship-based approach to interaction with patients, includes the ability to assist patients with complexity receive integrated physical health, mental health, and substance use disorder services without cross-disciplinary handoffs. However, it is also designed in such a way that it evaluates and incorporates action steps in the social and health system domains, both of which create barriers to improved health outcomes in their own right. It does this through the use of complexity assessment technology, the adult (IM-CAG) and pediatric (PIM-CAG) INTERMED-Complexity Assessment Grid, imported from Europe (de Jonge, Hoogervorst, Huyse, & Polman, 2004; de Jonge, Huyse, Stiefel, Slaets, & Gans, 2001; Huyse, de Jonge, Lyons, Stiefel, & Slaets, 1999; Huyse, Lyons et al., 1999; Latour, Huyse, de Vos, & Stalman, 2007; Stiefel et al., 1999; Stiefel et al., 2006), which has been adapted for application in health systems throughout the world.

The program goes far beyond linking physical and mental health needs. It more accurately focuses on uncovering and equally addressing barriers to improved health outcomes in complex patients in multiple domains. Put simply, patients who are candidates for case management, regardless of whether they have *only* general medical problems, *only* mental health or chemical dependence problems, or *both,* can be helped using the single evaluation and assistance paradigm taught in this manual.

Additional positive features available through use of the integrated case management framework of care include the following:

- The incorporation of practical high-risk case finding and enrollment procedures as a first step in value-based case management programs
- A systematic strategy in performing assessments with the stratification of actionable items
- The ability to assess, develop care plans, and provide integrated case management for complex children, adolescents, and adults
- An outcome-oriented method to estimate the number of cases that a case manager can carry and still perform effective case management
- An approach for case managers to document progress in overcoming barriers to health for the patients with whom they work
- A mechanism to measure clinical, functional, financial, quality of life, and satisfaction performance for patients, providers, and health managers—individually and in aggregate
- Steps to case closure
- A means to measure the value brought to populations or to purchasers through integrated case management using complexity assessment grid (CAG) technology.

Those studying this manual will come from diverse health care backgrounds. Many will be nurses, but not all. Many will have backgrounds in which the majority of their prior clinical activity has been provided to general medical patients. Others will have devoted most of their time to the development of skills related to the care of patients with mental health or substance use disorders. The chapters of the integrated case management manual have been created with this in mind. They are intended to provide the basics needed, regardless of the reader's background, to initiate the practice of cross-disciplinary case management.

MANUAL STUDY

The number of hours needed by integrated case management professionals to master the knowledge base found in the manual will vary based on their prior training, background, and experience. In addition to the manual, however, there are also supplemental readings suggested in the text. These supplementary materials facilitate the development of the skills needed to gain cross-disciplinary information about the health conditions of their patients. This, along with the face-to-face application of learned information about integrated case management, is considered a core feature of the learning process.

Those with more extensive health system and case management experience will find that the manual expands their understanding of health complexity and approaches that improve complex patient outcomes. For those with experience in both the medical and psychiatric health sectors, some of the material will already be familiar. For none, however, will it be possible to initiate integrated case management practices without studying the manual because all will need to: (a) understand how to link open-ended questions with cells in the IM-CAG and PIM-CAG, (b) know how to use CAG anchor points to complete patient assessments, (c) know how to connect CAG scores from items in its four domains to concrete actions and to create care plans, and (d) be able to systematically work with patients through health improvement while documenting health change for patients and value to the health system. That is information currently found only in this manual.

For those intending to use the knowledge base derived from manual study, the CMSA has developed a face-to-face training course designed to allow case managers to consolidate their understanding of the integrated case management approach, practice asking questions outlined in the manual in typical case management mock scenarios under the supervision of certified integrated case management trainers, score the IM-CAG and PIM-CAG using established anchor points, and initiate integrated case management procedures. Those completing the adult and pediatric course will receive a certificate of completion through CMSA. Case management supervisors, working in developed programs specializing in case management, will have the opportunity to become certified trainers for personnel working in their system through a train-the-trainer course offered through CMSA.

For those taking a course in integrated case management through accredited academic programs, it is anticipated that the manual course would be accompanied by practicum application in the clinical setting before integrated case management training would be considered complete. Ultimately, it is anticipated that integrated case management will become an area of nursing and social work practice with advanced certification requirements.

INTEGRATED PEDIATRIC CASE MANAGEMENT

One of the most consistent recommendations of those participating in the beta testing of the adult integrated case management manual and training program was that a pediatric version of integrated case management ought to be developed. In this manual, a pediatric version is introduced, which has been developed through the collaborative efforts of pediatricians, child psychiatrists and child psychologists, pediatric case managers, and investigators who were involved in the development of the adult integrated case management program. While the pediatric version does not yet have the same depth of research supporting its use in children and adolescents that the adult version does, readers will recognize the parallel between the adult and pediatric versions yet readily appreciate the differences. The PIM-CAG contains five additional items—that is, cognitive development, adverse developmental events, caregiver/parent health and function, caregiver/family support, and school functioning—in addition to alteration of the content of several items in the IM-CAG to make it pertinent to children and youth (e.g., in the social/family domain "Job and Leisure" is changed to "School and Community Participation").

Pediatric integrated case management is in its infancy but it can draw on the 15 years of experience with the IM-CAG and the expertise of clinicians who recognize the challenges of children and youth with health complexity. The authors of the first edition of this book are fully aware of the need for formative research using this approach to improve care for children and adolescents who present challenges to their many treating practitioners due to a complicated interplay of personal, health, social, and health system factors that will predictably lead to poor short- and long-term outcomes. Nonetheless, they felt that one of the ways in which research could be facilitated would be to develop the starting pediatric methodology based on experience from the adult setting. Health complexity

does not appear to differentiate among populations of different ages. Children and adolescents with complex presentations are as likely as adults to demonstrate treatment resistance, symptom persistence, personal and social impairment, and high health care service use as adults. It just did not make sense to delay the availability of integrated case management for them while waiting for basic research to be completed.

Importantly, there is little downside to introducing the pediatric version at this point. Experience with adult integrated case management suggests that children exposed to a pediatric equivalent should do better than those who are not exposed. Treating providers will be supported in their care and potentially have better outcomes for their patients. Finally, since children and adolescents with health complexity will be targeted for intervention, purchasers of care and those who distribute health resources to providers of care should see a reduction in total health care spending. Improved health of their highest-cost enrollees should lead to lower total health care service use.

Since pediatric integrated case management has a number of additional training variables that require attention as its clinical implementation is rolled out, additional face-to-face training, offered by CMSA after completion of the face-to-face adult training, will be necessary to obtain a pediatric certificate of completion. Those completing the pediatric training program will be equipped to address the needs of children and adolescents as well as their adult caregivers/parents. While they may choose to focus clinical attention on children/youth and the family unit, with the combined training they will be able to recognize when they are able to address the case management needs of the family unit and when the caregiver/parent may require referral to obtain their own case management support. As with adult integrated case management, a pediatric integrated case management training course will be offered for supervisors of developed pediatric case management training programs.

INTERNATIONAL APPLICATION OF INTEGRATED CASE MANAGEMENT PRINCIPLES AND PRACTICE

The principles of integrated case management delineated in the "Integrated Case Management" section above can be applied in health systems throughout the world. While this manual is primarily written for a U.S. case manager readership, with adaptation, case managers in many clinical settings, who provide services in other cultures and countries, can use the core integrated case management principles to better respond to the needs of their complex patients. Health complexity, as defined by the INTERMED system

(Huyse & Stiefel, 2006), which will be discussed in detail in following chapters, creates barriers to improvement in a small percentage of all peoples regardless of nationality, culture, or health system organization. Changing practice, based on the principles laid out in this manual, can thus improve health, reduce disability, and lower the total cost of care in some of the most difficult to treat and costly patients in virtually all health systems.

With this in mind, those reading this manual who live in other countries and work in health care environments that have different strengths and weaknesses than those found in the United States are encouraged to focus on the core components of integrated case management found in this manual that would bring value to patients seen in their clinical settings and health systems. For some this may mean altering the mechanism used to identify patients for assistance through integrated case management. For others, it may mean altering the items included in the Complexity Assessment Grid or the actions related to item anchor points. For still others, it may mean altering job descriptions of key case management personnel so that they can take a longitudinal view as they work with complex patients in their system.

Many of the recommendations in this manual regarding components of integrated case management are concrete and specific and often relate to health practices commonly used in the U.S. system of care. By providing this type of structure, it helps those studying integrated case management procedures to build a mental picture of what integrated management would look like in operation. In the United States, however, there are many variations in the approach to care. Thus, though the examples may relate to care delivery situations in the United States, even in the United States, program customization is usually required. We encourage readers in other countries and cultures to do the same.

BASELINE KNOWLEDGE AND FUTURE GROWTH

The integrated case management manual and face-to-face implementation training are designed to provide the basics in working with patients with health complexity. Both knowledge-based and operational aspects are considered essential components for the initiation of integrated case management activities in a clinical setting. U.S. and international case management practices vary widely. For this reason, we consider that adherence to the basic principles of integrated case management set forth in this manual and its accompanying training course is necessary in order for the programs adopting it to consistently bring value to their patients and health system.

Solidification of knowledge and skills, however, occurs as case managers start working with real patients. After reading and studying the manual and learning to apply its principles, the next stage of training occurs at the case manager's worksite through case conferences, supervisory relationships (both medical and psychiatric), continuing education, and staff level cross-fertilization. Those who invest themselves well and have support through their place of employment will find that they become more and more proficient in assisting most patients with complex and comorbid general medical and mental conditions. By the third to fourth month of initiating the use of integrated management practices, most case managers will feel comfortable in the use of the CAG and cross-disciplinary service to patients. Importantly, they will understand where their limitations lie and know where to find answers for the interesting and perplexing challenges their patients present.

Welcome to the next generation of case management. We hope you appreciate the value that you will bring to the patients you encounter using integrated approaches to case management assistance. Perhaps more importantly, we hope you derive as much pleasure as we have in assisting some of the most complicated patients in our health system recapture their humanity through return to health stability.

REFERENCES

de Jonge, P., Hoogervorst, E. L., Huyse, F. J., & Polman, C. H. (2004). INTERMED: A measure of biopsychosocial case complexity: One year stability in multiple sclerosis patients. *General Hospital Psychiatry, 26*(2), 147–152.

de Jonge, P., Huyse, F. J., Stiefel, F. C., Slaets, J. P., & Gans, R. O. (2001). INTERMED—A clinical instrument for biopsychosocial assessment. *Psychosomatics, 42*(2), 106–109.

Huyse, F. J., de Jonge, P., Lyons, J. S., Stiefel, F. C., & Slaets, J. P. (1999). INTERMED: A tool for controlling for confounding variables and designing multimodal treatment. *Journal of Psychosomatic Research, 46*(4), 401–402.

Huyse, F. J., Lyons, J. S., Stiefel, F. C., Slaets, J. P., de Jonge, P., Fink, P., et al. (1999). "INTERMED": A method to assess health service needs. I. Development and reliability. *General Hospital Psychiatry, 21*(1), 39–48.

Huyse, F. J., & Stiefel, F. C. (Eds.). *Integrated care for the complex medically ill.* [Special issue.]. Medical Clinics of North America, 90 (2006).

Latour, C. H., Huyse, F. J., de Vos, R., & Stalman, W. A. (2007). A method to provide integrated care for complex medically ill patients: The INTERMED. *Nursing Health Science, 9*(2), 150–157.

Stiefel, F. C., de Jonge, P., Huyse, F. J., Guex, P., Slaets, J. P., Lyons, J. S., et al. (1999). "INTERMED": A method to assess health service needs. II. Results on its validity and clinical use. *General Hospital Psychiatry, 21*(1), 49–56.

Stiefel, F. C., Huyse, F. J., Sollner, W., Slaets, J. P., Lyons, J. S., Latour, C. H., et al. (2006). Operationalizing integrated care on a clinical level: The INTERMED project. *Medical Clinics of North America, 90*(4), 713–758.

CHAPTER 1

Case Management, Integrated Case Management, and Complexity Assessment Grids

- To review health system changes that led to the development of the specialty of case management
- To differentiate the types of care management, of which case management is one
- To summarize the 2010 *Standards of Practice for Case Management*
- To describe the difference between the application of traditional versus integrated case management
- To introduce concepts related to Complexity Assessment Grid (CAG) methodology
- To discuss the synergy between the goals of integrated case management and use of CAG methodology

INTRODUCTION

Before health care became big business and was recognized to have a major effect on national economies, the focus of medical practice for most physicians was to assist patients in the process of healing. For some this meant cure from an acute illness, for some stabilization of a chronic illness, and for others support through the progression of an ultimately fatal condition. For all, however, the physician-patient encounter addressed more than the illness of the patient. It was a pact in which all of the issues contributing to a patient's potential improvement were factored into the therapeutic relationship. Telling the patient about his or her illness and its consequences; involving the patient's significant others in discussions about treatment; ensuring ways to get medications and get to appointments; discussing life stresses; addressing communication barriers; and dealing with the patient's emotional state were all a part of this pact. The doctor and patient were conspirators in a quest to maximize the patient's health.

This changed when national health systems began looking for ways to streamline patient-doctor encounters to reduce costs. In an attempt to efficiently use limited health care resources given by high-cost health care providers during the past 25 years, medical visits have been transformed. Addressing so-called illness issues and delivering specific health-related services has become the center of the doctor-patient interaction. Discussions about physical and mental health findings, test results, and treatment options form content during 7- to 15-minute clinic appointments. Physician throughput has become as large a goal as patient improvement and is often mandated by hospital or clinic administrators dedicated to maximizing clinical service income.

For 70% of patients, this change has led to no disruption in health because they are healthy, have uncomplicated or readily treatable disease, or have sufficient intellect or personal resources to make it through their illness episode (left side of **Figure 1.1**). For the 30% of patients with chronic disease or the complex interactions of illness and life situations, however, the transition has led to more difficulty in managing their health, higher clinical care service use, and more disability for conditions that may have been less impairing in years past.

This problem initiated the development of a new industry, the care management industry, in which clinical, health system-savvy personnel assist the 20% of patients/clients (hereafter referred to as patients) that use four-fifths of health care services, as well as those who are at risk of falling into this group of patients in the future. These professionals try to help their patients understand their illnesses, overcome biopsychosocial and health system barriers to improvement, adhere to their providers' recommended treatments, and navigate health systems that have become so complicated and fragmented that many patients do not even know who to ask for help, let alone for what to ask.

FIGURE 1.1 Health care cost savings opportunity.

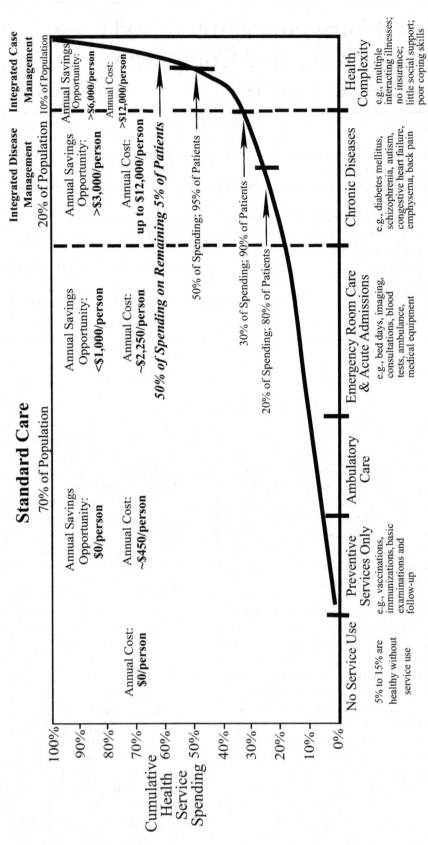

Average Annual Per Capita Health Care Costs: $6,100 in 2007 US$

Adapted with permission from Minnesota Medical Association, Physicians' Plan for a Healthy Minnesota: The Minnesota Medical Association's Proposal for Health Care Reform. Supplement to Minnesota Medicine, March 2005, p. 9.

CARE MANAGEMENT

The term *care management* has many definitions within the health care industry. In this book, we have chosen to define it as the use of trained health personnel (mostly nurses, but also social workers, psychologists, rehabilitation counselors, and other health professionals, including some physicians) to work directly with selected populations of patients in an attempt to improve their health and thus contain their health-related costs. Care managers do not treat patients. Rather, they collaborate with patients to facilitate healthy behaviors and improve health outcomes in those at risk for developing or who already have health complexity or illness combinations. Care managers are described by a variety of names (**Exhibit 1.1**). These names portray the locations in which the care managers work and the populations that they serve.

At the prevention end, there are health coaches and wellness counselors. They assist those at risk for poor outcomes unless healthy behaviors are adopted. The thrust for these coaches and counselors is to foster healthy eating habits, exercise, and preventive measures known to reduce the onset of illness or illness progression. For those with specific chronic illnesses, there are disease managers. Disease managers educate the patients that they work with about their illness or illnesses and treatments (e.g., diabetes, depression, kidney disease, etc.). In some settings, disease managers also help patients learn strategies and skills designed to help them stabilize symptoms and prevent progression. At the illness acuity/severity end, disease managers may actively evaluate and assist patients with obtaining disease-specific, evidence-based practices from their treating providers. When evidence-based services are not being delivered, the disease manager collaborates with the patient in overcoming disease-specific barriers to improvement (e.g., adherence to recommended treatment, documentation of clinical outcome variables, attendance at appointments, seeking second opinions from other specialists, etc.).

For employees who develop a medical condition that is either the result of a work-related event (workers' compensation) or merely interferes with an employee's ability to perform at work (disability/rehabilitation), there are managers who facilitate efficient use of the medical system and advocate, on behalf of the employee, for effective medical support. Employee assistance programs (EAPs) provide another form of care management. While focusing on worksite issues, such as personnel conflicts, jobsite reentry after an illness, and so forth, they also often help employees get needed health services, such as through substance use disorder programs or company-sponsored health fairs. Some even provide time-limited situational counseling or crisis intervention.

Notably absent from those included among care managers are managers with the primary responsibility of adjudicating whether a requested health service is covered or meets medical necessity criteria (utilization managers). These individuals, who most often work for health plans, more correctly manage claims rather than patients. While there is always some utilization management activity associated with most forms of care management, it is easy to separate the two because utilization managers spend little time talking with patients and virtually none in helping them overcome barriers to improvement. They primarily interact with providers and delivery system personnel.

EXHIBIT 1.1   **Types of Care Managers**

Health care coaches: Professionals who assist clients at risk for complications from health conditions unless a healthy lifestyle is adopted

Employee assistance counselors: Professionals who help employees address workplace, family, financial, and health issues to maximize happiness, health, and workplace productivity

Workers' compensation managers: Professionals who help ensure that employees get the health care support they need while recovering from a workplace injury

Disability managers: Professionals who help ensure that employees get the health care support they need while on disability benefits

Disease managers: Health care professionals who assist patients to maximize care for specific illnesses—for example, diabetes, depression, and asthma

Assertive community treatment (ACT) team managers: Health professionals who assist patients with chronic mental health conditions to function within the community setting

Case managers: Health care professionals who assist patients with chronic illnesses or with health complexity to maximize improvement and stabilize their health

CASE MANAGEMENT

Case management falls within the rubric of care management. These managers assist patients with health complexity or those whose illness control is worse than expected given the level of acuity/severity. On the general medical side, most often these professionals are nurses, though clinicians from other disciplines are also represented. On the mental health side, case managers, such as those who assist seriously and persistently mentally ill patients, provide management services as a part of assertive community treatment (ACT) teams. Mental health case managers often include social workers, psychologists, and substance use disorder counselors, in addition to nurses.

Case managers usually work with the 2%–5% of the population who use a third to a half of health care resources (far right side of **Figure 1.1**). According to the 2010 *Standards of Practice for Case Management* (Case Management Society of America [CMSA], 2010) delineated by the CMSA, the following is used to define case management: "Case management is a collaborative process which assesses, plans, implements, coordinates, monitors and evaluates options and services to meet an individual's health needs through communication and available resources to promote quality cost-effective outcomes." (CMSA, 2010).

Principal case manager functions include:

- Conducting a comprehensive assessment of the patient's health needs
- Educating the patient and members of the health care delivery team about case management, identified barriers to health improvement, community resources, insurance benefits, and so forth, so that informed decisions can be made
- Developing and carrying out a care plan collaboratively with the patient, the patient's family, the primary care physician/provider, other health care providers, the payer, and/or the community that maximizes health, quality of life, appropriate use of health services, and conservation of health care resources
- Facilitating communication and coordination among members of the patient's biological and psychological health care teams to minimize fragmentation and maximize evidence-based care delivery
- Involving the patient in the decision-making process
- Problem solving and exploring options for improving care
- Considering alternative plans, when necessary, to achieve desired outcomes
- Striving to improve the quality of care and maintain cost effectiveness on a case-by-case basis

- Assisting patients in safely transitioning their care information and needed procedures among care settings (e.g., inpatient, outpatient, nursing facility, rehabilitation center, etc.)
- Advocating for patients to receive quality care, the health care team to be supported in providing quality services, the payer to conserve health resources, and the purchaser to minimize disability and impairment at an affordable cost
- Encouraging the patient to similarly self-advocate

Activities associated with these functions make up the current *Standards of Practice for Case Management,* summarized in **Exhibit 1.2**. For the first time since *Standards of Practice for Case Management* were defined by CMSA in 1995, case manager responsibilities include the coordination of biological, psychological, social, and health system barriers to improvement as core activities. With the patient at the center, working as a team with the case manager, the two collaborate in coordinating resources from the community, the patient's health care team, and those who pay to foster health in an attempt to reverse the life circumstances that have led to their health complexity (**Figure 1.2**).

Locations in which case management is offered are quite diverse. They include but are not limited to: hospitals and integrated care delivery systems, ambulatory care clinics, corporations, public and private health insurance programs, independent case management companies, government-sponsored programs, provider agencies and facilities, geriatric services facilities, telephonic triage and call centers, life care planning programs, and disease management companies. Since case management is provided in such a wide range of settings

FIGURE 1.2   Case management model.

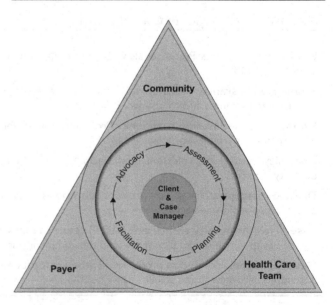

EXHIBIT 1.2   Case Management Standards of Practice

Case managers with active licensure and up-to-date competence in their specialty area of practice should be able to:

- Supervise high-risk case identification procedures
- Obtain appropriate and informed patient consent
- Provide complete, comprehensive, culturally and linguistically sensitive assessments
- Identify actionable barriers to improvement in multiple domains
- Create a prioritized short-, medium-, and long-term culturally and linguistically diverse care plans
- Monitor progress related to the care plan
- Move toward, document, and measure patient outcomes
- Satisfy a patient's need for case management assistance and close the case
- Facilitate the coordination, communication, and collaboration among the patient's providers
- Assist patients in getting quality care while attempting to conserve scarce health resources
- Advocate for patients and teach them to advocate for themselves
- Use the ethical principles of beneficence, nonmaleficence, autonomy, justice, and fidelity in fulfilling case management activities
- Adhere to applicable local, state, and federal laws
- Preserve a patient's privacy and confidentiality

Adapted from Case Management Society of America, Standards of Practice for Case Management, *2010, p. 7.*

and to populations with varied needs, approaches to case management in various settings require customization so that parochial needs are met; however, the standards of practice should remain the same.

INTEGRATED CASE MANAGEMENT

To date, traditional case management has largely been separated into that provided by management personnel with backgrounds in general medical care and that provided by those with backgrounds and training in mental health and substance use disorders, the combination of which will hereafter be known as mental conditions. Case managers with medical backgrounds concentrate their efforts almost entirely on biological factors that contribute to poor physical health. Only occasionally are social factors, such as difficulty in getting to appointments or paying for medications, or unhealthy behaviors, such as dietary indiscretion or smoking, that contribute to treatment resistance and symptom persistence addressed. Conversely, case managers associated with mental health programs only target assistance with the diagnosis and treatment of mental conditions and unhealthy behaviors that predict poor mental health outcomes. Rarely do case managers coming from one or the other background choose to address health issues outside of their area of practice contributing to a patient's poor health situation, other than perhaps to refer for cross-disciplinary care when blatant symptoms become too prominent to ignore.

Integrated case management, until now mostly performed by individual clinicians dedicated to working at the interface of physical and mental health, is

an approach proposed as a replacement for traditional case management. To date, reimbursement barriers and limited knowledge about practical models for implementation of integrated practices have impeded its growth. This has changed as more has been learned about the destructiveness of health service fragmentation, the need for a patient-centered approach to care, and the negative impact of concurrent medical and psychiatric illness (Institute of Medicine, Committee on Crossing the Quality Chasm: Adaptation to Mental Health and Addictive Disorders, 2006; Institute of Medicine, Committee on Quality of Health Care in America, 2001; Kathol, Saravay, Lobo, & Ormel, 2006; President's New Freedom Commission on Mental Health, 2003). Further, integrated case management has been facilitated by a better understanding of health complexity and how to measure it (Huyse & Stiefel, 2006).

Integrated case management is designed to topple general medical and mental condition silos by training professionals from both the physical health and mental health sectors in techniques that will allow them to provide interdisciplinary assistance, using the 2010 *Standards of Practice for Case Management,* to patients with health complexity. This is possible because case managers by definition do not treat patients. Rather, they assist their patients in getting outcome-changing care—that is, stabilizing health by using their understanding of health and the health system to guide them through the health care maze. Case managers with physical health backgrounds do not have to know how to diagnose and treat depression, psychotic illness, or eating disorders. They use their understanding of illness, treatment, and the components of care that prevent improvement to help the patient get and follow through on care from his or her treating providers. Likewise, case managers with mental health backgrounds do the same.

This does not mean that it is unnecessary for case managers from either sector to know something about cross-disciplinary illnesses and treatments. A basic reciprocal understanding is necessary for members of both groups. This is why this manual has been written and the integrated case management training program has been developed by CMSA. All case managers who choose to extend their capabilities by providing integrated case management need to develop the skills required to assist patients with concurrent and treatment-resistant physical and mental illness in overcoming the challenges they face in getting the type of care that will return them to health or at least to stable control of their disorders. Examples of the type of cross-disciplinary information needed by case managers using integrated case management techniques are provided in Chapters 5 and 6. Perhaps the first and most difficult challenge for a case manager who is considering entry into integrated case management is deciding that he or she is willing to put forth the effort to learn new techniques that can improve the health of his or her patients.

INTEGRATED PEDIATRIC CASE MANAGEMENT

There are clearly special skills needed to work with children and adolescents and their caregivers/parents as a part of the case management process. While the *Standards of Practice for Case Management* remain the same, there are unique challenges faced by case managers who choose to assist children/youth and their families with health complexity because they must deal with a different set of illnesses and practitioners, both general medical and mental health. Moreover, they must consider the contributions of caregivers/parents, teachers, coaches, and peers in their assessments and care plan development. Finally, they often must include assistance not only to the child/youth, but also to caregivers/parents and teachers involved with the child/youth before outcome change and health stabilization can be expected.

Since children/youth are at as great, if not greater, risk for multiple factors contributing to health complexity than are adults, an approach to integrated pediatric case management has been added to this manual that parallels the approach that is taken in adults. This will allow case management programs that understand the importance of correcting mental health issues as a means of reversing persistent physical symptoms to include a child/youth component in their case management services, particularly if they have already decided to provide adult integrated case management and have a child/youth population to serve as well.

INTERMED METHODOLOGY

It is with integrated case management that INTERMED methodology enters the scene. The INTERMED, the formal name used by the European developers for this method of complexity assessment, approach was designed to reconnect siloed factors in the health system that influence health outcomes for a patient. It has been undergoing development, standardization, and validation in seven languages (English, French, German, Spanish, Italian, Dutch, and Japanese) for the past 15 years (de Jonge, Bauer, Huyse, & Latour, 2003; de Jonge, Hoogervorst, Huyse, & Polman, 2004; de Jonge, Latour, & Huyse, 2003; Huyse, Stiefel, & de Jonge, 2006; Lyons, 2006; Stiefel et al., 2006) with a focus on health complexity. Health complexity includes two components: complexity of the patient (the case) as well as complexity of the health system (the care; de Jonge, Huyse, & Stiefel, 2006). For instance, diabetes is complicated by depression. Depression, in turn, negatively influences adherence to diabetes management (a case characteristic). It also necessitates communication between physical and mental health service providers (a care characteristic). The INTERMED method addresses both the case and the care components.

Health complexity can be defined as the interference in standard care by biological, psychological, social, and health system factors, which require a shift from standard (biomedical) care to individualized (integrated) support for care in order for patient outcomes to improve. Individualized support for care is largely delivered through the services of case managers.

Until now, the field of case management focused on identifying patients at risk for future poor outcomes. While these patients could be uncovered using health plan claims databases, predictive modeling schema, health risk assessments, or clinical characteristics of hospitalized or high service using outpatients in general medical or surgical settings, discovery procedures did little to suggest a systematic way to reveal, disentangle, and overcome barriers to improvement. Once patients were identified, case managers assisted them by maximizing illness understanding and fostering adherence to treatment for primary and secondary, but mainly *physical health,* conditions. The hope was that such assistance would decrease medical/surgical complications and reduce health care service use. Indeed, studies suggest that it does so to some extent for specific health conditions (Goetzel, Ozminkowski, Villagra, & Duffy, 2005). Interventions included instructing patients about their general medical disorders, altering factors that led to treatment nonadherence, and, in the more robust case management programs, confirming that progress toward recovery was occurring.

In these programs, the greatest, if not exclusive, attention was given to factors affecting appropriate general medical diagnostic assessments and treatment. To the extent that personal and social issues were revealed during unstructured interviews and led to nonadherence with medical intervention, they were included in case management activities. In most patients, psychological aspects were actively avoided because they were considered outside the purview of general medical health—that is, they were carved out of the process. Health system components entered into the case management process mainly when medical necessity decisions were required or, occasionally, when case managers were allowed to flex insurance benefits.

With the introduction of the INTERMED integrated system of case management, attention to the physical health domain (general medical disease) lost its position of dominance. It took its place alongside psychological, social, and health system factors as a shared set components that influence health and outcomes. Thus, through INTERMED methodology, *complexity* became defined as a composite of interacting historical, current state, and vulnerability health risks and health needs from each of these four domains in which barriers to care could arise.

The INTERMED was developed based on the assumption that return to health is dependent on altering factors in all four domains that interfere with patients' ability to get better. This includes such things as whether significant family members agree with the diagnosis and treatment; whether the patient has a co-occurring, adherence-altering depression; whether the patient has transportation to an appointment and the money to fill prescriptions; or whether the patient knows how and has the energy to find a specialist in her provider network to treat her complicated general medical and psychiatric conditions.

Inherent in the INTERMED system is the understanding that an uncomplicated and otherwise easily treatable physical illness could be made complex by the presence of one or more factors in other domains in a patient's life. For instance, pneumococcal pneumonia in most patients can be controlled by the administration of penicillin. However, if the patient lives on an Indian reservation and has a cultural aversion to taking oral medication or the patient has paranoid psychosis and is concerned about being poisoned, a simple course of antibiotics becomes much more complicated. Cultural and mental health factors must be considered to effectively treat an otherwise uncomplicated, yet potentially serious, health problem. All that may be required to effectively treat the Native American would be a shot of benzathine (long-acting) penicillin. The paranoid patient, on the other hand, may require admission with supervised administration. The concept

of health complexity, using the INTERMED system, paints a more complete picture of the patient so that assistance in all domains is brought to the patient, not in isolation, but in relation to each other.

In order to optimize the effects of the health risks and needs assessment, the INTERMED is designed to be clinically relevant—that is, it leads the case manager to ask, "How should I act based on this score?" It also enhances communication between and among the patients and their providers. Improved clinical relevance and the communimetric, rather than psychometric, approach are synergistic since together they allow the case manager and patient to immediately understand and address the question, "Is action needed and how intensively?" (Lyons, 2009). All the health risks and needs assessed with the INTERMED method are translated into scores, which lead to: immediate action (red, level 3), treatment administration or the development of a treatment plan (orange, level 2), monitoring or prevention (yellow, level 1), or no action (green, level 0) for the patient. Enhanced communication is supported by the organization of risks and needs into a grid, that is, the Complexity Assessment Grid (CAG), in which the seriousness of the risks or needs is visualized with colors and thus easily communicated once interpretation of the grid is understood (see **Table 1.1** for an example of the grid without color indicators). This is covered in greater detail in Chapter 3 and within the color insert section.

In this introduction to integrated physical and mental condition case management, the authors have taken lessons learned from the development of the INTERMED, adapted them for use by case managers in most national health systems, including the United States, and renamed the resulting tool the INTERMED-Complexity Assessment Grid (IM-CAG). For this reason, the case management adaptation found in this manual is very similar to the approved European INTERMED Foundation version. Viewing both Appendix 6 and Appendix 15 allows a head-to-head comparison. For children/youth, a pediatric version of the IM-CAG (the PIM-CAG) has been developed. The pediatric version contains 25 cells yet uses the same domain and anchor point system (**Table 1.2**). It has been adapted to reflect complexity items, such as family and school, which affect and are affected by the child's/youth's health and function. The structure and approach to uncovering complexity and linking it to actions in children and adolescents, however, are similar to those in the adult version.

For convenience, an abbreviation system uses corresponding letters from the grid headings to represent IM-CAG complexity items and to denote their place on the grid (see **Table 1.3**). In this system the first letter of the time frame (**H**istorical, **C**urrent state, or **V**ulnerability) is followed by the first letter(s) of the domain

TABLE 1.1	INTERMED-Complexity Assessment Grid

	Health risks and health needs		
	Historical	Current state	(Future) Vulnerability
Biological domain	1. Chronicity 2. Diagnostic dilemma	1. Symptom severity/impairment 2. Diagnostic/therapeutic challenge	Complications and life threat
Psychological domain	1. Barriers to coping 2. Mental health history	1. Resistance to treatment 2. Mental health symptoms	Mental health threat
Social domain	1. Job and leisure 2. Relationships	1. Residential stability 2. Social support	Social vulnerability
Health **S**ystem domain	1. Access to care 2. Treatment experience	1. Getting needed services 2. Coordination of care	Health system impediments

Adapted from Huyse et al., 1999.

TABLE 1.2	Pediatric INTERMED-Complexity Assessment Grid

	Health risks and health needs		
	Historical	Current state	(Future) Vulnerability
Biological domain	1. Chronicity 2. Diagnostic dilemma	1. Symptom severity/impairment 2. Diagnostic/therapeutic challenge	Complications and life threat
Psychological domain	1. Barriers to coping 2. Mental health history 3. Cognitive development 4. Adverse developmental events	1. Resistance to treatment 2. Mental health symptoms	Learning/mental health threat
Social domain	1. School functioning 2. Relationships 3. Caregiver health	1. Residential stability 2. Child/youth support 3. Caregiver/family support 4. School and community participation	Family/school/social system vulnerability
Health **S**ystem domain	1. Access to care 2. Treatment experience	1. Getting needed services 2. Coordination of care	Health system impediments

title (**B**iological, **P**sychological, **S**ocial, or **H**ealth system). If there are multiple complexity items within a grid box, a corresponding number is placed at the end of the abbreviation. For instance, the complexity item "Chronicity" is located within the Historical time frame in the **B**iological domain and it is the 1st option within that box; therefore, it is abbreviated "HB1." "Coordination of care" is a **C**urrent state item of the **H**ealth system domain and it is the 2nd option, thus it is abbreviated "CHS2." Since there is only one **V**ulnerability item for each domain, no number is added for the four items relating to **V**ulnerability. For example, "Mental health threat" is abbreviated "VP" (**V**ulnerability time frame; **P**sychological domain) and "Health system impediments" uses the "VHS" abbreviation (**V**ulnerability time frame; **H**ealth system domain). When first learning the abbreviation system, it may be convenient to think of a football (gridiron) metaphor. The sequence of letters is *"T-D"* for both the abbreviation system *"Time frame"-"Domain"* and

the football score of touchdown (T-D). Abbreviations for the PIM-CAG complexity items parallel the IM-CAG abbreviation system; however, there are five extra complexity items (HP3, HP4, HS3, CS3, and CS4). An example of these additional items is "CS3" for "Caregiver/family support," which corresponds to the **C**urrent state time column, the **S**ocial domain row, and the 3rd item in this box on the pediatric complexity assessment grid.

While the IM-CAG and PIM-CAG are designed to provide an overall picture of the needs, risks, and vulnerabilities of complex patients with actionable steps related to each cell, they are constructed with the understanding that the relationship between the patient (and family) and the case manager is what drives the achievement of goals and leads to health improvement. They are, therefore, patient-centered and further enhanced by the use of motivational interviewing techniques when gathering information and developing and implementing care plans collaboratively with

TABLE 1.3 **Abbreviation System for IM-CAG**

Abbreviation	Time Frame	Domain	Option Number	Name Of Item
HB1	**H**istorical	**B**iological	1	Chronicity
HB2	**H**istorical	**B**iological	2	Diagnostic dilemma
CB1	**C**urrent state	**B**iological	1	Symptom severity/impairment
CB2	**C**urrent state	**B**iological	2	Diagnostic/therapeutic challenge
VB	**V**ulnerability	**B**iological	–	Complications and life threat
HP1	**H**istorical	**P**sychological	1	Barriers to coping
HP2	**H**istorical	**P**sychological	2	Mental health history
CP1	**C**urrent state	**P**sychological	1	Resistance to treatment
CP2	**C**urrent state	**P**sychological	2	Mental health symptoms
VP	**V**ulnerability	**P**sychological	–	Mental health threat
HS1	**H**istorical	**S**ocial	1	Job and leisure
HS2	**H**istorical	**S**ocial	2	Relationships
CS1	**C**urrent state	**S**ocial	1	Residential stability
CS2	**C**urrent state	**S**ocial	2	Social support
VS	**V**ulnerability	**S**ocial	–	Social vulnerability
HHS1	**H**istorical	**H**ealth **S**ystem	1	Access to care
HHS2	**H**istorical	**H**ealth **S**ystem	2	Treatment experience
CHS1	**C**urrent state	**H**ealth **S**ystem	1	Getting needed services
CHS2	**C**urrent state	**H**ealth **S**ystem	2	Coordination of care
VHS	**V**ulnerability	**H**ealth **S**ystem	–	Health system impediments

patients. The IM-CAG and PIM-CAG help guide the case manager to determine the greatest needs and the domains in which complexity is introduced. Most importantly, identified complexity immediately translates into actionable steps mutually taken by the case manager and patient to improve health.

REFERENCES

Case Management Society of America. (2010). *(CMSA) Standards of Practice for Case Management*. Retrieved April 18, 2010, from http://www.cmsa.org/portals/0/pdf/memberonly/Standards OfPractice.pdf

de Jonge, P., Bauer, I., Huyse, F. J., & Latour, C. H. (2003). Medical inpatients at risk of extended hospital stay and poor discharge health status: Detection with COMPRI and INTERMED. *Psychosomatic Medicine, 65*(4), 534–541.

de Jonge, P., Hoogervorst, E. L., Huyse, F. J., & Polman, C. H. (2004). INTERMED: A measure of biopsychosocial case complexity: One year stability in multiple sclerosis patients. *General Hospital Psychiatry, 26*(2), 147–152.

de Jonge, P., Huyse, F. J., & Stiefel, F. C. (2006). Case and care complexity in the medically ill. *Medical Clinics of North America, 90*(4), 679–692.

de Jonge, P., Latour, C. H., & Huyse, F. J. (2003). Implementing psychiatric interventions on a medical ward: Effects on patients' quality of life and length of hospital stay. *Psychosomatic Medicine, 65*(6), 997–1002.

Goetzel, R., Ozminkowski, R., Villagra, V., & Duffy, J. (2005). Return on investment in disease management: A review. *Health Care Financing Review, 26*(4), 1–19.

Huyse, F. J., de Jonge, P., Lyons, J. S., Stiefel, F. C., Slaets, J. P. (1999). INTERMED: a tool for controlling for confounding variables and designing multimodal treatment. *Journal of Psychosomatic Research* (Vol. 46, pp. 401–2).

Huyse, F. J., & Stiefel, F. C. (Eds.). Integrated care for the complex medically ill. [Special issue.]. *Medical Clinics of North America,* 90 (2006).

Huyse, F. J., Stiefel, F. C., & de Jonge, P. (2006). Identifiers, or "red flags," of complexity or need for integrated care. *Medical clinics of North America, 90*(4), pp. 703–712.

Institute of Medicine, Committee on Crossing the Quality Chasm: Adaptation to Mental Health and Addictive Disorders. (2006). *Improving the quality of health care for mental and substance-use conditions.* Washington, DC: National Academies Press.

Institute of Medicine, Committee on Quality of Health Care in America. (2001). *Crossing the quality chasm: A new health system for the 21st century.* Washington, DC: National Academies Press.

Kathol, R. G., Saravay, S., Lobo, A., & Ormel, J. (2006). Epidemiologic trends and costs of fragmentation. *Medical Clinics of North America, 90*(4), pp. 549–572.

Lyons, J. S. (2006). The complexity of communication in an environment with multiple disciplines and professionals: Communimetrics and decision support. *Medical Clinics of North America, 90*(4), 693–701.

Lyons, J. S. (2009). *Communimetrics: A communication theory of measurement in human service settings.* New York: Springer.

Minnesota Medical Association. (2005). Physician's Plan for a Healthy Minnesota: The Minnesota Medical Association's Proposal for Health Care Reform, (p. 9). Minneapolis: Minnesota Medical Association.

President's New Freedom Commission on Mental Health. (2003). *Achieving the promise: Transforming mental health care in America.* Retrieved April 18, 2010 from http://www.mentalhealthcom mission.gov/reports/FinalReport/toc.html

Stiefel, F. C., Huyse, F. J., Söllner, W., Slaets, J. P., Lyons, J. S., Latour, C. H., et al. (2006). Operationalizing integrated care on a clinical level: The INTERMED project. *Medical Clinics of North America,* 90, pp. 713–758.

CHAPTER 2

Overview of Health Complexity and the Interaction Between Physical Health and Mental Conditions

OBJECTIVES

- To define "health complexity" and "mental conditions" and their importance in case management
- To describe the adverse interaction of physical and common comorbid mental conditions in patients with health complexity
- To discuss the difficulty in getting concurrent physical and mental condition treatment and its impact on health and cost outcomes
- To review illness multimorbidity in children and adolescents
- To summarize the potential value of physical and mental condition health service integration

INTRODUCTION

Procedures described in this integrated case management manual are applicable for all forms of care management (see **Exhibit 1.1**); however, emphasis is on the development of integrated management skills for managers who perform case and, to some extent, disease management since these are the areas of management practice with the greatest opportunity for health, function, and economic performance enhancement. Case managers, as defined in Chapter 1, work primarily with patients having high health complexity. Disease managers work with patients having chronic illnesses. Up to a half of these individuals will have multiple chronic conditions, and some will have health complexity. Patients in disease management programs, on average, necessarily require less health support and intensity of assistance by management personnel.

Disease managers, however, either work closely with case managers or assume what would appropriately be considered case management activities when the small but significant percentage of their patients experience increased complexity during the course of their targeted condition. For this reason, the activities described in this manual are directly applicable and can bring value to those performing both case and disease management. For purposes of simplicity, the term "case management" will henceforth encompass both case and disease managers working with complex patients.

Although the manual focuses on case manager activities, it does not diminish the potential value of using integrated case management techniques and tools for patients assisted by wellness, employee assistance, disability management, or workers' compensation programs. Populations served by these programs will necessarily have lower complexity than patients found in case management programs. Nonetheless, the principles of integrated case management apply equally to patients with less complexity, plus there will continue to be a small percentage from these populations that exhibit poorly controlled health problems. In these patients, the integrated case management approach should be considered for implementation either by a subset of managers trained in integrated management skills or by referral to a management group that uses them. The only reason not to utilize an integrated management approach for all patients supported through these programs is that the return on investment decreases as complexity decreases. Strategically, therefore, it makes the most sense to target the most complex first and work down the complexity scale as resources and personnel become available.

Chapter 2 of the manual assists case managers, regardless of their backgrounds, training, or clinical activity, in understanding the concepts of health complexity, mental conditions and how they relate to general medical problems, and the impact that the interaction of the two have on health and cost outcomes. It emphasizes the importance of uncovering and assisting with both medical and psychiatric contributions to patient problems. Perhaps more importantly, however, it attempts to demonstrate the need for coordination of physical and mental condition services for patients so affected in an attempt to maximize clinical, functional, and economic outcomes.

HEALTH COMPLEXITY

As described in Chapter 1, health complexity is defined as the interference with standard care by the interaction of biological, psychological, social, and health system factors. It includes two components, case and care complexity, and requires a shift from standard (biomedical) care to individualized (integrated) care in order for patient outcomes to improve (de Jonge, Huyse, & Stiefel, 2006). Patient-based case complexity is manifest in many clinical situations, such as when patients experience adverse medication events or drug interactions or when symptoms overlap from multimorbid illness (e.g. chronic lung disease and anxiety or hypothyroidism and depression). Health system-based, care complexity is manifest by the way that health services are supported by the system, delivered by practitioners, and available to the patient. For instance, patients experience care complexity when delays in care occur with long wait lists, translation services are not available, or clinicians providing care do not talk with each other and coordinate services.

It is important to realize that support for health services is often prioritized by the degree to which there is research evidence to document value in the current care delivery environment. While this manual argues that evidence-based practices should be used when they are available, most outcome studies documenting clinical service value are performed in pure, noncomorbid populations. Thus, even when studies are available, they may not generalize to complex, multimorbid patients. Rather than taking a nihilistic attitude in these complicated, high-cost patients—that is, providing no care because evidence-based interventions are not available—case managers need to become comfortable in supporting best practice approaches when evidence is limited. Interfering factors are the rule rather than the exception in these patients, thus results of existing research need to be adjusted to maximize benefit to patients.

FIGURE 2.1 Health complexity requiring individualized physical and mental condition care integration.

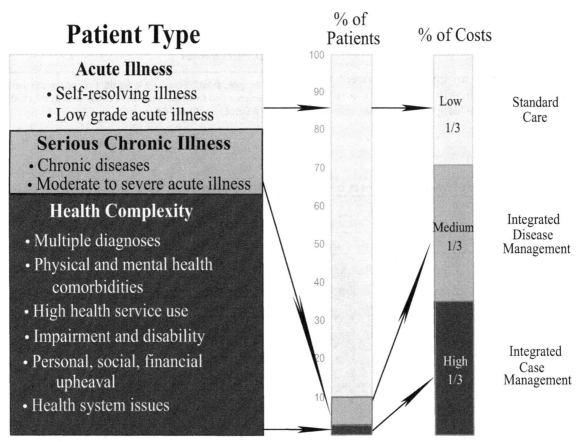

Adapted from Meier DE, National Blue Cross Blue Shield Association Presentation, 2002.

"Individualized care" means that health professionals, such as integrated case managers (**Figure 2.1**), help patients with health complexity bring their illnesses under control using health system navigation and advocacy techniques. These augment patients' capabilities to access best practice care, to improve exposure to evidence-based care, and to adhere to the outcome-enhancing treatments recommended by their doctors.

In the current health care system, there is a tendency to equate complexity with acuity and severity, often harbingers of complications related to physical or mental illness. While acuity and severity are clearly components of complexity, the concept of complexity used in this manual includes psychological, social, and health system risks and needs, which can also create barriers to and challenges for health. For instance, essential hypertension in most patients can be controlled by antihypertensive medications. However, if a patient has coexisting memory impairment, has an influential family member who believes that medications poison a person's body, or speaks little English but must order his or her prescriptions by mail, then easily treatable hypertension becomes treatment refractory. It leads to unnecessary medication additions/alterations and/or hypertensive complications. Psychological, social, and health system factors in such patients trump the acuity and severity of the physical illness, which is low in hypertensive patients, in making them treatment nonresponsive.

Health complexity is an important concept that expands on acuity and severity by helping to identify the small percentage of patients who use the majority of health resources (**Figure 2.2**; Zuvekas & Cohen, 2007). Predictive modeling elements, such as those published by Monheit and summarized in **Table 2.1** (Monheit, 2003) can be used to uncover patients at risk for future health needs and high service use. The Case Management Society of America (CMSA) *Standards of Practice for Case Management* also contain a list of risk factors associated with poor outcomes (CMSA, 2010). While these are useful to efficiently screen for those who might be candidates for case management, it is through the measurement of

TABLE 2.1	Predictive Modeling for Future High Service Use		
Patient features		**Marginal effect**	**p value**
Over 75 years of age		9.9	< .05
"Fair to poor" health		18.4	< .01
Prior high service use		20.7	< .01
White, non-Hispanic		5.8	< .05
Having the following illnesses:			
Mental health disease		11.0	< .01
Cancer		9.9	< .01
Infectious disease		9.0	< .01
Diabetes mellitus		7.7	< .05

Adapted from "Persistence in Health Expenditures in the Short Run: Prevalence and Consequences," by A. C. Monheit, 2003, Medical Care, 41(7 Suppl.) pp. III-60–61.

FIGURE 2.2   **Percent of health care costs used by complex patients.**

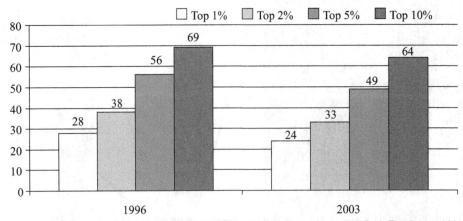

Adapted from "Prescription Drugs and the Changing Concentration of Health Care Expenditures," by S. H. Zuvekas and J. W. Cohen, 2007, Health Affairs, 26(1). p. 251.

health complexity, learned in this manual, that specific barriers to care and the actions needed to change them can be identified.

MENTAL HEALTH CONDITIONS

Mental health disorders and subthreshold symptoms, which lead to impairment by altering emotions, thinking, or behavior in the absence of mind-altering substances, and *substance use disorders*, which lead to impairment by altering emotions, thinking, or behavior in relation to substances known to affect mental function, will together be described by the term "mental conditions" in this manual. Just as with any general medical condition, the key factor is that those affected by a mental condition suffer, lose personal effectiveness, and benefit from intervention (**Exhibit 2.1**; unexplained physical complaints references: Hansen, Fink, Frydenberg, & Oxhoj, 2002; Inouye, Bogardus, Williams, Leo-Summers, & Agostini, 2003; Katon, Russo, et al., 2006; Katon, Unutzer, et al., 2006; Parthasarathy, Mertens, Moore, & Weisner, 2003; Rost, Kashner, & Smith, 1994; Smith, Monson, & Ray, 1986; Toft, 2004) whether it is the mental health or substance use disorder difficulty or a combination of the two that cause symptoms.

Some consider problems with chemical dependence in a separate category from other mental disorders because they are the result of inappropriate use of mind-altering substances (i.e. conditions created by the patients themselves). While the two have differing etiologies, it does not follow that those who are impaired because of substance use disorders do not need or deserve treatment. Data now demonstrate that patients with drug abuse problems exposed to evidence-based treatment have less impairment, better function, and ultimately lower total health care costs (Fleming et al., 2002; Holder & Blose, 1992; Parthasarathy & Weisner, 2005).

If one took the argument that those with chemical dependence should not be treated since they were volitionally responsible for their symptom onset to its logical conclusion, then the health system should also refuse treatment for obese patients with diabetes or heart disease, for smokers with chronic obstructive lung disease or lung cancer, and for promiscuous individuals with sexually transmitted diseases, including HIV and cervical cancer. There is no logical rationale for doing so since it would be associated with substantial suffering and ultimately higher health care costs as patients would seek treatment for more extensive and life-threatening diseases resulting from substance use disorder-related physical and mental health complications.

Another misconception about mental conditions is that they are untreatable. This is something that has changed dramatically in the past 30 years. The science of mental condition treatment for many illnesses

---

EXHIBIT 2.1   **Health Care Delivery-Based Integration Improves Outcomes and Lowers Costs**

- **Depression and diabetes:** 2 months fewer days of depression/year; projected $2.9 million/year lower total health costs/100,000 diabetic patients[a]
- **Panic disorder in primary care:** 2 months fewer days of anxiety/year; projected $1.7 million/year lower total health costs/100,000 primary care patients[b]
- **Substance use disorders with medical compromise:** 14% increase in abstinence; $2,050 lower annual health care cost/patient in integrated program[c]
- **Delirium prevention programs:** 30% lower incidence of delirium; projected $16.5 million/year reduction in inpatient costs/30,000 admissions[d]
- **Unexplained physical complaints:** no increase in missed general medical illness or adverse events; 9% to 53% decrease in costs associated with increased health care service utilization[e]
- **Health complexity:** halved depression prevalence; statistical improvement of quality of life and perceived physical and mental health; 7% reduction in new admissions at 12 months[f]

Summarized from:

[a] *"Cost-Effectiveness and Net Benefit of Enhanced Treatment of Depression for Older Adults With Diabetes and Depression,"* by W. Katon, J. Unutzer, M. Y. Fan, J. W. Williams, Jr., M. Schoenbaum, E. H. Lin, et al., 2006, Diabetes Care, 29.

[b] "Incremental Cost Effectiveness of a Collaborative Care Intervention for Panic Disorder," by W. J. Katon, J. Russo, C. B. Sherbourne, M. Stein, M. Craske, M.Y. Fan, P. Roy-Byrne, 2006, Psychological Medicine, 36.

[c] *"Utilization and Cost Impact of Integrating Substance Abuse Treatment and Primary Care,"* by S. Parthasarathy, J. Mertens, C. Moore, and Weisner, C., 2003, Medical Care, 41(3).

[d] *"The Role of Adherence on the Effectiveness of Nonpharmacologic Interventions: Evidence From the Delirium Prevention Trial,"* by S. K. Inouye, S. T. Bogardus, Jr., C. S. Williams, L. Leo-Summers, and J. V. Agostini, 2003, Archives of Internal Medicine, 163(8).

[e] *Summary of eight experimental/control outcome studies (references in text).*

[f] *"Effects of a Multifaceted Psychiatric Intervention Targeted for the Complex Medically Ill: A Randomized Controlled Trial,"* by F. C. Stiefel, C. Zdrojewski, F. Bel Hadj, D. Boffa, Y. Dorogi, A. So, et al., 2008, Psychotherapy Psychosomatics, 77(4).

is now on par with that of physical health conditions (**Table 2.2**). Importantly, in no discipline do all conditions have effective (evidence-based) treatments. Some are partially treatable. For others, palliation is all that is available. The same is true for mental health disorders.

Understanding that many common mental conditions are as treatable as general medical disorders allows the case manager to project a sense of optimism to the patient. Even in patients who have illnesses with worse prognoses, many of whom come to the attention of case managers, recognizing that interventions that maximize function and/or provide palliation is as important as identifying interventions that lead to recovery for both physical and mental conditions. Case managers who assist with noncurative interventions can also bring great comfort to their patients.

Case managers support patients in getting the right evaluations from an appropriate provider in a timely fashion and in helping them follow through on treatment recommendations. Components that contribute to effective case management can be found in **Exhibit 2.2**.

GENERAL MEDICAL AND MENTAL CONDITION COMORBIDITY, TREATMENT, AND INTERACTION

The Venn diagram in **Figure 2.3** illustrates the little-acknowledged fact that 85% of mental conditions are seen primarily in the general medical sector. Importantly, in the current health care environment, virtually all mental health dollars are targeted to assist the 15% of patients seen in the mental health sector (the dark gray sliver) in an artificially designed and independently managed behavioral health system. Mental conditions for patients seen in the general medical sector are either not treated (65%) or are ineffectively treated by primary and specialty medical practitioners (Kessler et al., 2005). This is true in virtually all countries and cultures (Demyttenaere et al., 2004). Only 13% of mental health patients have been shown to receive minimally effective mental health treatment in the non-mental health setting (Wang et al., 2005; Wang, Demler, & Kessler, 2002). This

---

TABLE 2.2	**Mental Conditions Are as Treatable as Physical Illnesses**

MENTAL CONDITIONS	PHYSICAL ILLNESSES
Conditions That Have Highly Effective Treatments	
■ Affective/anxiety disorders	■ Peptic ulcers
■ Delirium	
■ Acute psychoses	■ Pneumonia
	■ Kidney stones
Conditions That Have Less Effective Treatments	
■ Attention deficit hyperactivity disorders	■ Common colds
	■ Diabetes
■ Eating disorders	■ Back pain
■ Alcoholism	
Conditions That Respond Poorly to Treatment	
■ Dementia	■ Pancreatic cancer
■ Antisocial/borderline personality disorder	■ Amyotrophic lateral sclerosis
■ Paranoid disorder	■ Completed stroke

EXHIBIT 2.2	**Requirements for Effective Assistance Through Case Management**

Patient's responsibilities:

1. Be willing to form a relationship with the case manager; maintain trust
2. Learn about and participate in illness stabilization/recovery
3. Initiate agreed upon treatments and recommendations
4. Participate actively and diligently in the improvement process
5. Give feedback on the success, failure, and problems with treatment

Case manager's responsibilities:

1. Build a relationship with the patient; maintain positive regard
2. Provide an adequate understanding of illnesses
3. Identify and reverse of barriers to improvement
4. Facilitate outcome-changing interventions
5. Confirm improvement; adjust based on treatment nonresponse (follow up with patient and providers)

FIGURE 2.3 **FIGURE 2.3**   Mental condition treatment in the general medical sector.

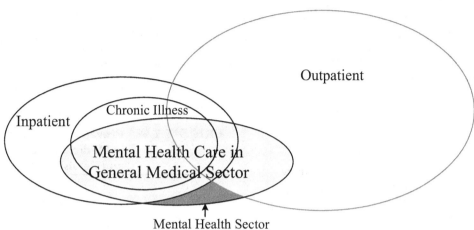

- 85% of mental health patients are seen in the physical health sector
- 65% receive no mental condition treatment
- Primary care physicians give 70% of mental condition treatment
- Only 13% of those treated by primary care physicians get evidence-based care

- 3% of mental health providers work in the general medical sector
- 80% of expenses for patients with mental conditions are from medical benefits, half of which are for additional physical health services
- Not treating patients with mental conditions shifts costs for mental health patients from the mental health to the general medical budget with higher total expenditures

is associated with doubling of total health care costs, the majority of which are for medical services (Kathol et al., 2005)

It is no longer acceptable from a health and cost perspective to continue independent, and to a large degree segregated, general medical and mental health assessment and treatment. In addition to the fact that this division perpetuates the stigma of having a mental health problem, projected estimates suggest that to continue to divide services in this way will lead to net system-wide additional costs for complex patients with mental conditions in the trillions of dollars during the next decade in the United States alone (**Exhibit 2.3**; Kathol, Melek, Bair, & Sargent, 2008). Reversing even a portion of this anticipated health system loss requires the adoption of business practices in which mental condition treatment would become incorporated as a basic component of general medical care at each level of the health industry. Integrated case management is one of the first steps possible in this transition process. Case managers taking part in this training program, who actually implement integrated care practices, will be frontrunners for the next generation of health care.

COMORBIDITY AND TREATMENT

The prevalence of psychiatric illness in patients with physical disorders and especially those with chronic medical illnesses has been documented to be high in a number of studies. The international actuarial firm of Milliman, Inc. recently summarized this data for a number of chronic medical conditions (**Exhibit 2.4**; Aina & Susman, 2006; Anderson & Horvath, 2004; Bayliss, Steiner, Fernald, Crane, & Main, 2003; Kessler, Ormel, Demler, & Stang, 2003). Further analyses of the literature, in fact, demonstrates an interaction between the apparent level of general medical morbidity and the frequency of concurrent psychiatric illness (Kroenke & Rosmalen, 2006). When community samples are assessed for the point prevalence of psychiatric illness, approximately one-tenth of the population is affected. For patients seen in the outpatient general medical clinic setting, the prevalence increases to approximately one-fourth (Cole, Saravay, & Hall, 1997). Medical inpatients, however, show the highest prevalence of comorbid psychiatric illness, with an average of two-fifths showing some form of mental condition symptoms (Hansen et al., 2001; Silverstone, 1996).

EXHIBIT 2.3   **Accumulated Data About the Top 5% of Patients Using 50% of Health Resources**

- ~60% to 80% have comorbid mental conditions[a]
- ~70% to 85% receive no mental health treatment[a]
- ~80% to 90% of those with mental conditions see no mental health specialists[a]
- ~5% to 15% get mental health treatment that would be expected to improve outcomes[a]
- ~$2 trillion is the projected U.S. health system additional spending for patients with mental conditions during the next 10 years if mental health management is not integrated with general medical management[b]

---

[a]*From Cartesian Solutions, Inc., unpublished medical and mental health claims review for multiple health plan clients.*
[b]*From S. Melek, Milliman, Inc., personal communication and "Chronic Conditions and Comorbid Psychological Disorders" by S. Melek & D. Norris, 2008.*

EXHIBIT 2.4   **Mental Condition Comorbidity in Patients With Physical Illness**

Condition	Prevalence
Neurological	37.5%
Heart disease	34.6%
Chronic obstructive pulmonary disease	30.9%
Cancer	30.3%
Arthritis	25.3%
Diabetes	25.0%
Hypertension	22.4%

From Melek S., Milliman presentation at the Milliman Healthcare Symposium, March, 2006 (summary of four studies, see references in text).

EXHIBIT 2.5   **Prevalence of Medical Disorders in Medicaid Patients with Serious and Persistent Mental Illness**

	Prevalence
Pulmonary	31%
Heart disease	22%
Gastrointestinal disease	25%
Skin and connective tissue	19%
Metabolic	15%
Diabetes	12%
Any medical illness	75%
Two or more medical illnesses	50%

Adapted from "Prevalence, Severity, and Co-occurrence of Chronic Physical Health Problems of Persons with Serious Mental Illness," by D. R. Jones, C. Macias, P. J. Barreira, W. H. Fisher, W. A. Hargreaves, and C. M. Harding, 2004, Psychiatric Services, 55(11), p. 1253.

While patients with some illnesses or in some clinical settings have much greater propensity for the co-occurrence of general medical and psychiatric illness, such as those with burns or those admitted to medical or surgical intensive care units, the presence of chronic or persistent physical conditions also puts patients at greater risk (Harter et al., 2007). Other factors, besides the presence of a medical illness, also contribute to the risk of concurrent general medical and mental health conditions. Some of these factors include preexisting psychiatric illness, multiple medications, increased age, poor social support, the involvement of numerous physicians, low socioeconomic status, and others. Consideration of these factors is important when triaging populations of patients in the medical setting, to identify those who are not more likely to benefit from the assistance of case management (see Appendix 2; Huyse, Stiefel, & de Jonge, 2006).

Since the majority of patients with mental conditions are seen in the general medical setting, it does not mean that concurrent illness is any less likely to be seen nor any less important in the mental health sector (Jones et al., 2004). Seventy-five percent of patients with serious and persistent mental illness, such as schizophrenia, eating disorders, or bipolar illness, have been shown to have at least one medical illness. Multiple medical illnesses are found in 50% (**Exhibit 2.5**). For instance, bipolar patients experience twice as much heart disease, migraines, and asthma and have mortality rates 1.5 to 2 times community standards, excluding suicide and homicide as causes of death (McIntyre et al., 2006). Even patients with less severe psychiatric illness are at double or more the risk for medical comorbidity.

If the point prevalence of mental conditions in patients seen in the physical health setting and general medical disorders in the mental health setting is as high as the preceding data suggest, it is important to understand the level of access that patients with concurrent illness have to treatment for both conditions regardless of setting. For this, there is now excellent data showing that only a third of patients with mental conditions in the medical setting receive any form of

FIGURE 2.4 Treatment of mental conditions in the general medical sector.

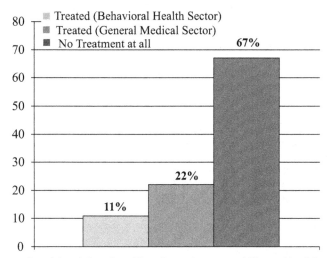

Consolidated data from "Prevalence, Severity, and Unmet Need for Treatment of Mental Disorders in the World Health Organization World Mental Health Surveys," by K. Demyttenaere, R. Bruffaerts, J. Posada-Villa, I. Gasquet, V. Kovess, J. P. Lepine, et al., 2004, Journal of the American Medical Association, 291(21). "Prevalence and Treatment of Mental Disorders," by R. C. Kessler, O. Demler, R. G. Frank, M. Olfson, H. A. Pincus, E. E. Walters, et al. 2005, New England Journal of Medicine, 352(24), and Kessler et al, AGP 62:617–627, 2005.

EXHIBIT 2.6 The Quality of Treatment for Depression

Statistics on the percentage of patients with depression receiving at least minimally effective treatment:
48% of those treated in mental health setting
13% of those treated in medical setting
8% of all patients based on prevalence
Many patients receive no treatment at all

Adapted from "The Epidemiology of Major Depressive Disorder: Results From the National Comorbidity Survey Replication (NCS-R)," by R. C. Kessler, P. Berglund, O. Demler, R. Jin, D. Koretz, K. R. Merikangas, et al., 2003, Journal of the American Medical Association, 289(23), p. 3102.

treatment (**Figure 2.4**; Demyttenaere et al., 2004; Kessler et al., 2005). Even in those who receive treatment, minimally effective care occurs in only 13% (**Exhibit 2.6**; Kessler, Berglund, et al., 2003). This bodes poorly for patients in terms of health and cost outcomes, as we will see in the discussion of the interaction of physical and mental conditions that follows.

Patients with mental conditions fare no better with regard to access to general medical assessments and

TABLE 2.3 Barriers to Treatment of General Medical Disorders in Mental Health Patients

	Psychotic disorders (N = 592)	Bipolar disorder (N = 511)	Major depression (N = 1,828)
	Adjusted odds ratio		
Source of regular primary care	0.55	0.74	0.97
Delayed care due to cost concerns	2.56	4.15	3.75
Unable to get needed care	4.01	6.37	4.46
Unable to get prescription for medication	4.83	5.45	4.80

Adapted from "Access to Medical Care Among Persons With Psychotic and Major Affective Disorders," by D. W. Bradford, M. M. Kim, L. E. Braxton, C. E. Marx, M. Butterfield, and E. B. Elbogen, 2008, Psychiatric Services, 59(8), p. 850.

intervention. In a comparison of medical care for patients with schizophrenia to a community sample, 39% of patients with schizophrenia received no treatment compared to 17% of those without schizophrenia (Vahia et al., 2008). These findings are supported in another study showing that barriers to treatment are substantially more likely for those with mental health difficulties (**Table 2.3**; Bradford et al., 2008). Importantly, poor access to treatment has significant consequences in terms of morbidity and mortality (**Figure 2.5**; Miller, Paschall, & Svendsen, 2006).

In a series of studies in different populations (end-stage renal disease, diabetes mellitus, multiple sclerosis, rheumatoid arthritis, back pain, general internal medicine [inpatient], and psychiatric consultation [inpatient]) performed in Europe using the INTERMED method, it was possible to illustrate the importance of the medical and mental health interaction (de Jonge, Bauer, Huyse, & Latour, 2003; de Jonge, Ruinemans, Huyse, & ter Wee, 2003; Fischer et al., 2000; Hoogervorst et al., 2003; Koch et al., 2001; Stiefel et al., 1999). In fact, using this approach, the proportion with health complexity—that is, those who would benefit from individualized, integrated care—could be defined. In all the studies, an INTERMED assessment was performed at baseline, and then clinical, quality of life, and health care utilization outcomes were documented. Patients with increased health complexity in terms of baseline INTERMED scores were consistently sicker, more impaired, and incurred higher cost than those with lower

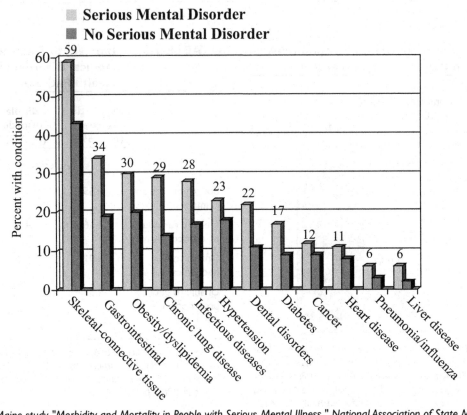

From report on Maine study "Morbidity and Mortality in People with Serious Mental Illness," National Association of State Mental Health Program Directors (Parks J., Svendsen D., Singer P., Foti M.E. [Eds.]), October 2006.

FIGURE 2.6   Relationship of complexity to clinical context and health outcomes.

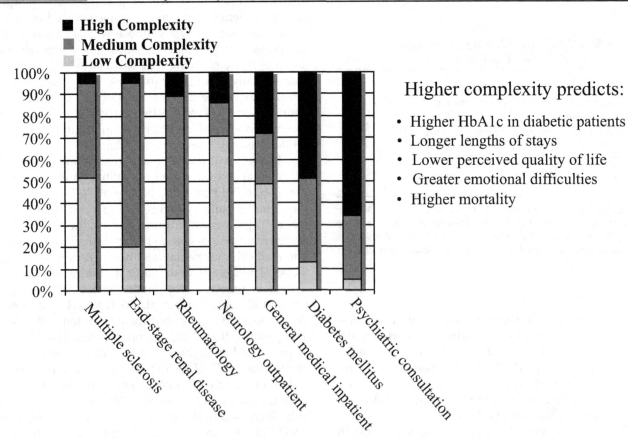

Higher complexity predicts:

• Higher HbA1c in diabetic patients
• Longer lengths of stays
• Lower perceived quality of life
• Greater emotional difficulties
• Higher mortality

Courtesy of Dr. Frits Huyse.

scores. There was also a remarkable variation among populations (**Figure 2.6**). Using an INTERMED cut-off score of 21, only 17% of multiple sclerosis patients qualified as complex, while nearly 70% of patients with diabetes mellitus did. Thus, the INTERMED approach to risk and needs assessment has internal validity as a predictor of future poor health outcomes and can be used to identify medical and mental health populations at greatest risk.

Part of the reason that patients with concurrent general medical and mental health problems have difficulty in receiving effective and coordinated physical and mental health care is that the general medical and mental health systems are segregated, both clinically and financially. A significant challenge for case managers, using integrated case management techniques, therefore, will be to help patients bridge this divide. Currently, segregated case management systems (independent physical and mental health) use management approaches that essentially throw patients over the wall so that general medical managers will not be accountable for outcomes in the mental health domain and vice versa (**Figure 2.7**). Since such handoffs rarely occur and when they do most often lead to little health enhancement, independent management practices contribute to health care cost shifts mainly in the form of increased medical service use (**Figure 2.8**) in large part due to psychiatric illness nontreatment (Rosenheck,

Druss, Stolar, Leslie, & Sledge, 1999). With integrated case management using IM-CAG methodology, the clinical and financial disconnect can be attenuated.

IMPACT OF COMORBIDITY ON HEALTH AND COST OUTCOMES

Perhaps the best way to appreciate the massive impact of concurrent general medical and mental health conditions, particularly in patients with chronic illness or health complexity, is to review the difference in health care expenditures (health care service use) for those with and those without mental condition comorbidity. Several studies now demonstrate that patients grappling with mental health and chemical dependence issues use twice the health care resources of those who don't have such issues (**Figure 2.9**; Kathol et al., 2005; Thomas et al., 2005). Of significant note, the majority of health care resource use is for medical and pharmacy claims, not for behavioral health assessment and treatment. In fact, in the numerous populations in which these findings have been reported to date, the amount used for additional physical health services (over the general medical service use baseline seen in those without mental conditions) far exceeds the total spent for behavioral health services. For instance, in the Thomas et al. study (**Figure 2.9**), extra medical spending on patients with mental conditions

---

FIGURE 2.7   Barriers in care created by the segregated reimbursement system.

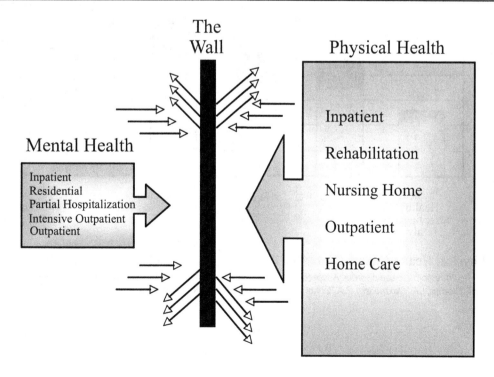

FIGURE 2.8   Physical and mental health pots of gold.

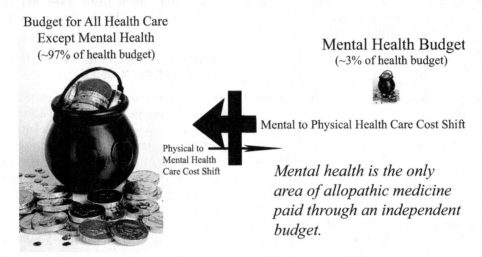

Budget for All Health Care
Except Mental Health
(~97% of health budget)

Mental Health Budget
(~3% of health budget)

Mental to Physical Health Care Cost Shift

Physical to
Mental Health
Care Cost Shift

*Mental health is the only
area of allopathic medicine
paid through an independent
budget.*

FIGURE 2.9   Claims expenditures for 6,500 Medicaid patients with and without mental condition service use.

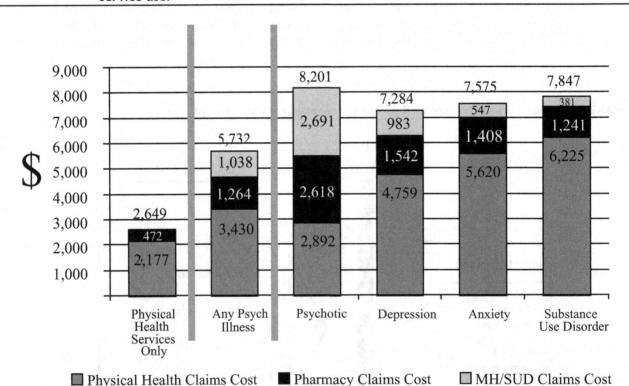

MH/SUD = Mental health/substance use disorder. Adapted from "Prevalence of Psychiatric Disorders and Costs of Care Among Adult Enrollees in a Medicaid HMO," by M. R. Thomas, J. A. Waxmonsky, P. A. Gabow, G. Flanders-McGinnis, R. Socherman, and K. Rost, 2005, Psychiatric Services, 56(11), p. 1397.

was $2,045 ($4,694 [$1,264 + $3,430] – $2,649), nearly double the total amount spent on mental condition treatment ($1,038). What this says is that for those who have mental health service needs, the potential for cost savings through improved mental condition care occurs more through reduction in spending on the general medical side than on the mental health side. This points to the importance of connecting physical and mental health support through integrated case management.

From the perspective of integrated case management, it is useful to understand the dynamic of the physical and mental health interaction and the importance of connecting general medical and mental condition services while assisting patients with return to or stabilization of health. Perhaps the best way to do this is to review the effect of depression—a health comorbidity seen in approximately 30% of patients with diabetes mellitus—on diabetic symptoms, treatment, and outcomes. **Figures 2.10** through **2.13** and **Tables 2.4** and **2.5** demonstrate that depression associated with diabetes: (a) increases the odds for physical complaints associated with diabetes, (b) puts the patient at greater risk for nonadherence to diabetic treatment recommendations, (c) leads to increased risk for diabetic complications and poor diabetic control, and (d) is associated with work impairment and disability (Egede, 2004; Katon, Simon, et al., 2004; Katon, von Korff, et al., 2004; Katon, Lin, et al., 2004; Lin et al., 2004; Ludman et al., 2004)

GENERAL MEDICAL AND MENTAL HEALTH INTERACTION IN CHILDREN AND ADOLESCENTS

Recent studies demonstrate that physical and mental health multimorbidity in children has similar consequences to that found in adults (Hysing, Elgen, Gillberg, Lie, & Lundervold, 2007; McDougall et al., 2004; Waters, Davis, Nicolas, Wake, & Lo, 2008). Nearly 7% of children and adolescents drawn from a school-based epidemiologic sample had four or more combined general medical and mental health conditions (Waters et al., 2008). This was associated with significantly greater child/youth impairment of health and well-being on 8 of 12 Child Health Questionnaire domains even when compared to children/youth with three or fewer conditions.

Children/youth with chronic conditions, such as asthma and cystic fibrosis, are at greater risk for poor outcomes than those without (Hysing et al., 2007). Of particular concern is the finding that these children/youth not only have worse health but that they are less able to participate in age-appropriate activities (McDougall et al., 2004).

VALUE OF INTEGRATED PHYSICAL AND MENTAL HEALTH CASE MANAGEMENT

We are in the early stages of initiating case management practices that attempt to integrate physical and mental

---

FIGURE 2.10 **Relationship of depression to diabetic symptoms.**

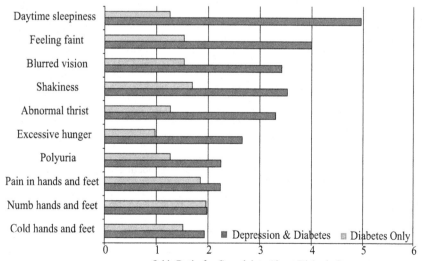

Adapted from "Depression and Diabetes Symptom Burden," by E. J. Ludman, W. Katon, J. Russo, M. Von Korff, G. Simon, P. Ciechanowski, et al., 2004, General Hospital Psychiatry, 26(6), p. 433.

FIGURE 2.11 Medication adherence in patients with diabetes.

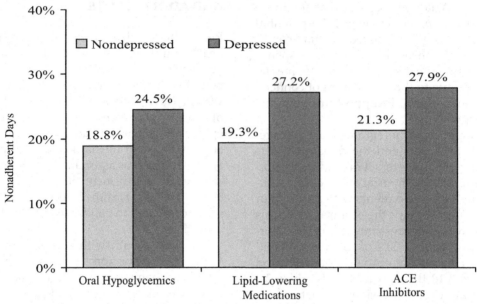

Data from "Relationship of Depression and Diabetes Self-Care, Medication Adherence, and Preventive Care," by E. H. Lin, W. Katon, M. Von Korff, C. Rutter, G. E. Simon, M. Oliver, et al., 2004, Diabetes Care, 27(9), p. 2158.

FIGURE 2.12 Depression effect on cardiac risk factors in diabetic patients.

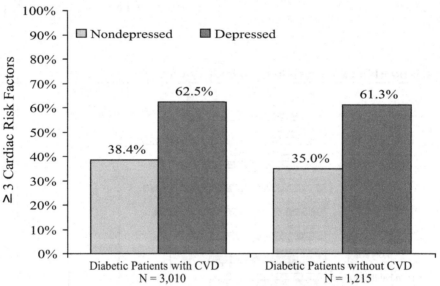

Data from "Cardiac risk factors in patients with diabetes mellitus and major depression," by W. J. Katon, E. Lin, J. Russo, M. von Korff, P. Ciechanowski, G. Simon, et al., 2004, Journal of General Internal Medicine, 19(12), p. 1195.
CVD = cardiovascular disease.

FIGURE 2.13   **Depression effect on HbA1c control in diabetic patients.**

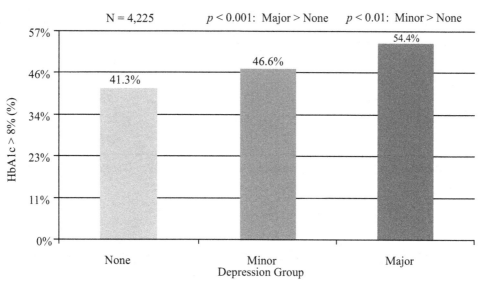

Adapted from "Behavioral and Clinical Factors Associated With Depression Among Individuals With Diabetes," by W. Katon, M. von Korff, P. Ciechanowski, J. Russo, E. Lin, G. Simon, et al., 2004, Diabetes Care, 27(4), p. 916.
Adjusted for demographics, medical comorbidity, diabetes severity, diabetes type and duration, treatment type, and clinic.

TABLE 2.4   **Depression Effect on Self-Care in Diabetic Patients**

Self-care activities (past 7 days)	No major depression	Major depression	Odds ratio	95% CI
Healthy eating ≤ 1 time/week	8.8%	17.2%	2.1	1.59–2.72
5 servings of fruit/vegetables ≤ 1 time/week	21.1%	32.4%	1.8	1.43–2.17
High fat foods ≥ 6 times/week	11.9%	15.5%	1.3	1.01–1.73
Physical activity (>30 min) ≤ 1 time/week	27.3%	44.1%	1.9	1.53–2.27
Specific exercise session ≤ 1 time/week	45.8%	62.1%	1.7	1.43–2.12
Smoking: Yes	7.7%	16.1%	1.9	1.42–2.51

Adapted from "Relationship of depression and diabetes self-care, medication adherence, and preventive care," by E. H. Lin, W. Katon, M. von Korff, C. Rutter, G. Simon, M. Oliver, et al., 2004, Diabetes Care, 27(9), p. 2157.

health assistance in care plans, thus a limited amount can be said of the potential clinical and economic value that they bring to improved health and function for patients with health complexity. On the face of it, one would expect that the integration of physical and mental condition case management would bring significant improvement, both in health and cost. In fact, that is what existing studies show for the few patients who have been assisted using early forms of integrated case management.

In the clinical setting, strong evidence exists for improved outcomes through the integration of care management capabilities for depressed elderly patients and for patients with depression and diabetes mellitus (**Figure 2.14**; Katon & Seelig, 2008; Seelig & Katon, 2008; Unutzer et al., 2002). The same was found in a European study in which diabetic and rheumatoid arthritis patients were selected based on their complexity. Care management interventions in these patients led to improved depressive symptoms and lower

TABLE 2.5	Annual Work Days Lost and Disability Days for Depression and Diabetes			
	Neither	**Diabetes**	**Depression**	**Both**
Work days lost	4.5	6.3	13.2	13.1
Odds ratio	(1.0)	(1.5)	(3.08)	(3.25)
Disability bed days				
Employed	2.2	3.5	7.9	23.4
Unemployed	6.5	8.5	23.2	45.8
Odds ratio	(1.0)	(1.63)	(4.0)	(5.61)

Adapted from "Effects of Depression on Work Loss and Disability Bed Days in Individuals With Diabetes," by L. E. Egede, 2004, Diabetes Care, 27(7), p. 1752.

FIGURE 2.14   **Integrated treatment of patients with diabetes improves depression and lowers cost.**

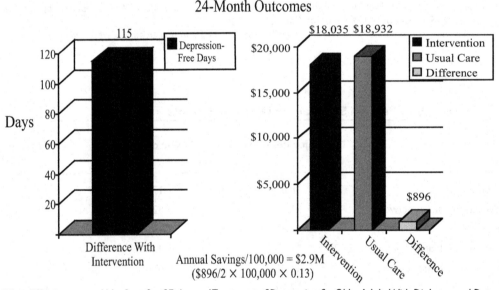

Adapted from "Cost-Effectiveness and Net Benefit of Enhanced Treatment of Depression for Older Adults With Diabetes and Depression," by W. Katon, J. Unutzer, M. Y. Fan, J. W. Williams, Jr., M. Schoenbaum, E. H. Lin, et al., 2006, Diabetes Care., 29(2), p. 268.

hospitalization rates (Stiefel et al., 2008). Long-term follow-up now indicates that early clinical improvement and further cost reduction persists up to 4 to 5 years (Katon et al., 2008; Simon et al., 2007; Unutzer et al., 2008).

In the health plan setting, integrated case management for complex patients has demonstrated value in a small Medicaid health plan in Colorado (**Exhibit 2.7**). More recent data from a national health plan, which initiated an integrated general medical and depression disease management program, has also been able to show positive clinical (**Table 2.6**) and economic

(**Exhibit 2.8**) results. While these data represent early findings of the integration of general medical and psychiatric case management practices, they are encouraging for the future of an integrated case management industry. In fact, the claims cost differential between those with and those without concurrent mental conditions in general medical patients suggests that much greater health-improving and cost savings opportunities are yet on the horizon since current integrated case management practices do not systematically address the social and health system factors that are found in this manual's integrated case management approach.

EXHIBIT 2.7	Net Savings with ColoradoAccess Care Integration

- Office visits: 22% decrease
- Emergency room visits: 26% decrease
- Hospital admissions: 72% decrease
- Hospital days: 76% decrease
- Medical and pharmaceutical costs: 24% decrease

Total net savings $400 (per member, per month)

Adapted from "Big Picture," by J. Miller, 2005, Managed Healthcare Executive, http://www.managedhealth careexecutive.com/coloradoaccess

EXHIBIT 2.8	Net Savings with Integrated Depression/Medical Case Management

Medical costs:	$175 to $222 PMPM decrease
Inpatient care:	$129 to $170 PMPM decrease
Pharmacy costs:	$21 to $40 PMPM increase
Antidepressant:	$8 to $11 PMPM increase)
Net cost:	**$136 to $201 PMPM decrease**
Net medical cost reduction with return on investment (ROI)	3:1
Average work days gained per month:	3.95
Improvement in work performance:	11.2%

From Un H:Aetna—www.academyhealth.org/2006/tuesday/611/unh.ppt
Data acquired from member responses to intake and discharge questions.
PMPM = per member, per month.

TABLE 2.6	Integrated Depression/Medical Case Management: Clinical Outcomes

Mental health survey			
Condition	**Intake**	**Discharge**	**Outcome**
Depression	79%	44%	35% drop in depression
Energy level	49%	75%	26% increase in energy
Work limitations	63%	29%	34% drop in work limitations
Social limitations	71%	41%	30% drop in social limitations

Physical health survey			
Condition	**Intake**	**Discharge**	**Outcome**
General health	5%	9%	4% increase in general health
Work limitations	61%	48%	13% drop in work limitations
Does less work	64%	45%	19% increase in work
Bodily pain	12%	5%	7% decrease in bodily pain

From Un H:Aetna-www.academyhealth.org/2006/tuesday/611/unh.ppt
Data acquired from member responses to intake and discharge questions.

EXHIBIT 2.9	**Net Annual Cost of Unchecked Dis-Integrated Care**

Population	Annual additional cost (in billions)
Commercial	$83.4–$241.2
Medicare	$49.2–$109.8
Total	**$132.6–$351.0**

From "Chronic Conditions and Comorbid Psychological Disorders," by S. Melek and D. Norris, 2008, Seattle, WA: Milliman. Based on Medstat claims database, 2005–2006.

Perhaps the most sobering factor that supports the adoption of integrated case management procedures, however, is the estimated cost of doing nothing. Actuaries from Milliman, Inc., recently published a report on the cost of maintaining the status quo in patients with 10 common chronic or acute physical illnesses (Melek & Norris, 2008). In the report, they projected that the cost to the U.S. in additional health service use for patients with a chronic illness and concurrent mental health conditions in commercial and Medicare programs alone would be between $136 and $351 billion annually (**Exhibit 2.9**). It is at least in part through the use of integrated case management procedures in complex patients that this cost gap can be closed.

REFERENCES

Aina, Y., & Susman, J. L. (2006). Understanding comorbidity with depression and anxiety disorders. *Journal American Osteopathic Association, 106*(5 Suppl. 2), S9–S14.

Anderson, G., & Horvath, J. (2004). *Chronic conditions: Making the case for ongoing care. September 2004 update.* Baltimore, MD: Johns Hopkins University and Robert Wood Johnson Foundation.

Bayliss, E. A., Steiner, J. F., Fernald, D. H., Crane, L. A., & Main, D. S. (2003). Descriptions of barriers to self-care by persons with comorbid chronic diseases. *Annals Family Medicine, 1*(1), 15–21.

Bradford, D. W., Kim, M. M., Braxton, L. E., Marx, C. E., Butterfield, M., & Elbogen, E. B. (2008). Access to medical care among persons with psychotic and major affective disorders. *Psychiatric Services, 59*(8), 847–852.

Case Management Society of America. (2010). *(CMSA) Standards of Practice for Case Management.* Retrieved April 18, 2010, from http://www.cmsa.org/portals/0/pdf/memberonly/Standards OfPractice.pdf

Cole, S., Saravay, S., & Hall, R. C. (1997). *Mental health disorders in general medical practice: Adding value to health care through consultation-liaison psychiatry.* Dubuque, IA: Academy of Psychosomatic Medicine.

de Jonge, P., Bauer, I., Huyse, F. J., & Latour, C. H. (2003). Medical inpatients at risk of extended hospital stay and poor discharge health status: Detection with COMPRI and INTERMED. *Psychosomatic Medicine, 65*(4), 534–541.

de Jonge, P., Huyse, F. J., & Stiefel, F. C. (2006). Case and care complexity in the medically ill. *Medical Clininics North America, 90*(4), 679–692.

de Jonge, P., Ruinemans, G. M., Huyse, F. J., & ter Wee, P. M. (2003). A simple risk score predicts poor quality of life and non-survival at 1 year follow-up in dialysis patients. *Nephrology Dialysis Transplantion, 18*(12), 2622–2628.

Demyttenaere, K., Bruffaerts, R., Posada-Villa, J., Gasquet, I., Kovess, V., Lepine, J. P., et al. (2004). Prevalence, severity, and unmet need for treatment of mental disorders in the World Health Organization World Mental Health Surveys. *Journal of the American Medical Association, 291*(21), 2581–2590.

Egede, L. E. (2004). Effects of depression on work loss and disability bed days in individuals with diabetes. *Diabetes Care, 27*(7), 1751–1753.

Fischer, C. J., Stiefel, F. C., De Jonge, P., Guex, P., Troendle, A., Bulliard, C., et al. (2000). Case complexity and clinical outcome in diabetes mellitus. A prospective study using the INTERMED. *Diabetes & Metabolism, 26*(4), 295–302.

Fleming, M. F., Mundt, M. P., French, M. T., Manwell, L. B., Staufacher, E. A., & Barry, K. L. (2002). Brief physician advice for problem drinkers: Long-term efficacy and benefit-cost analysis. *Alcoholism: Clinical & Experimental Research, 26*(1), 36–43.

Hansen, M. S., Fink, P., Frydenberg, M., Oxhoj, M., Sondergaard, L., & Munk-Jorgensen, P. (2001). Mental disorders among internal medical inpatients: Prevalence, detection, and treatment status. *Journal of Psychosomatic Research, 50*(4), 199–204.

Hansen, M. S., Fink, P., Frydenberg, M., & Oxhoj, M. L. (2002). Use of health services, mental illness, and self-rated disability and health in medical inpatients. *Psychosomatic Medicine, 64*(4), 668–675.

Harter, M., Baumeister, H., Reuter, K., Jacobi, F., Hofler, M., Bengel, J., et al. (2007). Increased 12-month prevalence rates of mental disorders in patients with chronic somatic diseases. *Psychotherapy Psychosomatics, 76*(6), 354–360.

Holder, H. D., & Blose, J. O. (1992). The reduction of health care costs associated with alcoholism treatment: A 14-year longitudinal study. *Journal of Studies on Alcohol, 53*(4), 293–302.

Hoogervorst, E. L., de Jonge, P., Jelles, B., Huyse, F. J., Heeres, I., van der Ploeg, H. M., et al. (2003). The INTERMED: A screening instrument to identify multiple sclerosis patients in need of multidisciplinary treatment. *Journal of Neurology Neurosurgery & Psychiatry, 74*(1), 20–24.

Huyse, F. J., Stiefel, F. C., & de Jonge, P. (2006). Identifiers, or "red flags," of complexity or need for integrated care. *Medical clinics of North America.* 90, pp. 703–712.

Hysing, M., Elgen, I., Gillberg, C., Lie, S. A., & Lundervold, A. J. (2007). Chronic physical illness and mental health in children. Results from a large-scale population study. *Journal of Child Psychology & Psychiatry, 48*(8), 785–792.

Inouye, S. K., Bogardus, S. T., Jr., Williams, C. S., Leo-Summers, L., & Agostini, J. V. (2003). The role of adherence on the effectiveness of nonpharmacologic interventions: Evidence from the delirium prevention trial. *Archives Internal Medicine, 163*(8), 958–964.

Jones, D. R., Macias, C., Barreira, P. J., Fisher, W. H., Hargreaves, W. A., & Harding, C. M. (2004). Prevalence, severity, and co-occurrence of chronic physical health problems of persons with serious mental illness. *Psychiatric Services, 55*(11), 1250–1257.

Kathol, R. G., McAlpine, D., Kishi, Y., Spies, R., Meller, W., Bernhardt, T., et al. (2005). General medical and pharmacy claims expenditures in users of behavioral health services. *Journal of General Internal Medicine, 20*(2), 160–167.

Kathol, R. G., Melek, S., Bair, B., & Sargent, S. (2008). Financing mental health and substance use disorder care within physical health: A look to the future. *Psychiatric Clinics of North America, 31*(1), 11–25.

Katon, W. J. MD, Lin, E. H. B. MD, MPH, Russo, J. PhD, Von Korff, M. ScD, Ciechanowski, P. MD, MPH, Simon, G. MD, MPH, Ludman, E. PhD, Bush, T. PhD, Young, B. MD, MPH. Cardiac Risk Factors in Patients with Diabetes Mellitus and Major Depression. *Journal of General Internal Medicine,* 2004; 19:1192–1199.

Katon, W. J., Russo, J., Sherbourne, C., Stein, M. B, Craske, M., Fan, M. Y., et al. (2006). Incremental cost-effectiveness of a collaborative care intervention for panic disorder. *Psychological Medicine, 36*(3), 353–363.

Katon, W. J., Russo, J. E., Von Korff, M., Lin, E. H., Ludman, E., & Ciechanowski, P. S. (2008). Long-term effects on medical costs of improving depression outcomes in patients with depression and diabetes. *Diabetes Care, 31*(6), 1155–1159.

Katon, W. J., & Seelig, M. (2008). Population-based care of depression: Team care approaches to improving outcomes. *Journal of Occupational & Environmental Medicine, 50*(4), 459–467.

Katon, W. J., Simon, G., Russo, J., Von Korff, M., Lin, E. H., Ludman, E., et al. (2004). Quality of depression care in a population-based sample of patients with diabetes and major depression. *Medical Care, 42*(12), 1222–1229.

Katon, W. J., Unutzer, J., Fan, M. Y., Williams, J. W., Jr., Schoenbaum, M., Lin, E. H., et al. (2006). Cost-effectiveness and net benefit of enhanced treatment of depression for older adults with diabetes and depression. *Diabetes Care, 29*(2), 265–270.

Katon, W. J., von Korff, M., Ciechanowski, P., Russo, J., Lin, E., Simon, G., et al. (2004). Behavioral and clinical factors associated with depression among individuals with diabetes. *Diabetes Care, 27*(4), 914–920.

Kessler, R. C., Berglund, P., Demler, O., Jin, R., Koretz, D., Merikangas, K. R., et al. (2003). The epidemiology of major depressive disorder: Results from the National Comorbidity Survey Replication (NCS-R). *Journal of the American Medical Association, 289*(23), 3095–3105.

Kessler, R. C., Demler, O., Frank, R. G., Olfson, M., Pincus, H. A., Walters, E. E., et al. (2005). Prevalence and treatment of mental disorders, 1990 to 2003. *New England Journal of Medicine, 352*(24), 2515–2523.

Kessler, R. C., Ormel, J., Demler, O., & Stang, P. E. (2003). Comorbid mental disorders account for the role impairment of commonly occurring chronic physical disorders: Results from the National Comorbidity Survey. *Journal of Occupupational & Environmental Medicine, 45*(12), 1257–1266.

Koch, N., Stiefel, F., de Jonge, P., Fransen, J., Chamot, A. M., Gerster, J. C., et al. (2001). Identification of case complexity and increased health care utilization in patients with rheumatoid arthritis. *Arthritis & Rheumatism, 45*(3), 216–221.

Kroenke, K., & Rosmalen, J. G. (2006). Symptoms, syndromes, and the value of psychiatric diagnostics in patients who have functional somatic disorders. *Medical Clinics North America, 90*(4), 603–626.

Lin, E. H., Katon, W. J., Von Korff, M., Rutter, C., Simon, G. E., Oliver, M., et al. (2004). Relationship of depression and diabetes self-care, medication adherence, and preventive care. *Diabetes Care, 27*(9), 2154–2160.

Ludman, E. J., Katon, W., Russo, J., Von Korff, M., Simon, G., Ciechanowski, P., et al. (2004). Depression and diabetes symptom burden. *General Hospital Psychiatry, 26*(6), 430–436.

McDougall, J., King, G., de Wit, D. J., Miller, L. T., Hong, S., Offord, D. R., et al. (2004). Chronic physical health conditions and disability among Canadian school-aged children: A national profile. *Disability & Rehabilitation, 26*(1), 35–45.

McIntyre, R. S., Konarski, J. Z., Soczynska, J. K., Wilkins, K., Panjwani, G., Bouffard, B., et al. (2006). Medical comorbidity in bipolar disorder: Implications for functional outcomes

and health service utilization. *Psychiatric Servon, 57*(8), 1140–1144.

Melek, S., & Norris, D. (2008). *Chronic conditions and comorbid psychological disorders.* Seattle, WA: Milliman.

Miller, B. J., Paschall, C. B., 3rd, & Svendsen, D. P. (2006). Mortality and medical comorbidity among patients with serious mental illness. *Psychiatric Services, 57*(10), 1482–1487.

Miller J. (2005). Big Picture. Managed Healthcare Executive, Retrieved April 18, 2010 from http://www.managedhealthcare executive.com/coloradoaccess

Monheit, A. C. (2003). Persistence in health expenditures in the short run: Prevalence and consequences. *Medical Care, 41*(7 Suppl.), III53–III64.

Parthasarathy, S., Mertens, J., Moore, C., & Weisner, C. (2003). Utilization and cost impact of integrating substance abuse treatment and primary care. *Medical Care, 41*(3), 357–367.

Parthasarathy, S., & Weisner, C. M. (2005). Five-year trajectories of health care utilization and cost in a drug and alcohol treatment sample. *Drug & Alcohol Dependence, 80*(2), 231–240.

Rosenheck, R. A., Druss, B., Stolar, M., Leslie, D., & Sledge, W. (1999). Effect of declining mental health service use on employees of a large corporation. *Health Affairs (Millwood), 18*(5), 193–203.

Rost, K., Kashner, T. M., & Smith, R. G., Jr. (1994). Effectiveness of psychiatric intervention with somatization disorder patients: Improved outcomes at reduced costs. *General Hospital Psychiatry, 16*(6), 381–387.

Seelig, M. D., & Katon, W. (2008). Gaps in depression care: why primary care physicians should hone their depression screening, diagnosis, and management skills. *Journal of Occupational & Environmental Medicine, 50*(4), 451–458.

Silverstone, P. H. (1996). Prevalence of psychiatric disorders in medical inpatients. *Journal of Nervous & Mental Disease, 184*(1), 43–51.

Simon, G. E., Katon, W. J., Lin, E. H., Rutter, C., Manning, W. G., Von Korff, M., et al. (2007). Cost-effectiveness of systematic depression treatment among people with diabetes mellitus. *Archives of General Psychiatry, 64*(1), 65–72.

Smith, G. R., Jr., Monson, R. A., & Ray, D. C. (1986). Psychiatric consultation in somatization disorder. A randomized controlled study. *New England Journal of Medicine, 314*(22), 1407–1413.

Stiefel, F. C., Zdrojewski, C., Bel Hadj, F., Boffa, D., Dorogi, Y., So, A., et al. (2008). Effects of a multifaceted psychiatric intervention targeted for the complex medically ill: A randomized controlled trial. *Psychotherapy Psychosomatics, 77*(4), 247–256.

Stiefel, F. C., de Jonge, P., Huyse, F. J., Guex, P., Slaets, J. P., Lyons, J. S., et al. (1999). "INTERMED": A method to assess health service needs. II. Results on its validity and clinical use. *General Hospital Psychiatry, 21*(1), 49–56.

Thomas, M. R., Waxmonsky, J. A., Gabow, P. A., Flanders-McGinnis, G., Socherman, R., & Rost, K. (2005). Prevalence of psychiatric disorders and costs of care among adult enrollees in a Medicaid HMO. *Psychiatric Services, 56*(11), 1394–1401.

Toft, T. (2004). *Managing patients with functional somatic symptoms in general practice.* Aarhus, Denmark: University of Aarhus.

Un, H.: Presentation at the Carter Center. Retrieved April 18, 2010 from www.cartercenter.org/resources/pdfs/health/mental.../panel2-09-un.ppt

Unutzer, J., Katon, W., Callahan, C. M., Williams, J. W., Jr., Hunkeler, E., Harpole, L., et al. (2002). Collaborative care management of late-life depression in the primary care setting: A randomized controlled trial. *Journal of the American Medical Association, 288*(22), 2836–2845.

Unutzer, J., Katon, W. J., Fan, M. Y., Schoenbaum, M. C., Lin, E. H., Della Penna, R. D., et al. (2008). Long-term cost effects of collaborative care for late-life depression. *American Journal of Managed Care, 14*(2), 95–100.

Vahia, I. V., Diwan, S., Bankole, A. O., Kehn, M., Nurhussein, M., Ramirez, P., et al. (2008). Adequacy of medical treatment among older persons with schizophrenia. *Psychiatric Services, 59*(8), 853–859.

Wang, P. S., Berglund, P., Olfson, M., Pincus, H. A., Wells, K. B., & Kessler, R. C. (2005). Failure and delay in initial treatment contact after first onset of mental disorders in the National Comorbidity Survey Replication. *Archives General Psychiatry, 62*(6), 603–613.

Wang, P. S., Demler, O., & Kessler, R. C. (2002). Adequacy of treatment for serious mental illness in the United States. *American Journal of Public Health, 92*(1), 92–98.

Waters, E., Davis, E., Nicolas, C., Wake, M., & Lo, S. K. (2008). The impact of childhood conditions and concurrent morbidities on child health and well-being. *Child Care, Health & Development, 34*(4), 418–429.

Zuvekas, S. H., & Cohen, J. W. (2007). Prescription drugs and the changing concentration of health care expenditures. *Health Affairs (Millwood), 26*(1), 249–257.

CHAPTER 3

The Organization of Integrated Case Management Environments and Work Processes

OBJECTIVES

- To provide a high-level view of the integrated case management process
- To describe the personnel, training, and organizational needs for effective integrated case management
- To review patient triage, stratification, and prioritization
- To define the duties of enrollment specialists and integrated case managers
- To summarize case manager activities in the integrated management process, initiation through graduation

INTRODUCTION

Integrated case management is only as successful as the system in which integrated case management techniques are used. For instance, since the patients who are candidates for and would benefit from case management often have concurrent general medical and mental conditions that introduce barriers to health outcomes, programs in which physical and mental health management personnel have geographically discrete service locations will have greater difficulty in bringing value to patients and their health care operation than those in which cross-disciplinary access and interaction is expected and immediate. Other factors, such as how patients are triggered as candidates for case management, how integrated case managers are trained, how interdisciplinary documentation is recorded, and so forth play significant roles, which augment or reduce effectiveness. Managers who work in settings that are not organized to facilitate appropriate patient case finding and allow the implementation of outcome-changing management practices cannot be expected to be as effective in improving health and generating a return on investment as those who work in settings that do have these qualities, even if the case managers form excellent relationships with their patients and use exemplary integrated case management techniques.

This chapter is designed to discuss critical ingredients in the organization and administration of effective integrated case management programs. Training managers and developing effective organizational structures for integrated management programs that serve patients with lower levels of health complexity, such as disease management or wellness programs, are just as appropriate and important. The operational descriptions discussed in this chapter, however, do not specifically cover programs focused on less complex patients. On the other hand, it does provide an understanding of the principles of how integrated management programs should be structured, regardless of the targeted population or management location, thus it can provide guidance even for programs serving populations with lower-intensity needs or those with a mixture of management services offered.

THE INTEGRATED CASE MANAGEMENT PROCESS: THE BIG PICTURE

Integrated case management can be provided by individual nurses or social workers working in an outpatient clinic, by small groups of case managers who address the needs of patients admitted to or being discharged from a hospital, or by large cadres of managers providing telephonic management services for tens of thousands or millions of patients covered by health plans, a subset of which will have health complexity. In the current chapter, a framework for the construction of integrated case management services in a medium-to-large general medical health plan is presented. It will provide organizational principles that can be used regardless of the number of managers involved or the service location. To obtain an overview, a series of graphical illustrations summarizing the complete health plan-based telephonic integrated case management process has been developed. To see a consolidated overview, the reader should visit Appendix 1 at the back of the manual.

The illustration in Figure 3.1 depicts the development of integrated interdisciplinary case manager pods—five to nine closely connected and personally interacting case management professionals working in discrete units—as a core methodology in creating integrated services for larger organizations. The same methodology would not be appropriate when one or two case managers work in a multispecialty medical clinic, but it would be appropriate for managers working in small groups, such as for regional assertive community treatment (ACT) teams or in hospital-based case management services. Adjustments to the model are appropriate based on personnel, service location, the target population, and the goals of the program.

RELATIONSHIP OF CASE MANAGEMENT OBJECTIVES TO CORE INTEGRATED CASE MANAGEMENT ACTIVITIES

At the onset, it should be noted that the objectives of those who purchase or administer the services of case management personnel differ. For instance, case managers working for clinic systems typically target management activities that improve the efficiency and outcomes related to care for patients being treated by practitioners within their system. In such settings, targeted activities likely include patient education, treatment adherence measures, and assistance with clinic-related priorities (e.g., ensuring that Health Effectiveness Data and Information Sets [HEDIS] guidelines are followed, reducing clinic costs, etc.). Further, the management goals may focus only on the illness or illnesses addressed within a particular clinic, such as checking cardiac medication refills or ensuring rehabilitation participation. Typically, the role of the case manager is time limited and focused on factors related to the clinic visit and specific illness episode. The goal of the clinic is to maximize clinic-related outcomes, both clinical and financial. Overall health is not necessarily an action-stimulating priority.

The motives to support case managers for hospitals may be to improve the efficiency of discharge planning; for health plans, it may be to reduce claims costs;

for employers, it may be to increase work performance and decrease disability; and for case management vendors, it may be to generate return on investment for purchasers through the administration of efficient and extensive management services. There is nothing wrong with multiple organizations supporting case management activities or even having targeted goals for the managers that work for them. It is, however, important to understand these goals and objectives and how they affect outcomes for those exposed to case management services. Core integrated case management activities (**Exhibit 3.1**) are designed to maximize benefit to patients with health complexity. If work processes dictated by administrators of the case management program vary greatly from these core activities, predicted outcomes resulting from integrated case management techniques will necessarily change.

For instance, there is nothing wrong if case managers who work for hospitals focus on discharge planning for patients with complex postdischarge needs. Typically, however, after discharge arrangements have been made, managers disengage and move on to other patients. Focused management activity, such as this, may decrease denials for medically unnecessary extended stays and potentially reduce readmission rates, but it has not been shown to alter postdischarge adverse events, like medication death (Moore, Cohen, & Furberg, 2007), to improve health stability, or to lower long-term health costs. Achieving these additional goals would require taking a more longitudinal view by following through on and reversing elements of complexity on behalf of the patient even after discharge, as suggested by the core integrated case manager activities (**Exhibit 3.1**).

Core integrated case management activities are necessary for predicted health and cost outcomes to unfold as expected. For this reason, one of the most important considerations in putting together integrated case management programs in any setting is to align as closely as possible the focal organizational approach with core integrated case management practices. If more than one stakeholder (e.g., physicians, hospitals, and health plans) would benefit from the integrated case management activity, then collaboration among

---

EXHIBIT 3.1   **Core Integrated Case Manager Activities**

- Establishes a person-to-person relationship with the patient
- Takes a longitudinal view (weeks, months, or years)
- *Always* works primarily with the patient or patient's guardian, but also with the family, clinicians, and so forth
- Systematically assists patients in overcoming physical, psychological, social (biopsychosocial), and health system barriers
- Follows through and follows up
- Works toward patient problem resolution, stabilization, and case management graduation

business partners should drive the attempt to maximize outcomes for patients, sharing costs and profits among those contributing.

INTEGRATED CASE MANAGEMENT PERSONNEL AND ORGANIZATIONAL STRUCTURE

INTEGRATED CASE MANAGEMENT TEAMS

The development of integrated case management programs requires special attention to the recruitment of personnel interested in providing integrated management, the background and training of the personnel, and the way that they work with each other. Most health systems have been dis-integrated for so long that infrastructure reorganization requires the recruitment of personnel interested in working with the whole patient, willing to learn and apply new skills, and having the personal attributes needed to work on integrated management teams (**Figure 3.1**). The good news is that there are many health professionals who fall into the category of those interested in providing integrated services, such as nurses and social workers.

What cannot be done is to *force* a group of discrete physical and mental health case managers, invested in the management practices that they are currently providing, to change to new management practices, with or without integrated management training. While a significant subset of case managers will want to provide integrated services when additional training is provided, some managers wish to stick with the management practices to which they have become accustomed. It is important to recognize this fact and make a clean transition, providing training to those willing to give integrated practices a try.

In the health plan setting, there may be 40 or 50 case managers performing case or disease management on behalf of members at the greatest risk for poor outcomes—that is, complex patients. Depending on the population served, the objectives of the management process, and the percentage of the population exposed to integrated and nonintegrated case management, such large groups of managers should be divided into pods of seven to nine managers and a supervisor (**Figure 3.1**). Each of the integrated management pods will be composed of a combination of complementary personnel with mixed general medical and mental health backgrounds. Likely, most will be nurses because medical knowledge and sophistication will be necessary to assist complicated physically and mentally comorbid patients. Managers from other disciplines, such as social work, rehabilitation counselors, and so forth, however, may also be represented and can be very effective as long as they are willing to learn.

These pods will work together as educational and support units. While the patients that each case manager is assigned will remain with him or her through the course of management activity (a primary case manager model), pod members will educate and support each other in providing the best and most appropriate assistance to their patients through direct intrapod communication. This arrangement is particularly important as integrated services are being initiated because most team members will come from either general medical or mental health backgrounds, but not both. Managers will need assistance from cross-disciplinary team members as they work through interactive physical and mental condition problems for the first time. When pod team members mature in integrated care support, they will find that they need less ongoing help. Nevertheless, they will continue to give and receive advice long into the future for complex patients with complicated problems.

In addition to education and support derived from other pod members, integrated case managers are also expected to maintain a close working relationship with a supervising physician or physician team (general medical and psychiatric specialists), such as medical directors, to ensure that there is progression toward health barrier resolution with each complex patient. While more will be said about this later, this interaction largely takes place during weekly or biweekly systematic case reviews and is considered a critical component to ensure the application of coordinated and evidence-based general medical and mental health intervention.

In contrast to case managers employed through health plans or management vendors, who have a well-developed network of colleagues to support them in their work, clinical case managers working in inpatient general hospital settings often do not have more than one or two others providing such services for their hospitals. Further, more often than not, case managers are departmental or clinical site employees working in relative isolation and with limited backup. These traditional inpatient case management services, just as those in the health plan setting, require rethinking if they are going to bring value to patients, their hospitals, the professionals caring for the patients, and the health system in terms of improved outcomes and reduced health service use. For instance, a cadre of inpatient integrated case managers may be supervised by consultation-liaison psychiatrists, who specialize in mental health care for general medical patients, or physicians with combined general medical and psychiatric training. This physician group, which has an understanding of the medical and mental health interaction, sees a high percentage of patients with health complexity. Thus, they would be a logical group to support and

FIGURE 3.1   Integrated case management team formation and training.

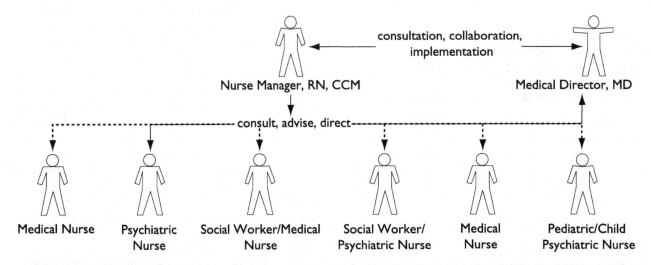

Skills
• Manager (RN, CCM)—preferably with background in general medical and mental health nursing, otherwise cross-training (CCM; certificate—integrated CM, motivational interviewing)
• Medical Director, MD—this is either a physician having comfort with assessment and treatment of physical and mental health problems or a collaborative team including a primary care physician and psychiatrist.
• Staff (CCM or working toward CCM; certificate—integrated CM with basic cross-training in the discipline from which they do not come); team size can vary by 1 or 2 either way

Cross-Training—basics started in integrated CM manual and onsite training (extra training required for child/youth integrated CM)
• Three weeks didactics in cross-discipline
• Three weeks direct mentoring in cross-discipline
• Case management vignettes
• Special integrated case management issues—legal, documentation standards, care coordination; emergency procedures (medical, psychiatric, and pediatric)

Shift Work
• During the first 4 months, there will always be staff from both disciplines available for consultation
• Team composition ratios adjusted based on clinical needs of the population served

Case Responsibility
• Full indirect, nonclinical assistance for patient needs (physical and mental condition care coordination, authorization, etc.) with advice from cross-trained teammates when needed
• Initial assignment should take into account the CM's case load composite IM-CAG or PIM-CAG-based health complexity level
• Few handoffs

Continuing Educational Enhancement
• Integrated CM grand rounds; complicated case reviews; news and views handouts on common problems, member outcomes, obstacles, successes; consultation with medical director (special arrangements for child/youth CM)

Expert Backup
• Team member collaboration
• Medical directors—general medical, psychiatric, pediatric
• Expert consultant specialists

to supervise case management activities in inpatient general hospital programs (Kathol et al., 2009).

In hospital systems and clinics, integrated case management may more effectively be supported at the organizational level (i.e., as a part of a public or private hospital and clinic system, an academic medical center, the local Veterans Administration health operation, etc.) rather than at a departmental or hospital unit level. If a clinical case management program is designed, which follows complex patients through their treatment and illness episodes in multiple locations throughout the delivery system, there is greater opportunity for long-term clinical change and cost reduction for those entering case management. In addition, organizing integrated case management services for complex patients on a system-wide basis would allow closer fidelity to the case management teams described for health plans and management vendors.

CASE MANAGEMENT WORKFLOWS

The activities in which case managers are involved greatly influence the workflow design and training needs for the managers involved. For instance, the preceding health plan example specifically relates to the longitudinal services of case managers using telephonic communication. Such an arrangement would not be necessary for ACT team managers because they provide onsite services to patients, primarily those with chronic and persistent mental illness. An alternative model would be to create a design with a smaller number of members in each pod and greater representation by professionals with mental health backgrounds on each team. On the other hand, general medical disorders are common in patients with complex, serious mental health problems, so team members with physical health backgrounds remain indispensable (Druss & von Esenwein, 2006; Jones et al., 2004). Further, the intent would be for case managers with mental health backgrounds to follow and assist with both mental condition and physical health issues without handing the patient to someone else. With one or more case management colleagues with general medical backgrounds on the ACT team in addition to physician support, cross-fertilization and medical supervision should allow this to happen most of the time.

Another example in which an alternative workflow model would be required is if an integrated case manager worked specifically for a discrete clinical service, such as on a complexity intervention unit (Kathol et al., 2009). In this situation, the case manager would need to marshal his or her own backup support from service personnel connected with the clinical service. This can sometimes be a challenge when the clinical location is connected to a discrete general medical or

mental health operation or is located at a distance from other health services. In these integrated case management settings, the case manager, her or his supervisor, and the system in which case management services are being delivered should form an alliance in setting up the support network that is needed to do integrated case management. This is particularly important if the case manager has only a general medical or mental health background.

There are unlimited combinations and permutations of clinical service delivery contexts, each of which requires customization of integrated case management work processes to meet organizational needs. Rather than approach this problem on an individual program basis, however, we prefer for those who are involved in developing such programs to become fluent enough in the principles of integrated case management to be able to adapt their own clinical settings such that they will deliver outcome-changing and cost-reducing management services. The basic principles related to this process are found in this manual.

CASE MANAGEMENT PERSONNEL TRAINING

Integrated case management team members should be drawn from both physical and mental health backgrounds; however, the expectation is that regardless of the background of the case manager, he or she will receive sufficient training and have professional colleague and medical director backup so that he or she will be able to address needs for both general medical and mental health barriers to improvement in the same patient. General skills of case managers are learned during basic case management training. They are described in the case management Standards of Practice (Exhibit 1.2; CMSA, 2010) and are the subject of a number of books on the topic (Fattorusso & Quinn, 2007; Mullahy & Jensen, 2004; Powell, Tahan, & CMSA, 2008; Weed & Berens, 2009). Training specific to integrated case management is summarized in **Exhibit 3.2**.

Integrated case management requires the development of cross-disciplinary skills. While some may think that the manual would focus primarily on common cross-disciplinary conditions, in fact, this is only a piece of the training process. It is important but by no means overriding. In addition, the managers must learn to deal with unfamiliar emergent situations, differing admissions processes and policies, divergent medical necessity criteria, legal reporting requirements, cross-disciplinary community resources, autonomous payment practices, and other issues. To some, this may seem daunting. Experience, however, shows that those who are willing become comfortable with

---

EXHIBIT 3.2   Cross-Disciplinary Integrated Case Manager Training

General (use integrated care vignettes—e.g., diabetic crises, suicidal, medically compromised eating disorder)

- Case management standards (see CMSA Standards of Practice: Section 2 and www.cmsa.org)—for example, assessment, planning, facilitation, and advocacy
- Standards of care (e.g., identification of patient's need for case management services), problem identification, planning, monitoring, evaluating, outcomes measurement, case closure
- Interpersonal skills, coping skills training
- Interviewing techniques—for example, development of a relationship, use of open-ended questions, knowledge of when and how to share personal information, use of motivational interviewing techniques
- Assessment of physical and mental condition insurance coverage limitations and exclusions
- Documentation processes—for example, check sheet for opening and closing cases, use of scripts, use of computer, here and now entry
- Follow-up—for example, how often should the patient be seen, how to work through prioritized actions
- Legal concerns—for example, HIPAA; privacy; physical, mental health, and child/youth consents; approach to confidentiality; objective documentation techniques
- Closing cases—for example, proper graduation processes with the patient, handling of medical records received, and so forth
- Use of Internet—for example, educational sites and social service and community resource links

From Psychiatric Background

- General medical disorders/problems update—for example, diabetes, hypertension, back pain, asthma, enuresis, congestive heart failure, emphysema, ischemic heart disease, dementia, head injury
- Community resources available for medically ill
- Basics on medical emergencies, medical admissions, placement, durable medical equipment procurement and use in the medical setting

From Medical Background

- General psychiatric disorders/problems update—for example, affective disorders, anxiety, eating disorders, schizophrenia, autism, delirium, somatoform disorders, chemical dependence
- Community resources available for psychiatrically ill
- Basics on psychiatric emergencies, admissions, and placement; payment issues in the psychiatric setting; levels of care (residential, partial hospitalization, intensive outpatient, etc.)

Pediatric Case Management

- Pediatric management practices—for example, working with parents/caregivers and children/youth
- Cross-disciplinary updates—for example, child psychiatry for those with medical backgrounds and medical for those with psychiatric backgrounds
- Pediatric resources and procedures—for example, foster homes, abuse reporting, guardianship

---

the added procedures do so within several months of initiating integrated work. Further, they take great pride in newly learned skills and the help that they bring to their patients.

The majority of work in integrated case management, and indeed in traditional case management as well, has taken place in the adult setting. For this manual, pediatric specialists have worked together to create a pediatric version of integrated case management in response to a recognized need. The authors feel strongly that supplementary training will be required to perform pediatric integrated case management in

addition to manual study and adult certificate completion because it is a specialized skill set. Those who perform pediatric integrated case management will not only be working with children/youth; they will also be interacting with caregivers/parents, many of whom may be in as great a need for case management support as their child/youth. Two chapters (Chapter 8 and Chapter 14) are devoted to pediatric integrated case management. For those wishing to utilize their integrated pediatric case management knowledge base, supplemental specialized onsite pediatric training will be available through CMSA.

CONNECTING GENERAL MEDICAL AND MENTAL HEALTH CASE MANAGEMENT

Physical and mental conditions interact to create treatment failure scenarios for patients, as discussed in Chapter 2. The integrated system changes the case management paradigm and requires training that will allow professionals with backgrounds focused on assisting patients with physical illness to develop the skills needed to also assist those with mental conditions, and vice versa. This will be covered in greater detail in Chapters 5 and 6.

Since cross-disciplinary skills cannot be expected to appear overnight, the integrated case management system, which incorporates complexity assessment grid methodology, also includes strategies to facilitate the transition from a segregated approach to an integrated one. Case managers coming from medical or surgical backgrounds will systematically learn the skills needed to identify and intervene for psychological and social factors that cause barriers to improvement. Likewise, using guidelines for the care of most common chronic and acute general medical conditions will become a daily part of professional activity for case managers with mental health backgrounds.

Since case managers are not involved in the treatment of the patients, their job is to use their backgrounds and experience in health, health care, and the health system to assist patients in receiving the best care possible, given the complicated nature of illness, let alone the system in which it is delivered. Thinking in simple terms, case managers might be likened to knowledgeable, concerned offspring helping his or her parent obtain the best care and thus have the greatest chance of maintaining good health and quality of life. Case managers, however, possess medical sophistication, have dedicated time to help the patient, are supported by cross-disciplinary colleagues, and receive physician-based supervision. Therefore, the opportunity for health improvement and decreased health service utilization is even greater than that resulting from the assistance of caring relatives.

Finally, unlike existing programs that attempt to integrate physical and mental health management through a system of handoffs, integrated case management, which includes INTERMED-Complexity Assessment Grid (IM-CAG) and Pediatric INTERMED-Complexity Assessment Grid (PIM-CAG) methodology, places great importance on the relationship between the case manager and the patient. For this reason, handoffs from physical health to mental health specialists are kept to a minimum. Rather, the primary case manager will seek additional direction about conditions that fall outside of his or her area of expertise from interdisciplinary colleagues and from physician supervisors. Once direction is received, the primary case manager continues to work directly with the patient in attempting to resolve barriers to improvement.

CASE MANAGER CASELOAD LIMITS

Case management, as defined in this manual, is an intense, service-oriented activity that requires time, expertise, and effort for each patient enrolled with the case manager. It brings its value by changing clinical, functional, and economic outcomes for the patients that are served. This can only be accomplished when sufficient time is available to educate, assist, and support patients through the crises they are encountering.

Based on the experience of programs that utilize outcome-oriented care management procedures, the number of cases carried by integrated case managers should not exceed one manager to 70 active complex cases (1:70). In some markets, such as in public programs where health complexity is usually higher, the number of patients served per case manager should be no more than 1:20. On average, benchmark standards for cases with health complexity per manager would be between 1:30 and 1:50 when the type of management described in this manual is used. Considering these metrics and the knowledge that highly complex patients may average from 3 to 6 months in case management, it is possible for an integrated case manager to service the needs of 60 to 200 highly complex patients per year.

Recently acquired patients will have many risks and needs creating barriers to health. Thus, initially they require regular and frequent calls, often more than one per day to the patient, to the patient's clinicians, to family members, to community resources, to law enforcement, to schools, and to many others. Patients who are nearing graduation, on the other hand, may be working with the case manager on stabilization techniques no more than once per month before transfer back to standard care. Regardless of where a patient is in the case management process, it is important for the case manager to have time to complete actions that will change outcomes.

Disease managers devote their efforts to assisting those with chronic illnesses, such as congestive heart failure, end-stage renal disease, asthma, chronic obstructive pulmonary disease, diabetes, depression, and so forth. Patients who are assisted using this form of care management typically have chronic, persistent low to high levels of health service use and frequently have concurrent mental conditions complicating their treatment (Kathol, Saravay, Lobo, & Ormel, 2006). As a result, integrated disease management, though technically not a part of case management, can be a significant contributor to improved outcomes by using the same principles that are used for case management—that is, disease managers provide multidomain, multi-illness support rather than just disease-specific assistance.

Since patients with illnesses assisted through disease management average lower levels of health complexity, benchmarks for the number of patients that disease managers can carry have higher ratios than in case management. Further, the average length of time that they would be expected to work with the average patient would be shorter. In the absence of extenuating circumstances, benchmarks for the number of cases that a disease manager could carry would not exceed 1:250. In some markets, the number carried may not exceed 1:100 depending on the level of complexity needed for entry into active, not just educational, disease management services. In addition, the number of patients each manager could carry would be influenced by the management expectations—for example, number of calls to the patient; health status indicator achievement, such as a targeted HbA1c level; or alterations in health service usage, such as fewer emergency room visits.

On average, benchmarks for cases per disease manager are between 1:150 and 1:400 if all levels of health complexity enter the program with a given chronic illness. The number of patients that disease managers can assist per year, however, also relates to the number in each complexity level that they are expected to assist (see the following section, "Determining the Number of Managers Needed for Populations Served"). For instance, managers of patients in at-risk pregnancy programs, the majority of whom have low-risk pregnancies, may be able to service the needs of more than 400 individual patients per manager, whereas the case load for managers working with patients having end-stage renal disease or congestive heart failure may be no more than 70 active patients at a given time.

It is not only the type of illness on which disease managers focus that determines their caseload; it is also what they do with and for the patients with whom they work. In some disease management programs, when patients reach a certain level of complexity, they are transferred to dedicated *case* managers so that they can receive more aggressive assistance. In other programs, disease managers are expected to address all levels of complexity within their caseload. Disease managers in the first scenario would be able to handle a larger caseload than in the second if clinical and financial outcome change is the desired result.

DETERMINING THE NUMBER OF MANAGERS NEEDED FOR POPULATIONS SERVED

Case management is built on the principle that by offering individualized assistance to patients with chronic and/or complex illness, it is possible to improve clinical outcomes, reduce impairment, and lower future health service needs. As long as managers are able to continue to operationally deliver outcome-changing case management services, the more chronic and complex patients that are managed, the greater the clinical benefit and ultimately the lower the total cost of health care that can be achieved. Given this principle, virtually all programs in which case management services are offered would bring clinical and financial benefit if they staffed to the level that could address the service needs for the top 0.5% to 2% of complex patients (Katon et al., 2008; Thomas, Waxmonsky, McGinnis, & Barry, 2006). These treatment-resistant, functionally handicapped patients, nearly 80% of whom have general medical and mental health comorbidity, expend up to a third of health resources (Figure 2.2; Zuvekas & Cohen, 2007). Projected absolute dollar savings and return on investment are virtually assured, but only if core management services can be delivered (**Exhibit 3.1**).

In fact, one could extend management services to other less ill populations than highly complex patients and still achieve clinical, functional, and financial benefit. Disease management programs have demonstrated value when assistance is provided to selected populations of chronically ill patients (Goetzel, Ozminkowski, Villagra, & Duffy, 2005; Goetzel et al., 2004). As the level of complexity decreases, however, the value brought to individual patients decreases, both clinically and financially. For instance, in patients with chronic illness and low complexity, less rigorous management activities, such as education about illness, promoting healthy behaviors, and prevention, provided by lower cost personnel serving in wellness and health care coaching programs, can still be cost effective and health enhancing depending on how they target patients and work with them. The major opportunity for health improvement and cost containment, however, lies with case management in those with the most complexity.

Determining how to put together management programs that provide value to patients and the health system at each level of the care management continuum is currently a challenge. Specifically with regard to case management programs, most programs do not have a consistent method to determine the number of cases a manager can effectively carry and yet maintain the ability to overcome barriers to improvement. The industry caseload benchmarks already described provide guidelines but are poor at directing individual organizations as they determine the number and type of patients that their case managers can/should handle.

Factors that go into such decisions vary widely from organization to organization. They include but are not limited to: (a) the population served (e.g., commercial vs. indigent), (b) the goals of case management (e.g., health improvement vs. re-admission prevention), (c) case manager success metrics (e.g., health improvement vs. the number of patient contacts made), (d) the level of complexity of patients encountered (e.g., high vs. mixed), and (e) the expected duration of management contact (e.g., during hospitalization vs. through illness episode vs. when complexity issues have been addressed). Each of these and many other factors influence the case manager-to-patient ratio and the expected actions of the case managers, yet there are no outcomes-oriented rules for making such decisions. It often ends up being a judgment call made by the case management supervisor or medical director.

The integrated case management approach found in this manual offers a convenient and consistent way to estimate the number of managers needed to serve specific populations and even provides a way to document the complexity level of the patients served. Whether a patient is being assessed and assisted by a case manager, a disease manager, or a care manager involved in another program, it is possible using the integrated case management paradigm to create a logical, outcome-oriented approach to staffing based on patient stratification, prioritization, and complexity level. How this is accomplished is covered in Chapter 9, "Change Measurement and Case Manager Caseload Estimation."

GOALS, TRIAGE FOR CASE MANAGEMENT PARTICIPATION, AND PATIENT INDUCTION

GOALS

Integrated case management, as defined in this manual, is patient centric. The central hypothesis is that in patients with health complexity, reversing or attenuating barriers to improvement found in the biological, psychological, social, and health system domains will be associated with health care cost reduction and lower impairment. As noted in Chapter 2 ("Value of Integrated Physical and Mental Health Case Management" section), preliminary studies confirm that this change happens when integrated practices are initiated (Thomas et al., 2006). The findings, however, are more robust when patients with greater complexity are targeted for management (Katon et al., 2008). Significantly, if

patients do not improve clinically, better fiscal and functional outcomes cannot be expected. That is why adherence to the integrated case management approach used in this manual is considered so critical.

TRIAGE FOR CASE MANAGEMENT PARTICIPATION

Case management *always* begins with population triage (Appendix 2). Without this step, valuable case managers will be utilizing their skills working with patients who are unlikely or less likely to derive benefit. As with all else in setting up case management practices, the population served and the goals of management will dictate triggers for inclusion and the process through which patients are identified using these triggers. For instance, in a health plan, claims data provide a convenient way to uncover patients at risk for poor outcomes. Health plans with sophisticated information technology (IT) systems may use predictive modeling algorithms either developed internally or purchased from an external vendor. Others may use acuity groupers, such as adjusted clinical groups (ACGs; Weiner et al., 1996) or diagnostic cost groups/hierarchical condition categories (DCGs/HCCs; Ash, Zhao, Ellis, & Schlein Kramer, 2001), as the risk assessment and identification methodology.

In the clinical setting, such as in hospital inpatient units or in multispecialty clinics, an alternative to administrative claims review is the clinical application of similar health service use risk parameters, often readily identified or known by the patients' doctors and their clinical staff. Virtually all administrative assessment systems use some combination of the triggers listed in Appendix 2, which readers should now take time to review in the Appendices. Regardless, the trick is to quickly, efficiently, and inexpensively identify patients at the highest risk for health complexity so that they can enter and benefit from the services of case managers (**Figure 3.2**).

Two major obstacles can complicate the triage process. First, the triggering system can identify complex patients well after the opportunity for health improvement and savings has passed. This is perhaps the greatest drawback of a claims-based system for identification, whether a predictive modeling tool is used or not. To improve the problems associated with the 3- to 6-month delay in uncovering patients with claims incurred but not reported (IBNR), health plan and vendor-based case management systems can also accept referrals for case management from utilization managers, from clinicians working with complex patients, or from social services systems. In fact, collaborating with health personnel, especially if they have been trained in the meaning of health risk and complexity, can be a

FIGURE 3.2 Integrated case manager care plan triggering and triage.

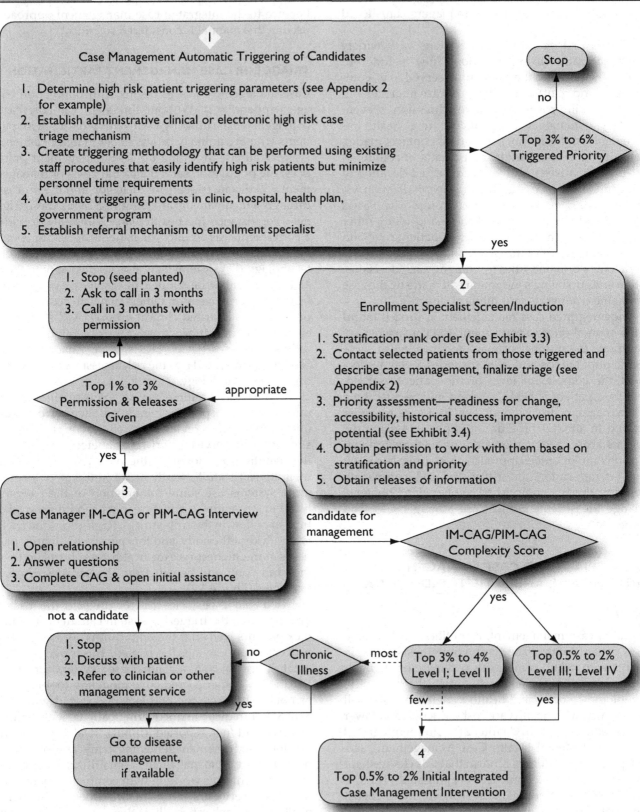

valuable strategy in catching high-risk patients before health problems grow in magnitude.

The second major obstacle is the mere time it takes in a system with high sensitivity but low specificity for health complexity to sort triggered patients that would benefit most from case management. The triggering system must be sufficiently discriminatory so that it moderates the candidate pool without involving much in the way of professional time.

The triggering algorithms and the process of efficiently narrowing patients to those who will be asked to participate in management activity is as important as the methods used by the managers once they have been assigned patients. As depicted in **Figure 3.2**, Step 1, the initial and preferably automatic triggering process should filter to the top 3% to 6% of candidates for case management, or a smaller percentage if the management program is designed or has staff to manage only 0.5% to 1% of the population served. Little in the way of staff time should be expended to get to the top 3% to 6%.

With a small number of initially triggered patients, an enrollment specialist should be able to efficiently stratify and prioritize (**Exhibit 3.3** and **Exhibit 3.4** or Appendix A, www.springerpub.com/kathol) remaining candidates and then obtain consent for participation from the 2% to 4% selected. Only after triage is complete do the more expensive and highly trained case managers become involved.

Additional patients will still be filtered during the initial case management assessment, using the adult or pediatric version of the CAG (**Figure 3.2**, Step 3). Most who reach this stage will still derive benefit from health barrier identification and suggestions from case managers related to items in the CAG. Less complex patients, as determined by IM-CAG and PIM-CAG scores, will not enter longitudinal case management. Rather, they will receive suggestions from the case manager about the things that they can do for themselves and with their personal clinicians to overcome identified barriers to improvement. In addition, they will be directed to other care management resources if they are available—for example, disease management. The patient's clinicians should receive a copy of the scored IM-CAG with an explanation of the scoring system and recommended goals and action items. Maintaining good relations with the triggered but not managed group is important because a number of them will reenter the system at a time when their need for case management may be greater or when the number of case managers expands.

The enrollment specialist considers a number of factors in the process of determining how many of the triggered patients will be candidates for case management. While most factors have to do with the characteristics of the patients and their willingness to participate, of equal importance is the number of managers available to take new cases, based on their current caseload. This is one of the benefits of IM-CAG methodology since it helps to document the total complexity level of the patient pool for each case manager. From this determination, it is possible to estimate desirable manager caseloads and the advisability of adding additional patients to the manager's list (see Chapter 9, "Change Measurement and Case Manager Caseload Estimation").

As a rule of thumb, a claims-based triggering system should uncover only two to three times the number of potential candidates for case management as the number of case manager slots available. This enables enrollment specialists to weed out those who do not wish to participate, to stratify and exclude triggered patients with less complexity, and to prioritize those most likely to benefit. Another factor that should be taken into consideration is whether patients with comparable complexity, but who have been directly referred should be given preference over those coming from a claims-based triggering process. Since directly referred patients, picked up earlier in the complexity/high service use spiral potentially have greater opportunity for improvement, they generally should be given more serious consideration for entry into case management.

PATIENT INDUCTION

Once patients are identified as part of the top 3% to 6% of those at risk for poor outcome, they are stratified (**Exhibit 3.3**) and then they are contacted (**Figure 3.2**, Step 2). Based on the stratification level, the enrollment specialist then contacts patients, shares information with them about the program, and answers questions (Appendix B, www.springerpub.com/kathol).

If the person remains interested, a readiness for change evaluation is performed (Appendix B, www.springerpub.com/kathol). This initiates the priority assessment to determine if a patient will be asked to enter case management (**Exhibit 3.4**). Those with motivation to change, a prior history of improvement through case management, the ability to engage with the manger either personally or through a significant other, and the potential for clinical benefit will be asked if they would be willing to work with a case manager. For those willing, information releases will be signed, preliminary administrative information will be obtained (**Exhibit 3.5**), and the patient will be directly transferred to a case manager. The administrative checklist is passed to the case manager for further information to be added as it becomes available.

Contact with the patient can be face-to-face, as might occur in an inpatient setting, in a healthcare clinic, at an ACT site, or at an employer's health center.

EXHIBIT 3.3   Stratification Levels*

LEVEL I

- **Little impact:** Minimal case management involvement (e.g., wellness, health care coaching), such as:
  - Education
  - Placement assistance
- **Anticipated time of involvement:** Days or less
- **Typical clinical situation:**
  - Coming out of a high health care cost activity, such as an inpatient stay, with anticipated rapid recovery and little follow-up need
  - Minimal interaction of medical and psychiatric illness and/or issues have already been addressed
- **Likely IM-CAG score:** Below 22

LEVEL II

- **Low impact:** Brief case management involvement (e.g., disease management, disability management), such as:
  - Education
  - Placement assistance
  - Referral to personal nurse or disease management
  - Assistance with workplace reentry (Employee Assistance Program [EAP] involvement)
  - Assistance with community programs
- **Anticipated time of involvement:** Days to weeks
- **Typical clinical situation:**
  - Coming out of high health care cost activity, such as inpatient stay, with anticipated persistent need for support to prevent delayed recovery and/or poor long-term outcome
- **Likely IM-CAG score:** 23 to 29

LEVEL III

- **Moderate impact:** Standard case management involvement, such as:
  - Identification of patient needs in the physical, social, behavioral, and health system domains
  - Development of a care plan
  - Assistance to the patient in understanding illnesses and health system factors that impede receiving appropriate care
  - Systematically working through the care plan
- **Anticipated time of involvement:** Weeks to months
- **Typical clinical situation:**
  - Inpatient and outpatient persistent service use and probability of further difficulties
  - Poorly treated psychiatric comorbidity in the face of serious subacute and/or chronic general medical illness, social challenges, and health system issues
  - Poorly treated medical comorbidity in the face of serious sub-acute and/or chronic psychiatric illness, social challenges, and health system issues
- **Likely IM-CAG score:** 30 to 35

LEVEL IV

- **High impact:** Extended case management involvement, as in Level III, however, problems are persistent, complex, and multiple, with long-term high service use or anticipated risk of high service use, thus longer term case management involvement warranted
- **Anticipated time of involvement:** Months or longer
- **Typical clinical situation:**
  - Complex, concurrent physical and mental conditions with inpatient and outpatient long-term service use
- **Likely IM-CAG score:** 36 or above

---

*"Stratification" of potential candidates for case management is based on a triggering process estimate by the enrollment specialist of a patient's service use pattern, which suggests persistent or worsening illness, functional impairment, and high health care service use.

EXHIBIT 3.4   **Priority Levels***

Priority Level Evaluation and Scoring

1. Motivation to change:

   a—none
   b—some
   c—good

2. Case management response history:

   a—poor
   b—never tried
   c—good

3. Ease of contact:

   a—nearly impossible
   b—complicated
   c—easy

4. Improvement potential:

   a—little
   b—some
   c—significant

Scoring system:

If no "a" responses and "c" for three or more: High priority
If no "a" responses and "c" for at least one: Medium priority
If any "a" response combination: Low priority

---

* *"Prioritization" of potential candidates stratified at a high level and in serious consideration for case management intervention relates to practical considerations about who are most likely to benefit, i.e., improvement potential, motivation to change, ease of contact, and prior case management outcome.*

EXHIBIT 3.5   Case Management Checklist

Patient Name: _____

Patient's DOB: _____ **Patient's Sex:** _____ **Case #** _____

Caregiver/Parent/Guardian Name: _____

Phone: _____

E-mail: _____

Primary Clinician Name: _____

Primary Clinician Phone #: _____

Insurance Company: _____

Insurance ID #: _____

Benefits Phone #: _____

Insurance Plan Provisions:

Copay _____; Deductible _____

General Medical Health Inpatient _____; Outpatient _____

Residential or Long-Term Care _____

Mental Health Inpatient _____; Outpatient _____; Day Treatment _____

Initiation Activities:

_____ Verbal and written consents obtained and on file

_____ Introductory phone call to patient made (document attempts)

_____ Introductory letter to patient sent (with business card)

_____ IM-CAG or PIM-CAG completed

_____ Primary clinician(s) offices contacted by case management

_____ Family contact information on file (if consents given)

_____ Patient added to case management log

It could be through a telephone call or a letter (Appendix B, www.springerpub.com/kathol, provides letter examples/templates), the approach commonly used by health plans and management vendors. Regardless of the method of contact, enrollment specialists, most often with less training than case managers, can become proficient at enrolling case management participants. Even when they are unsuccessful in recruiting the patient, they provide candidates with a business card or contact number. Should the patient's willingness to participate or health status change, they will have a way to contact the enrollment specialist for further information and potential induction.

Stratification and prioritization is a subjective activity; however, enrollment specialists soon recognize patterns of patient presentations that show the greatest need and potential for health improvement. Further, as outcomes of the management process are documented, enrollment specialists and the organizations they work for can use results from patients who have participated in integrated case management during future screening and enrollment to target similar patients who have demonstrated the most benefit.

In addition to facilitating appropriate enrollment of high-risk patients, the enrollment specialist also plays a critical role in collecting data elements on nonparticipating, high-risk controls that can be used for comparison to patients involved in active management. Specifically, the enrollment specialist should record patient identifiers, stratification and priority levels, and the reasons for nonparticipation, such as: (a) not asked (e.g., low stratification level or priority), (b) not reachable or has a language barrier, or (c) not interested in the program despite being offered (e.g., too busy, inertia, bad prior experience). Aggregate claims information for secondary outcomes from these patients will serve as comparative control data for those actively participating in the case management process.

INFORMED CONSENT

For convenience and expediency, informed consent for participation in integrated case management programs should be written into the patient's health insurance contract as a part of basic clinical care when health complexity arises. Contract language preferably would allow complex, high-cost patients to access case management services without additional consent and include unfettered communication among clinicians from all areas in which clinical services and service support is being provided—for example, between and among physical and mental condition providers; between and among health plan case managers and care managers in other sponsored programs, such as disease management; and between and among case managers and the patient's clinicians. (A *clinician* is defined as any clinical-based health care professional who assists the patient in receiving interventions that will lead to better health outcomes.)

Some contracts do not have language written into them that allows communication among all providers. When this is the case, it is possible to have the patient sign a universal consent (Appendix 3), which allows all clinicians, including mental condition practitioners, working with the patient to have equal access to information that would be helpful for them to know. Universal consent increases the ability for clinicians to communicate openly with other clinicians on the patient's behalf.

Informed consent for case managers to communicate with a patient's clinicians is often not written into health insurance contracts. Since case management is an augmentation of health plan and/or hospital/clinic services, consent for participation should be based on the patient's willingness to participate in the case management process (implied consent) rather than there being a requirement for formal written informed consent. This is called the opt out approach to patient participation. By using the opt out approach versus the opt in approach (written informed consent required by all participants), enrollment can jump from 10% to 80%.

PERSONAL HEALTH INFORMATION PRIVACY

Mental condition care is an integral part of health. Informed consent with regard to mental health care should be *no different* than between clinicians handling general medical problems—for example, an urologist treating erectile dysfunction, a gynecologist treating gonorrhea, and a family practitioner providing birth control pills to a sexually active minor. Special rules apply for psychotherapy process notes and for substance use disorder treatment programs in HIPAA (Health Insurance Portability and Accountability Act) laws in the United States, but these generally do not inhibit free communication among clinicians about personal health information (PHI) in most instances.

Moving forward, contract language related to mental health and substance use disorders should be changed so that it is handled as a part of physical health. PHI privacy should be protected from nonclinicians rigorously and equally for both physical and mental conditions. There should be no need for a distinction or separation of notes.

CASE MANAGEMENT PROCESS: INITIATION, CONTINUATION, AND DISCHARGE

Using the health plan scenario already mentioned, we have described an enrollment specialist who transfers identified management candidates that have consented to participate to a case manager (**Figure 3.2**, Step 3). Information related to using CAG integrated case management methodology will be discussed in detail in Chapters 7 through 10 of the manual. Before we move to a discussion of the complexity assessment and intervention process, however, it is important to have a picture of the case management process—from start to finish—thus only basic features and use of the CAG will be described here.

Essential to any form of integrated case management is the development of a relationship between the patient and the manager. This starts with the CAG interview and closes with the patient's graduation from case management assistance. At the completion of the initial CAG interview, which uses open-ended relationship-building questions, the case manager will have completed a grid, scoring the patient's level of complexity in 20 cells or content items representing four domains (25 cells in the pediatric version). Scores in each cell are based on standardized anchor points and are linked to the level of patient vulnerability and of action required, as described in **Table 3.1** (see page **i1** for the color version of this table).

Cells with red/dark gray and orange/less dark gray suggest the greatest need for action. Thus, in a completed grid representing the interview findings of Harold, a 57-year-old patient with Parkinson's disease, dementia, and psychosis from his medication (**Table 3.2**; see page **i1** for the color version of this table), it is apparent that he is at risk for poor outcome, as much due to the fact that he just lost his wife, has no family, and is without insurance as from the severity/acuity of his illnesses. Initial intervention would be directed to correcting barriers represented by cells with red/dark gray rectangles, followed by orange/less dark gray,

and so forth. A score of 42 (**Table 3.2**, upper left corner) indicates very high complexity.

Figure 3.3 provides a graphical illustration of how an initial care plan would be developed and used iteratively to guide case manager and patient activities after the initial interview using integrated case management techniques. For the patient Harold, who has an IM-CAG score of 42, there are no personal goals, because of his dementia. Further, it is not possible to rely on him for assistance in setting goals; however, there is a social worker at his nursing home and personal friends who recognize the need for assistance to Harold through this life transition. Harold's wife took care of her husband until about 6 months prior to her death. At that time, he was transferred to a nursing home since she could no longer individually handle his needs. Harold retired at 55 from a high paying job and had few financial needs until he failed to pay his health insurance premiums and lost his coverage.

Since Harold is at significant risk for poor physical and mental health outcomes and for high health care service use with no insurance support for his care, the case manager for the hospital to which Harold was admitted uses item scores on the IM-CAG to guide and prioritize assistance with his immediate needs. Red/dark gray and orange/less dark gray items in multiple domains are easily identified. Several can be connected as a care plan is created. Harold definitely requires involvement of both physical and mental health specialists; however, several non-medical barriers to improvement are in many ways as, if not more, important to his long-term health and financial stability. Consistent with an integrated case management care plan, the case manager initiates and follows up on actions on Harold's behalf, working with his clinicians, the nursing home, distant relatives, close friends, and his previous insurance company to identify options, maximize benefit, and help him stabilize health and recover dignity. The case manager recognizes that Harold's needs for individualized assistance will likely be iterative and measured in months, long after discharge from the hospital, in order for a guardian to be appointed, insurance reinstated, health stabilized, and financial security recovered. Thus, she uses the iterative process depicted in **Figure 3.3**. While the case manager works in the hospital, her salary is supported by a funding source that allows her to help Harold transition to a more stable health care situation.

Integrated case management, particularly in patients with significant health complexity, is intended to move toward case closure. The case manager starts by systematically reversing and attenuating the greatest barriers to improvement that are measured through CAG methodology—that is, items scored as 2 or 3. When these have been addressed, the case manager

TABLE 3.1	Complexity Assessment Grid Scoring		
Patient's risks or needs	CAG score	Associated color code	Actions facilitated by case manager
None	0; green		No need to act
Mild	1; yellow		Need for monitoring or prevention
Moderate	2; orange		Need for action or development of intervention plan
Severe	3; red		Need for immediate action or immediate intervention plan

TABLE 3.2	Harold's IM-CAG (Baseline)					
Baseline	**HEALTH RISKS AND HEALTH NEEDS**					
Harold	**HISTORICAL**		**CURRENT STATE**		**VULNERABILITY**	
Total Score = 42	Complexity Item	Score	Complexity Item	Score	Complexity Item	Score
Biological Domain	Chronicity **HB1**	2	Symptom Severity/Impairment **CB1**	2	Complications and Life Threat **VB**	2
	Diagnostic Dilemma **HB2**	1	Diagnostic/Therapeutic Challenge **CB2**	3		
Psychological Domain	Barriers to Coping **HP1**	1	Resistance to Treatment **CP1**	3	Mental Health Threat **VP**	2
	Mental Health History **HP2**	1	Mental Health Symptoms **CP2**	3		
Social Domain	Job and Leisure **HS1**	3	Residential Stability **CS1**	0	Social Vulnerability **VS**	2
	Relationships **HS2**	1	Social Support **CS2**	3		
Health System Domain	Access to Care **HHS1**	3	Getting Needed Services **CHS1**	3	Health System Impediments **VHS**	3
	Treatment Experience **HHS2**	1	Coordination of Care **CHS2**	3		

Comments
Significant dementia with psychosis from l-dopa used for Parkinson disease treatment; can't follow directions; wife who took care of him recently died suddenly; no family; no insurance; no primary or consistent physician.

Scoring System

Green	0	= no vulnerability or need to act
Yellow	1	= mild vulnerability and need for monitoring or prevention
Orange	2	= moderate vulnerability and need for action or development of intervention plan
Red	3	= severe vulnerability and need for immediate action or immediate intervention plan

Biological Domain Items		**Psychological Domain Items**	
HB1	Physical illness chronicity	HP1	Problems handling stress and/or problem solving
HB2	Historic problems in diagnosing the physical illness	HP2	Prior mental condition difficulties
CB1	Physical illness symptom severity and impairment	CP1	Resistance to treatment; nonadherence
CB2	Current difficulties in diagnosis and/or treatment if case management is stopped	CP2	Current mental condition symptom severity
VB	Risk of physical complications and life threat if case management is stopped	VP	Risk of persistent personal barriers or poor mental condition care if case management is stopped

Social Domain Items		**Health System Domain Items**	
HS1	Personal productivity and leisure activities	HHS1	Health system-related access to appropriate care
HS2	Relationship difficulties	HHS2	Experiences with doctors or the health system
CS1	Residential stability or suitability	CHS1	Logistical ability to get needed care at service delivery level
CS2	Availability of social support	CHS2	Communication among providers and coordination of care
VS	Risk of work, home, and relational support needs if case management is stopped	VHS	Risk of persistent poor access to and/or coordination of services if case management is stopped

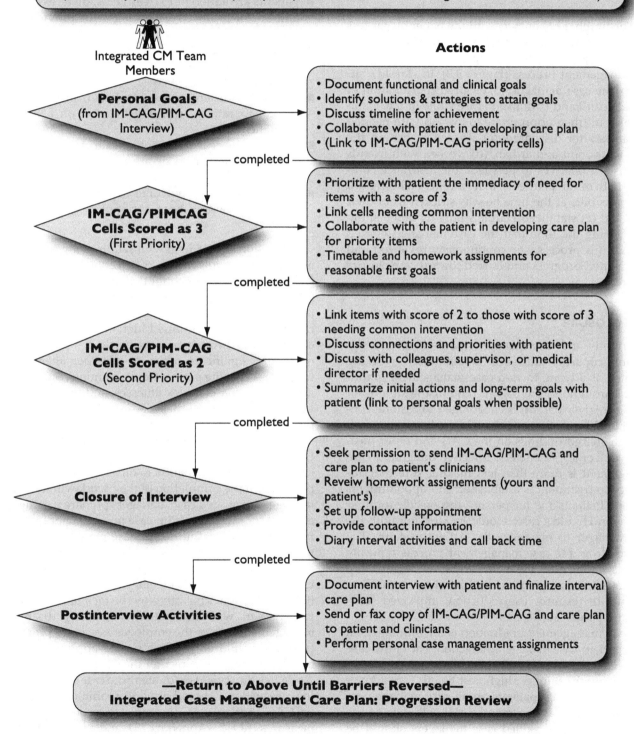

Initial & Iterative Case Management Intervention
(develop relationship and, with informed consent, share assessment results with patient, primary support persons, key providers, school (child/youth); send illness and case management educational materials)

Integrated CM Team Members

Actions

Personal Goals
(from IM-CAG/PIM-CAG Interview)

- Document functional and clinical goals
- Identify solutions & strategies to attain goals
- Discuss timeline for achievement
- Collaborate with patient in developing care plan
- (Link to IM-CAG/PIM-CAG priority cells)

— completed —

IM-CAG/PIMCAG Cells Scored as 3
(First Priority)

- Prioritize with patient the immediacy of need for items with a score of 3
- Link cells needing common intervention
- Collaborate with the patient in developing care plan for priority items
- Timetable and homework assignments for reasonable first goals

— completed —

IM-CAG/PIM-CAG Cells Scored as 2
(Second Priority)

- Link items with score of 2 to those with score of 3 needing common intervention
- Discuss connections and priorities with patient
- Discuss with colleagues, supervisor, or medical director if needed
- Summarize initial actions and long-term goals with patient (link to personal goals when possible)

— completed —

Closure of Interview

- Seek permission to send IM-CAG/PIM-CAG and care plan to patient's clinicians
- Reveiw homework assignments (yours and patient's)
- Set up follow-up appointment
- Provide contact information
- Diary interval activities and call back time

— completed —

Postinterview Activities

- Document interview with patient and finalize interval care plan
- Send or fax copy of IM-CAG/PIM-CAG and care plan to patient and clinicians
- Perform personal case management assignments

—Return to Above Until Barriers Reversed—
Integrated Case Management Care Plan: Progression Review

moves to those that require less immediate action. Case managers work with patients until barriers are overcome or are stabilized (maximum benefit) before graduation from the program is considered. They do this under the weekly or biweekly supervision/assistance of a physician or team of physicians that add clinical and administrative suggestions and interact directly with the patients' clinicians when needed.

The number of contacts with the patient is far less important than the outcomes that the manager and patient are able to generate during the iterative phase of the management process (**Figure 3.3**). In Harold's situation, the case manager: (a) ensured coordination of mental health and Parkinson's care while in the hospital, (b) confirmed appropriate follow-up with needed specialists after discharge, (c) assisted in getting the court to appoint a guardian, (d) worked with friends and distant relatives to persuade the insurance company (with minimal threats) that Harold had been unfit to pay his bills at the time he was stricken from their roles, and (e) stabilized Harold's nursing home situation. During the time that the case manager worked through this process, she continuously reviewed and documented progress and looked toward case closure (**Figure 3.4**).

CASE CLOSURE

Importantly, the case manager, the patient, and significant coparticipants are continuously working together, as a team, toward case management graduation. Throughout, the patient (and/or the significant other; caregiver/parent) is encouraged to assume control of health-related activity on his or her own behalf through shared findings on the CAG and other measured outcome parameters. Effective integrated case management is more than just making sure that adherence to treatment is established and appointments are kept. Patients and the persons responsible for their care, as in Harold's case, should be working with the case manager to maximize the patient's health. The rewards from the case management process typically take place long after the manager-patient relationship has closed. Success is measured by clinical stabilization, health resource use reduction, improved function, and patient satisfaction.

Case management graduation is the ultimate goal of the patient-case manager interaction. The entire case management process is one in which patients are assisted through complex, high cost health care service need. The time that patients are in case management will vary from days to months. All activities of the highly trained and skilled case managers should be directed toward resolution of complex issues, which are changeable, and the development of patient skills,

which allow them to better deal with health issues on their own through education about illness, outcomes, resources, and so forth. Indicators, recorded on the progression review (**Figure 3.4**), that patients are moving toward graduation include:

- Patients understand their illnesses and treatments
- Patients are adherent to treatments, diets, exercises, and so forth and are working with providers to achieve improved health and function
- Patients' biological, psychological, social, and health system (CAG cells) issues are stabilized, though they may not be resolved
- Patients' clinicians and other health professionals are collaboratively working together on behalf of the patient
- Patients' physical and mental health symptoms and signs have stabilized or are resolving at expected rates
- Case management outcome objectives and patient goals have largely been accomplished (maximum benefit)

Occasionally, patients will require long-term case management involvement (6 to 12 months or more). General guidelines for continued involvement include: (a) a persistent complex combination of illnesses that require special integrated input to prevent poor clinical outcomes and continued high cost service use, (b) cognitive impairment or psychiatric symptoms with no family, significant other, or provider alternative, which prevents the patient from assuming responsibility for his or her complex illnesses, and (c) potentially very high cost illness unless control is maintained (e.g., potential liver transplant in former alcoholic, etc.).

Since case management cases are by definition patients with high health complexity, they will often be candidates for participation in other care management programs at the completion of their work with the case manager. Integrated case managers prepare patients in advance for transition from case management to assistance by a personal nurse, disease manager, or other management staff, if it is available (**Figure 3.5**). Further, as case management procedures close, it is important to assist the patient with reentry into the workplace if that is an option. This can often be facilitated through involvement with the patient's company disability management firm or the employee assistance program (EAP). For children/youth, a similar approach would be taken to help them reenter the school setting.

When the patient graduates from case management, the case manager should provide a summary of the initial CAG, the final CAG, a completed record of outcome measures (ROM—Appendix 11), and an updated care plan measurement of progress (MP3—Appendix 12) to the patient (or guardian), the patient's providers, and

FIGURE 3.4 Integrated case manager care plan progression review.

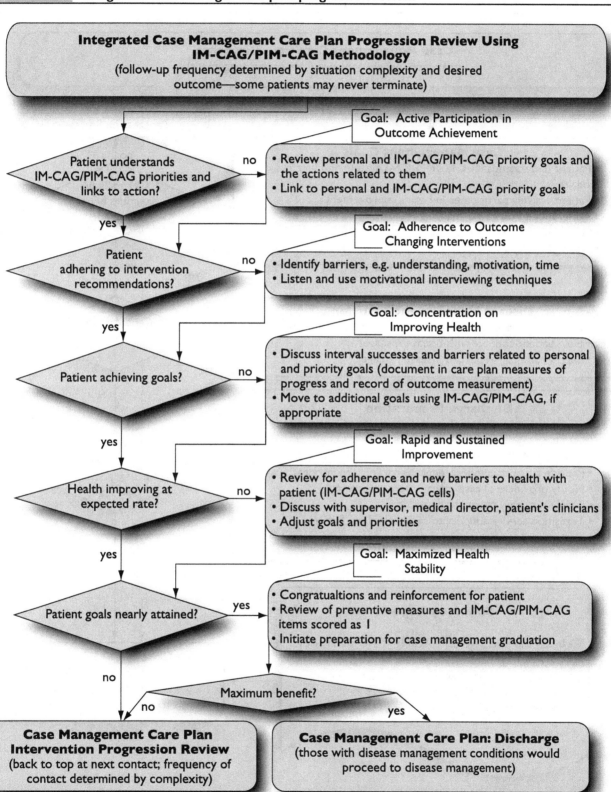

FIGURE 3.5   Integrated case manager care plan discharge.

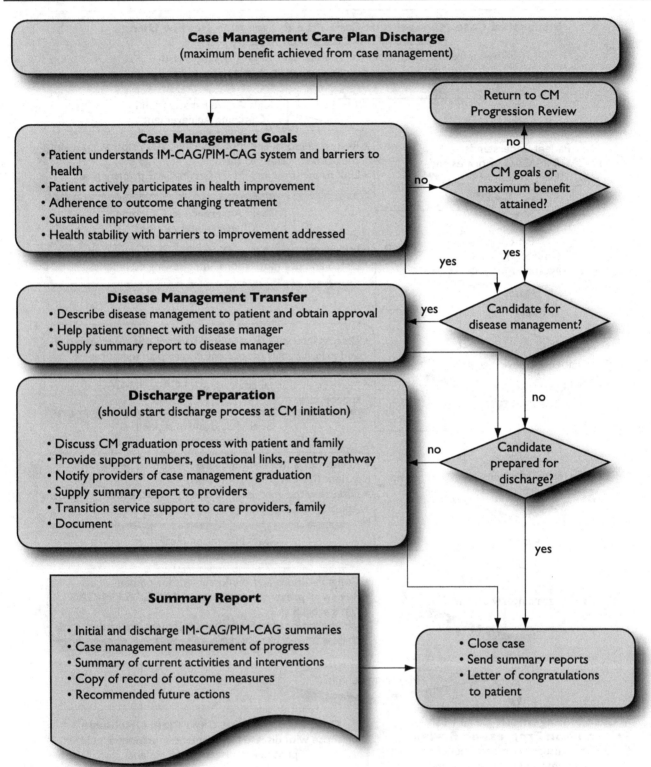

any care managers who will be assuming a role in assisting the patient, along with a narrative summary of the progress that has been made. Accompanying this summary should be ongoing interventions with recommendations about continued needs for the patient, based on the final CAG and goal statements. The patient should be informed whether the case manager is available to assist with needs in the future should they arise and, if so, should be given contact information.

SPECIAL ISSUES IN DEALING WITH COMPLEX PATIENTS

Harold's case was chosen purposely because it illustrates that despite best intentions, procedures recommended as a part of the integrated case management manual will not cover all situations. For instance, Harold has dementia and no nearby or involved relatives; therefore, it is not possible to form a case manager-patient relationship or even a relationship with a significant other in the conventional sense. Further, few of the open-ended questions designed to allow the case manager to fill in the CAG items and establish priorities for Harold (covered in Chapter 10) will be useable as data are gathered about Harold's biopsychosocial and health system situation. Rather, the case manager will need to establish Harold's level of complexity by contacting multiple informants, reviewing records, and making informed decisions. The situation can become even more complicated when working with children/youth, since multiple and conflicting information may arrive from various sources (e.g., the child/youth, each caregiver/parent, providers, the court, the school system, peers, etc.).

Nothing about working with complex patients is simple. First and foremost, case managers need to recognize that they are problem solvers. They adapt the procedures suggested in this manual to the individual patient with the ultimate goal of uncovering barriers to improvement and reversing their effect on the patient's health. To the extent that manual suggestions and procedures are inadequate or get in the way of accomplishing this task, they should be adapted to the patient so that the best result can occur.

Having said that, the core components of integrated case management should remain a central part of the case manager's actions. Even in Harold's situation, to the extent that the case manager can establish a relationship with Harold, it will be much easier to obtain cooperation with suggestions and adherence to treatment. Further, uncovering primary barriers to improvement remains central to the integrated case management process, as does a longitudinal approach to assistance.

FINANCING AND SUPPORTING INTEGRATED CASE MANAGEMENT

Seasoned case managers will recognize that integrated case management is very different than many common practices in traditional case management. It sees psychosocial and health system issues as a part of its accountability. It does not hand off the patients to another case manager when mental health issues contribute to complexity. It follows patients through multiple clinical settings and levels of care. It limits the number of cases that a case manager can carry, based on total patient panel complexity scores and the anticipated ability of the case manager to fulfill case management needs for assigned patients. It takes a longitudinal view of goals and objectives. It documents success in terms of clinical, functional, quality of life, and financial outcomes. With such a different paradigm, how can integrated case management be supported?

It is because integrated case management is a dramatically different approach to the care of complex patients that emphasis has been placed not only on learning the core components and procedures in this manual but also on reorganization of business practices and workflows that can be used to support integrated case management. Managers for nonintegrated traditional case management programs have marching orders to focus on problems in their own content areas, to maximize the number of patient contacts made, to assist patients using targeted short-term work processes, to document findings and suggestions in nonshared notes and data warehouses, to haphazardly communicate with others involved in the patient's care, and to measure success based on followed procedures (e.g., number of calls made, number of patients touched) rather than clinical and financial outcomes. These policies cannot be expected to change the known clinical and cost outcomes of complex multimorbid patients described in the Chapter 2 section "General Medical and Mental Condition Comorbidity, Treatment, and Interaction." Rather, an integrated case management system is needed.

REFERENCES

Ash, A. S., Zhao, Y., Ellis, R. P., & Schlein Kramer, M. (2001). Finding future high-cost cases: Comparing prior cost versus diagnosis-based methods. *Health Services Research, 36*(6 Pt. 2), 194–206.
Case Management Society of America. (2010). (*CMSA*) *Standards of Practice for Case Management.* Retrieved April 18, 2010, from http://www.cmsa.org/portals/0/pdf/memberonly/Standards OfPractice.pdf
Druss, B. G., & von Esenwein, S. A. (2006). Improving general medical care for persons with mental and addictive disorders: Systematic review. *General Hospital Psychiatry, 28*(2), 145–153.
Fattorusso, D., & Quinn, C. (2007). *A case manager's study guide: Preparing for certification* (3rd ed.). Sudbury, MA: Jones and Bartlett Publishers.

Goetzel, R. Z., Long, S. R., Ozminkowski, R. J., Hawkins, K., Wang, S., & Lynch, W. (2004). Health, absence, disability, and presenteeism cost estimates of certain physical and mental health conditions affecting U.S. employers. *Journal of Occupational Environmental Medicine, 46*(4), 398–412.

Goetzel, R. Z., Ozminkowski, R., Villagra, V., & Duffy, J. (2005). Return on investment in disease management: A review. *Health Care Financing Review, 26*(4), 1–19.

Jones, D. R., Macias, C., Barreira, P. J., Fisher, W. H., Hargreaves, W. A., & Harding, C. M. (2004). Prevalence, severity, and co-occurrence of chronic physical health problems of persons with serious mental illness. *Psychiatric Services, 55*(11), 1250–1257.

Kathol, R., Saravay, S., Lobo, A., & Ormel, J. (2006). Epidemiologic trends and costs of fragmentation. In F. Huyse & F. Stiefel (Eds.), *Medical Clinics of North America* (Vol. 90, pp. 549–572). Philadelphia: Elsevier Saunders.

Kathol, R. G., Kunkel, E. J., Weiner, J. S., McCarron, R. M., Worley, L. L., Yates, W. R., et al. (2009). Psychiatrists for the medically complex: Bringing value at the physical health and mental health substance use disorder interface. *Psychosomatics, 50*(March–April), 93–107.

Katon, W. J., Russo, J. E., Von Korff, M., Lin, E. H., Ludman, E., & Ciechanowski, P. S. (2008). Long-term effects on medical costs of improving depression outcomes in patients with depression and diabetes. *Diabetes Care, 31*(6), 1155–1159.

Moore, T. J., Cohen, M. R., & Furberg, C. D. (2007). Serious adverse drug events reported to the Food and Drug Administration, 1998–2005. *Archives of Internal Medicine, 167*(16), 1752–1759.

Mullahy, C. M., & Jensen, D. K. (2004). *The case manager's handbook* (3rd ed.). Sudbury, MA: Jones and Bartlett.

Powell, S. K., Tahan, H. A., & Case Management Society of America. (2008). *CMSA core curriculum for case management* (2nd ed.). Philadelpia: Lippincott Williams & Wilkins.

Thomas, M. R., Waxmonsky, J. A., McGinnis, G. F., & Barry, C. L. (2006). Realigning clinical and economic incentives to support depression management within a medicaid population: The Colorado Access experience. *Admistration & Policy Mental Health, 33*(1), 26–33.

Weed, R. O., & Berens, D. E. (2009). *Life care planning and case management handbook* (3rd ed.). Boca Raton: CRC Press.

Weiner, J. P., Dobson, A., Maxwell, S. L., Coleman, K., Starfield, B., & Anderson, G. F. (1996). Risk-adjusted Medicare capitation rates using ambulatory and inpatient diagnoses. *Health Care Financing Review, 17*(3), 77–99.

Zuvekas, S. H., & Cohen, J. W. (2007). Prescription drugs and the changing concentration of health care expenditures. *Health Affairs (Millwood), 26*(1), 249–257.

CHAPTER 4

Motivational Interviewing and Health Behavior Change in Complex Patients

With contributions by Jos Dobber, MSc

OBJECTIVES

- To define the principles and process of motivational interviewing in complex patients
- To clarify the importance of intrinsic motivation in the process of change
- To review the use of motivational interviewing in patients as a part of the case management process

INTRODUCTION

Multiple referral sources, such as payers, physicians, employee assistance programs, hospitals, and so forth contribute complex patients to case managers in hopes of getting assistance in turning around problem cases. Regardless of the source, each patient presents a challenge to case managers since they are typically suffering from several complicated and interacting general medical diseases (multiple high biological domain Complexity Assessment Grid [CAG] item scores). Some harbor low trust toward their doctors or have had difficulty with the health system, whether from long wait lists or care services that are not covered by insurance (high treatment experience and access to care scores). Still others have a history of having received well-intended but contradictory advice from different professionals (a high coordination of care score) that results in resistance or poor adherence to treatment (a high resistance to treatment score).

These patients seldom suffer only from physical health conditions. Sixty to eighty percent will also have a history of mental health difficulties (a high mental health history score) or present with current psychiatric symptoms (a high mental health symptoms score). The combination of physical and mental health problems contributes to a decreased ability to cope with family, work, or school stresses (a high barrier to coping score), which can lead to challenges in developing friendships (a high relationships score) and results in little availability of support when crises arise (a high social support score). In short, patients who are referred to case managers experience struggles in multiple domains that can contribute to persistence of poor health and function.

Using an integrated case management approach, of which adult and pediatric CAG methodology is a part, case managers can now disentangle factors that contribute to complexity and estimate the level of complexity through the overall CAG score—that is, they have a way to maximize benefit for the people with whom they work. Before they initiate case management, however, it is important to assess patient motivation since this is key to the actions patients will need to take on their own behalf. Such an assessment helps to determine whether patients will be considered for case management at all. It also provides a snapshot of the patient's initial level of motivation and the degree to which a motivational interviewing approach may be beneficial for those who are chosen and agree to enter case management.

Motivational interviewing skills, together with the development of a therapeutic relationship, are used to enhance the patient's own motivation to improve his or her health outcomes and associated functioning. There are many adaptations of motivational interviewing, often referred to as motivational enhancement therapy. This chapter will review the principles of motivational interviewing and how it can be applied in patients with health complexity as a part of the integrated case management process.

MOTIVATIONAL INTERVIEWING THEORETICAL CONSTRUCTS

Motivational interviewing is "a client-centered, directive method for enhancing intrinsic motivation to change by exploring and resolving ambivalence" (Miller & Rollnick, 2002, p. 25). There is growing evidence for the effectiveness of motivational interviewing, most of which has been summarized in a few systematic reviews (Burke, Arkowitz, & Menchola, 2003; Hettema, Steele, & Miller, 2005). Motivational interviewing builds on counselor effects that emphasize an empathic and nonconfrontational style. Case managers typically use this approach to facilitate change. Incorporating motivational interviewing within the case management paradigm requires that case managers use open-ended questions and complex reflections within the motivational interviewing spirit to evoke change talk from the patient. They learn to roll with resistance and to avoid confrontation and the giving of uninvited advice so they can enhance the patient's willingness to initiate action that will improve his or her health (Martino, Ball, Nich, Frankforter, & Carroll, 2008).

Starting a relationship with a new patient, the case manager takes some time to establish rapport, which is consistent with the integrated case management approach. Exploring previous patient experiences in the health care system, which may include confrontations with health care workers, is a part of this. Examples, such as negative communications with doctors or feeling forced into accepting treatment, can be acknowledged by suggesting that it is best for patients to be involved with treatment decisions (Kemp, David, & Hayward, 1996). Through skills such as reflective listening, case managers evoke change talk from patients (**Table 4.1**; Miller, Moyers, Amrhein, & Rollnick, 2006). This not infrequently leads to the development of commitment to a targeted behavior (e.g., adherence to treatment) if patients can be helped through their ambivalence about taking action. That is what motivational interviewing is designed to do.

Reading about motivational interviewing, viewing training tapes, or taking a motivational interviewing workshop can be a starting point for the development and implementation of motivational interviewing skills and putting them into practice. Proficiency is acquired through the application of learned knowledge and skill to patients under the supervision of a professional with experience in using motivational interviewing techniques (Hettema et al., 2005).

Traditionally, patients seek health care attention from doctors or other practitioners who diagnose or provide treatment for their condition or set of symptoms. While this basic component of health care is straightforward, diagnosing and effectively treating disorders is by no means simple. Symptoms of illness are often related to lifestyle choices (e.g., caloric intake, tobacco use, paucity of exercise, etc.). While lifestyle change is commonly part of the treatment of illness or impairment, many patients are not ready, are unwilling, or are unable to follow the lifestyle components of a treatment plan since it requires effort and change (Rollnick, 1999). The same is true for virtually all other activities related to health, whether it involves the patient's following through with diagnostic assessments or consistently taking medications. This is particularly true in patients with health complexity since the sheer number of things they have to do for themselves to maintain their health can overwhelm them.

According to motivational interviewing theory, readiness, willingness, and ability to change are three critical determinants of motivation (Miller & Rollnick, 2002). By practicing motivational interviewing, case managers purposefully influence these three components. They build supportive and empathetic therapeutic relationships. They explore arguments shared by the patient for and against change. It is the patient's reasons, needs, desires, and abilities to change that constitute the patient's change talk. With training in motivational interviewing, case managers can guide patients to change talk, using techniques such as reflective listening, asking open-ended questions, staying away from confrontation, and not overusing warnings about long-range dangers to change actions (**Table 4.2**; Miller, Moyers, Ernst, & Amrhein, 2008).

TABLE 4.1   Change Talk

Change talk: Statements in which the client talks about changing the direction of the target behavior

	Examples (target behavior: reduction of alcohol use)
Preparatory language (DARN):	
■ **D**esire statements	"I don't want to drink this much"
■ **A**bility statements	"I think I can drink less"
■ **R**easons statements	"I have to do this for my family"
■ **N**eed statements	"I need to stop drinking like this"
Commitment language	"I'm gonna end this drinking now"
Taking steps	"I didn't see my drinking friends at all last week"

TABLE 4.2   Examples of Responses Consistent With Motivational Interviewing

Consistent	Neutral	Inconsistent
■ Advice with permission	■ Facilitate	■ Advice without permission
■ Affirm	■ Filler	
■ Emphasize control	■ Giving information	■ Confront
■ Open-ended question	■ Closed-ended question	■ Direct
■ Reflect	■ Raise concern with permission	■ Raise concern without permission
■ Reframe		
■ Support	■ Structure	■ Warn

Case managers should avoid responses that are inconsistent with motivational interviewing technique, like confronting and directing the patient. Such efforts increase resistance and are related to poorer long-term outcomes (Miller, Benefield, & Tonigan, 1993). There are a few traps that also have to be avoided, such as asking closed-ended, single-answer questions (i.e., those in which the patient can give short answers like "yes," "no," or "maybe"). Six such traps are characterized in **Table 4.3** (Miller & Rollnick, 2002).

TABLE 4.3	Traps in Practicing Motivational Interviewing
Traps	**Description**
Question/answer trap	Case manager too active, patients too passive.
Trap of taking sides	Case manager argues in favor for change, instead of eliciting reasons for and against change from patients. If the case manager is arguing pro-change, this often results in patients wanting to show the other side of their ambivalence. They will argue against change and reinforce the negative.
Expert trap	Case manager taking the expert role and advising patients on the target behavior. This may force patients into a passive role in which they cannot explore (and resolve) their ambivalence.
Labeling trap	Case manager tells patients that they *are* something (the diagnosis), instead of that they are *doing* something (e.g., patients *are* noncompliant, instead of having difficulties in handling the prescriptions or having reasons not to act in conformance with the prescriptions).
Premature focus trap	Case managers want to focus on their own conception of the problem, while patients think that other concerns are more important to discuss.
Blaming trap	Talking about whose fault the problem is, instead of concentrating on present needs (i.e., complaints and concerns of patients and how they can be met).

"Willingness" refers to the patient's perspective on the importance of changing the target behavior. Miller and Rollnick use the term "discrepancy" to describe and understand the willingness of patients to move from their current state to their goals for the future (Miller & Rollnick, 2002). If there is just a small discrepancy between these two states, the patient's desires to change will probably also be small. The change does not seem important to the patient. To elicit change, the case manager's task will be to increase the level of discrepancy between current state and future goals and emphasize how this discrepancy affects patients' lives. If the patient experiences sufficient discrepancy between the current and the desired state, then change becomes more important. This enhances motivation for change.

It should be noted that many people feel ambivalent about changing. Ambivalence is a normal phenomenon, and case managers should not consider a patient with ambivalence as unmotivated. In patients with health complexity, for instance, ambivalence could originate from a patient's frustration with many prior but unsuccessful therapeutic trials. Such a patient may be nonplussed about another treatment, which they perceive as having no greater likelihood of success. By carefully exploring both sides of the ambivalence, case managers have the potential to uncover a core underlying issue that needs to be addressed (Miller & Rollnick, 2002).

"Ability" refers to the confidence patients have in their own personal resources to actually change a targeted behavior. Patients who are willing to change may not see a way to do so or have the strength to initiate the change. This commonly occurs with patients with weight problems where multiple attempts have been made but none have succeeded. In this situation, if patients discover a method to accomplish change that they think may be effective and that they can do (called self-efficacy), then the probability of their making efforts to change increases. If, on the other hand, they do not believe they have the personal resources to accomplish the change, attempts will not occur.

In complex patients whom case managers regularly assist, this problem can be complicated by low energy and fatigue from their underlying illnesses. A concurrent mental health issue, such as depression or anxiety, could also lower willingness to put forth effort to initiate change. In order to identify a patient's perception of his or her capacity to change, case managers must listen for statements suggesting that patients feel ill equipped to initiate the change process. If such feelings are uncovered, the focus of case management interventions would include exploring methods for change or assisting the patient in developing a change plan. None of this, however, may be possible until the patient's general medical and/or psychiatric condition improves. Thus, greater action on the part of the case manager as they begin working with the patient may be necessary, especially with attention to improving current clinical symptoms. Once these symptoms are under better control, patients may develop enough energy to do things for themselves. Witnessing a bit of success also boosts spirits and interest.

"Readiness" refers to the willingness and ability to identify areas of needed change and to set priorities about how to accomplish them. Is the patient ready to make the change now or are other things more important? Change will only occur if target behaviors have enough priority at the moment to initiate action. Because motivational interviewing aims to elicit intrinsic (long-lasting) motivation, it is important that the patients are ready to initiate change now, out of their own desire.

MOTIVATIONAL INTERVIEWING: A PATIENT-CENTERED PROCESS

Motivational interviewing is more than a collection of techniques. Rather, its foundation is based on the fundamental motivational interviewing principle that change occurs as a result of patient-practitioner collaboration, evocation of ways to change, and autonomy of decision (Miller & Rollnick, 2002). This means that case managers work with patients in partnership. Patients are the experts in their own lives. The role of case managers is to seek to understand the patients' perspectives, values, and goals concerning their own lives. These are also the source of intrinsic motivation for patients.

Thus, case managers do not assume the role of expert, giving advice and telling patients what to do. Rather, they reflect the patients' own thoughts about change and how it might occur. They emphasize the patients' control over the decision to change. When a decision is made, they actively support patients who have decided to change for their own reasons. Patients are personally responsible. Case managers facilitate, but then support. It is the patients who choose to change. They cannot be forced or goaded into doing so.

Four important case management activities promote the motivation to change (Miller & Rollnick, 2002):

1. Express empathy
2. Develop discrepancy
3. Roll with resistance
4. Support self-efficacy

EXPRESS EMPATHY

The case manager should build a therapeutic relationship in which acceptance, an active interest in

understanding the patient's perspective, collaboration with the patient, and an emphasis on the patient's autonomy is expressed. This is known as showing empathy (**Table 4.4**; Miller et al., 2008). It is not easy to do, but asking open-ended questions, using reflective listening, and avoiding judgment, criticism, and blame are key elements needed to establish an empathic relationship. Empathic statements, such as "That must have saddened you" or "That seems like a very frustrating situation" can help to let the patient know that the case manager understands how he or she must have felt in a disturbing situation.

TABLE 4.4   Empathetic Relationship Development

Dimension	Characterization
Acceptance	■ Warmth ■ Supportive ■ Respect ■ Unconditional positive regard

Empathy	■ Active interest to understand the patient's:
	  perception
	  situation
	  meaning
	  feelings
	■ Accurately following the patient's complex story or gently exploring the patient's complex story
	■ Reflective listening
	■ Communicating an understanding of the patient's perspective

Spirit of collaboration	■ Negotiating with the patient ■ Avoiding an authoritarian attitude ■ Avoiding persuasion ■ Focusing on supporting and exploring the patient's own concerns and ideas ■ Minimizing power differences ■ Establishing partnership
Spirit of evocation	■ Drawing out patient's perspective ■ Avoiding advice without permission ■ Actively helping patients tell themselves the reasons to change
Spirit of autonomy	■ Accepts the patient's choice to change or not to change ■ Does not press immediate commitment to change ■ Emphasizes the patient's control and freedom of choice ■ Exudes that change cannot be imposed by others

DEVELOP DISCREPANCY

Since motivational interviewing is a directive method, creating or increasing discrepancy enhances the perceived importance of the change. Motivational interviewing fosters intrinsic motivation of the patient; thus, it should be the patient, not the case manager, who brings up and articulates the arguments for change. No coercion or pressure should be used. Rather, open-ended questions and skillful reflections should assist the patient in defining his or her current situation and desired goals, recognizing his or her personal reasons for changing, understanding and expressing concerns about the effort that it will take to accomplish his or her goals, building confidence in his or her ability to complete a stepwise success plan, and establishing a commitment to try to change.

ROLL WITH RESISTANCE

Tension and disputes between the patient and a case manager should be avoided. The act of arguing itself allows the patient to consolidate the rationale for opposition to change while the case manager stresses the benefits. The result is that the patient becomes even more entrenched in current behavior. Further, the empathetic relationship between the patient and case manager could also be damaged. In motivational interviewing, case managers typically do not offer solutions for problems and questions. They preferably help patients come up with answers for themselves. In fact, comments suggesting resistance (argumentation) by a patient are signals that case managers should back off lest they root the patient even further in his or her inertia (Miller et al., 1993).

SUPPORT SELF-EFFICACY

The patients' confidence in their ability to change is a prerequisite for motivation. If case managers exude optimism about the patient's ability to change, this may become a self-fulfilling prophecy. Patients who are willing but not able to change usually minimize their desire to change and are not likely to undertake an effort to change. In this situation the case manager, therefore, should support the patient (e.g., by assisting in making a change plan).

STEPS IN USING MOTIVATIONAL INTERVIEWING

In motivational interviewing, case managers build a relationship and enter dialogue that fosters thought processes in patients that help them come to the realization that goal changes are reasonable, desirable,

and can be accomplished. The relationship between the case manager and the patient and the promotion of the internalization of an altered attitude in the patient about trying something different are the two processes that enhance motivation.

One of the best known models for applying these processes is the transtheoretical model (TTM) developed by Prochaska and DiClemente (DiClemente & Velasquez, 2002). The TTM conceptualizes the process of change in five stages: (a) precontemplation, (b) contemplation, (c) preparation, (d) action, and (e) maintenance. The challenge is to establish the patient's stage of change and then focus on motivational interventions accordingly. Once patients have succeeded in changing their behavior, procedures that address the possibility of relapse and/or the need to recycle through the stages of change may be invoked.

Using TTM, once a patient has entered case management, case managers judge and decide what to say based on the flow of the conversation. The intent, however, is to help the patient become increasingly motivated to try to alter the things that prevent the achievement of a desired goal. For example, in the situation presented in **Table 4.5**, the patient is in the precontemplation stage (i.e., he has not considered changing the way that he takes his antihypertensive medications). In this situation, the case manager establishes rapport with the patient, emphasizes the patient's control over his own situation, and starts enhancing the patient's perceived discrepancy.

During this interaction, the case manager moves the patient from precontemplation to contemplation. The stage is now set for action since the patient has identified in his own words that his current poor control of blood pressure is having more of an impact on his life than just being a bad number. The discrepancy between the current and desired goal has enlarged. The next step in the discussion would be uncovering ways to improve ease of taking medications (ability) and then setting the plan into action (commitment language). The strength and the frequency of commitment language is a predictor for behavior change (Amrhein, Miller, Yahne, Palmer, & Fulcher, 2003). Maintenance would involve reinforcement of changed behaviors. If problems arose (e.g., side effects from the medications), the case manager would encourage working with the patient's treating practitioner to adjust the dosage or change the medication.

There is no magic about this interaction, but it is important to note that the case manager does not use the terms "should" or "ought" and does not confront the patient with reasons for encouraging adherence to the blood pressure medications (i.e., to prevent heart disease or stroke). Instead, by asking open-ended questions and using complex reflections, the patient

TABLE 4.5	Working on Ambivalence and Developing Discrepancy

Target: to control blood pressure	Response types
Case Manager: *"Mr. Jones—so I understand that you really like to get down on the floor and give your grandkids piggyback rides."* (Response from earlier knowledge of Mr. Jones) **Mr. Jones:** *"Yes—it's a lot of fun and the kids really enjoy it. Lately, though I get headaches so quickly and the kids could go all day."*	Complex reflection
Case Manager: *"What do you think causes your headaches?"* **Mr. Jones:** *"Well, I am getting older, and I guess my blood pressure has been a little out of control lately."*	Open question
Case Manager: *"So your age and your high blood pressure cause headaches and the headaches interfere with your relationship with your grandchildren."* **Mr. Jones:** *"I guess that's true."*	Complex reflection
Case Manager: *"What are you doing to take care of your blood pressure?"* **Mr. Jones:** *"The doctor says to diet, get exercise, and take my medication. I do pretty good on the diet, and believe me, the kids give me the exercise, but remembering my pills . . ."*	Open question Taking steps to target behavior, two positive, one negative
Case Manager: *"I understand—you're managing well in two of three measures. But the medication, you seem to forget from time to time."* **Mr. Jones:** *"Yeah, well, forgetting and sometimes not wanting to take them but I know that I should talk with someone about that."*	Support; affirm; complex reflection Giving negative reasons[a]
Case Manager: *"What makes you not want to take your medication?"* **Mr. Jones:** *"Well you know, it's not natural to take pills all the time . . ."* **Case Manager:** *"I see."* **Mr. Jones:** *". . . and a lot of days, when I feel well, I just forget to take them."*	Open question Giving negative reason Facilitate Giving negative reason
Case Manager: *"So on one hand you don't want to take medications and feel that you don't need them all the time, and on the other hand you try to control your blood pressure by keeping your diet and staying active. Still your headaches seem to negatively impact your day to day life, like in the way you play with your grandchildren."* **Mr. Jones:** *"Yeah, I guess I must do more to handle my blood pressure."* **Case Manager:** *"You think you can do more."* **Mr. Jones:** *"Yeah, I want to do more."*	Complex reflection, (showing both sides of the ambivalence and working on discrepancy) Positive need statement[a] Complex reflection Positive desire statement[a]

[a] Positive: moving in the direction of the target behavior; Negative: moving away from the target behavior or keeping the status quo.

was helped to personally recognize the rationale for improving adherence to blood pressure control activities.

MOTIVATIONAL INTERVIEWING WITH ADOLESCENTS

Literature and research on motivational interviewing with young people primarily involves its use in adolescents. There are some reasons to expect that motivational interviewing would be a promising intervention for behavior change in adolescents. The motivational interviewing spirit fits with adolescents' developmental characteristics like autonomy and indi-

viduation (Baer & Peterson, 2002; Sindelar, Abrantes, Hart, Lewander, & Spirito, 2004). Since ambivalence is a common phenomenon in adolescence, an approach in which ambivalence is respectfully explored to enhance motivation fits well with this developmental stage (Baer & Peterson, 2002).

The research evidence on motivational interviewing with adolescents is limited. There are some small to medium effects on alcohol use, tobacco use, and dietary control, but, often, secondary effects like harm reduction and treatment adherence are the most important results (Baer & Peterson, 2002; Erickson, Gerstle, & Feldstein, 2005; Sindelar et al., 2004). Motivational interviewing seems to be more effective with adolescents with more severe problems (Baer & Peterson, 2002; Sindelar et al., 2004), such as alcohol or drug abuse or dependence, or with higher levels of ambivalence (Erickson et al., 2005). Often motivational interviewing is included as a part of a multicomponent intervention, which makes it hard to distinguish the specific motivational interviewing effects (Baer & Peterson, 2002; Erickson et al., 2005; Sindelar et al., 2004).

Adolescents with chemical dependence problems require an adapted motivational interviewing approach. With this group, case managers should invest extra time in developing a therapeutic alliance. Many adolescents with multifaceted difficulties tend to be more resistant, often in reaction to their past experiences with adults trying to tell them what to do. The case manager should distinguish him- or herself from those adults. A flexible attitude about conversational topics and the personal goals of the youth is important. It is also necessary to remain nonjudgmental and be prepared to interact when the adolescent is unwilling to talk (e.g., offering more structure, asking more close-ended questions). This helps case managers in building rapport with adolescents (Baer & Peterson, 2002).

CLOSING REMARKS

Motivational interviewing used in case management is not a standalone intervention but is a modality through which patients are helped to see the value of and take action in overcoming barriers to improvement. It should become a standard practice in dealing with patients, as case managers work with the complex and challenging problems with which such patients are confronted daily.

Those entering case management services can fall anywhere on the motivation continuum. Some will be highly motivated since they are so tired of being sick and impaired. They will try to do almost anything in an attempt to get better. Others, despite significant but reversible health difficulties, will not want to expend any extra energy to make things improve since it is such an effort just to stay afloat. For others, there may be some secondary gain associated with maintaining the sick and/or impaired role (e.g., retaining disability payments or getting the attention of caregivers).

Understanding motivational interviewing and using its techniques will increase the likelihood of change. Just as importantly, it will also help case managers recognize when motivational roadblocks to change are greater than efforts through the relationship and the motivational reframing can overcome. When pa-

tients are stuck at the precontemplation or contemplation level with little interest in moving to preparation and action, it is sometimes prudent to back off, accept that the patient is at maximum benefit, and move on to another more willing, ready, and able patient. As long as the seed of change has been planted, it is always possible to come back to the patient when he or she is more ready to participate in his or her own health improvement.

When working with patients who have health complexity, it is important to remember that their degree of illness alone can contribute to their level of motivation. For clinical and economic reasons, it is sometimes necessary for case managers to put in more effort than the patient as they initiate care plan procedures. As critical items in the care plan improve, often the patient or their caregivers (as in the case of children/youth and the elderly) recognize that the case manager truly cares (confirmation of a heartfelt relationship) and are more willing to become involved in the improvement process. In fact, this may influence the length of time that case managers retain their helper role. If patients and their caregivers become invested in moving to improved health but do not have health system knowledge or tools to maximize health, then several additional educational sessions may be required in an effort to help them develop the needed skills that can make the difference between early relapse and persistently stabilized health. Still, the case manager should avoid the expert trap in motivational interviewing and first ask permission of the client to give a brief explanation before providing education.

SUMMARY

Motivational interviewing is aimed at enhancing the patient's intrinsic motivation to change. It is inextricably bound with the patient's own values and meanings; therefore, in motivational interviewing, the case manager does not use pressure or coercion to achieve the change. Instead, the case manager builds an empathetic relationship and elicits patient change talk, in which the patient argues if, why, and how change can occur.

Motivational interviewing is not a technique that case managers occasionally pull out and use in the particularly difficult patient. Rather, it is a continuous and internalized way that effective case managers interact with patients. In virtually every patient with health complexity, assisting with motivation in one or more component of health change will be important. It is for this reason that understanding and developing skills in routine use of motivational interviewing techniques will improve the value that case managers can bring to their patients.

REFERENCES

Amrhein, P. C., Miller, W. R., Yahne, C. E., Palmer, M., & Fulcher, L. (2003). Client commitment language during motivational interviewing predicts drug use outcomes. *Journal Consulting Clinical Psychology, 71*, 862–878.

Baer, J. S., & Peterson, P. L. (2002). Motivational interviewing with adolescents and young adults. In W. R. Miller & S. Rollnick (Eds.), *Motivational interviewing. Preparing people for change.* New York: Guilford, pp. 320–332.

Burke, B. L., Arkowitz, H., & Menchola, M. (2003). The efficacy of motivational interviewing: A meta-analysis of controlled clinical trials. *Journal Consulting Clinical Psychology, 71*(5), 843–861.

DiClemente, C. C., & Velasquez, M. M. (2002). Motivational interviewing and the stages of change. In W. R. Miller & S. Rollnick (Eds.), *Motivational interviewing. Preparing people for change.* New York: Guilford, pp. 201–216.

Erickson, S. J., Gerstle, M., & Feldstein, S. W. (2005). Brief interventions and motivational interviewing with children, adolescents, and their parents in pediatric health care settings: A review. *Archives Pediatrics Adolescent Medicine, 159*(12), 1173–1180.

Hettema, J., Steele, J., & Miller, W. R. (2005). Motivational interviewing. *Annual Review Clinical Psychology, 1*, 91–111.

Kemp, R., David, A., & Hayward, P. (1996). Compliance therapy: An intervention targeting insight and treatment adherence in psychotic patients. *Behavioral and Cognitive Psychotherapy, 24*, 331–350.

Martino, S., Ball, S. A., Nich, C., Frankforter, T. L., & Carroll, K. M. (2008). Community program therapist adherence and competence in motivational enhancement therapy. *Drug Alcohol Dependence, 96*(1–2), 37–48.

Miller, W. R., Benefield, R. G., & Tonigan, J. S. (1993). Enhancing motivation for change in problem drinking: A controlled comparison of two therapist styles. *Journal Consulting Clinical Psychology, 61*(3), 455–461.

Miller, W. R., Moyers, T. B., Amrhein, P., & Rollnick, S. (2006). A consensus statement on defining change talk. *MINT Bulletin, 13*, 6–7.

Miller, W. R., Moyers, T. B., Ernst, D., & Amrhein, P. (2008). *Manual for the MISC 2.1.* Retrieved March 12, 2008 from http://casaa. unm.edu/download/misc.pdf

Miller, W. R., & Rollnick, S. (2002). *Motivational interviewing. Preparing people for change.* New York: Guilford.

Rollnick, S. M. (1999). *Health behavior change: A guide for practitioners.* Edinburgh, Scotland: Churchill Livingstone.

Sindelar, H. A., Abrantes, A. M., Hart, C., Lewander, W., & Spirito, A. (2004). Motivational interviewing in pediatric practice. *Current Problems Pediatric Adolescent Health Care, 34*(9), 322–339.

CHAPTER 5

Cross-Disciplinary Training for Integrated Case Managers

- To develop comfort in talking about health behaviors and emotional problems in the context of physical disease and vice versa
- To delineate differences in the way that mental health and substance use disorders (mental conditions) are addressed as compared to physical disorders
- To review how to handle special medical, psychiatric, and pediatric situations as a case manager
- To describe the knowledge and skill base needed for integrating assistance for common physical and mental conditions in case management

INTRODUCTION

Integrated case management is a process in which a single case manager assists patients with all barriers to health, including those related to physical illnesses or mental health and substance use disorders (mental conditions). Handoffs among managers are minimized, and total health outcomes for their patients are the responsibility of each individual case manager. Case assignment is based on the availability of a case manager with the time to initiate integrated management activities and the training needed to address issues in all domains that retard return to health. The specific clinical background of the case manager is relevant, not so much from the standpoint of the discipline in which they have clinical skills, as their understanding of the health system and the barriers it creates for patients. This requires that integrated case managers have:

- A sound understanding of case manager goals in working with the patient (**Exhibit 5.1**)
- Educational and work-related backgrounds that provide a basic grounding about physical and mental conditions (examples found in Chapter 6), the system in which health care is provided, and the value that integrated assistance brings when appropriately applied
- The management skills required to alter barriers to care in the domains in which they exist, with the patient as a partner

The primary purpose of this chapter is to equip: (a) case managers with backgrounds in physical health disorders with basic information about mental conditions, their assessments, and their treatments and (b) case managers with backgrounds in mental condition care with basic information about general medical illnesses, their assessments, and their treatments. By learning the information in this chapter, case managers with either background should be able to coordinate physical and mental health assistance to patients found to have a combination of general medical and mental condition problems.

The chapter first describes how to talk with patients about emotions, behaviors, and cognitions, whether they are related to difficult life circumstances or to mental health disorders in the context of their general medical illnesses and vice versa. It then discusses the differences between access to and payment for clinical services in the physical and mental health sectors; reviews the basics on handling general medical, psychiatric, and pediatric emergencies; and defines the training and capabilities of various mental health practitioners. Finally, it ties the unified management of general medical and mental conditions into a package for case managers in terms of total health for the patient.

In order to effectively provide integrated case management, personnel with general medical backgrounds do not need to be experts in mental conditions. In fact, there are few case managers with general medical backgrounds who could claim to be experts in more than a small number of the myriad of physical conditions for which they provide help to patients in the medical sector. Likewise, case managers with mental health backgrounds need not be experts in general medical disorders. Case managers assist patients in obtaining the type of treatment that improves the likelihood that they will get better but do not provide the treatment themselves. To give such assistance requires a mixture of common sense and basic illness understanding that allows them to work with patients who have little health care sophistication in hopes that they

---

EXHIBIT 5.1   **Integrated Case Manager Goals**

- To address issues of patients with physical illnesses, mental conditions, or both *without* handing off the patients
- To confirm the fidelity of patients' physical and mental health diagnoses with their symptom presentations, with the treatment they are receiving, and with the frequency and type of follow-up
- To support and collaborate with the patients' clinicians on behalf of the patients
- To assist patients with understanding their illnesses and the activities that they can do to facilitate the best outcomes (to educate)
- To overcome barriers to adherence with provider-directed appropriate intervention including biological, psychological, social, and health system components
- To motivate patients to maximize their health and productivity (to encourage healthy behaviors)
- To prevent unnecessary or potentially harmful care
- To coordinate case management services with those of other care managers and health resources

---

make better decisions related to the direction of their care. Case managers help reverse barriers to treatment and monitor progress toward recovery.

For instance, it is not necessary for a case manager who has spent the majority of her career in obstetrical nursing to know all of the medications and dosing regimes that could be used in patients with major depression or with end-stage renal disease. Nor is it necessary for her to know how the psychotherapies shown as effective for depression should be administered or to be aware of all the foods included in a diet for a patient with renal failure. The case manager, instead, must be familiar enough with the basics of common illnesses to know:

- Core symptoms (e.g., nine in the case of syndromatic depression)
- The common classes of medication with evidence of benefit for the patient's condition or how to look them up, if needed
- The types of additional therapies important for recovery other than medication (e.g., effective psychotherapies, such as cognitive behavioral therapy or problem-solving therapy for depression; physical therapy approaches for back pain)
- How often patients should be followed to ensure adherence and to monitor clinical improvement
- What can be used to document symptom change
- When symptom improvement typically starts and how symptoms resolve
- What to do when the patient is not improving

Likewise, it is not necessary for a case manager who has spent the majority of his or her career in assisting those with mental conditions to know all of the oral hypoglycemic medications and dosing regimens that could be used in a patient with type 2 diabetes. The case manager, instead, must be familiar enough with the basics about such illnesses as diabetes and its treatment to know:

- General interventions for type 1 and type 2 diabetes, such as oral hypoglycemics and insulin
- The levels of HbA1c that document control of diabetes and how to follow levels
- The types of complications patients with diabetes mellitus experience
- How often patients should be followed when diabetes is in poor control
- The approximate frequency of screening necessary for potential complications of diabetes (e.g., retinal examinations, kidney tests, diabetic foot care, etc.)
- General characteristics of diabetic diets and exercise regimens
- The need to pursue evaluation and get treatment for diabetic complications
- Parameters for the frequency of follow-up when diabetic complications are present
- The effect of depression and other mental conditions on diabetic control

Even with this base knowledge, seasoned case managers will have questions about assessment and intervention for selected patients. Thus good case managers, as any clinician, also know when to ask those with more expertise for help and how to look up information about the condition of concern.

Becoming familiar enough with cross-disciplinary conditions to provide effective assistance to complex patients seems like a daunting task, particularly for nurses who concentrated on either general medical or mental health issues during an extended career. Case managers without medical science backgrounds, such as social workers, psychologists, or pharmacists, would appear to be at an even greater disadvantage since they have even less understanding about many illnesses that their managed cases would be experiencing.

In order to address the angst associated with plunging into a world in which the case manager is accountable in multiple domains, including for physical and mental health conditions, integrated case management programs, as described in this manual, are encouraged to incorporate several supports that aid successful transition from focused and fragmentary to integrated case management with patients. First, as mentioned in Chapter 3, cross-disciplinary geographic pods of five to nine case managers, preferably composed of professionals from multiple disciplines, facilitate access to help while assisting patients with problems outside the case manager's individual area of expertise. Second, integrated case managers receive weekly to biweekly assistance and supervision from physicians that routinely review active cases. They educate, brainstorm, and troubleshoot with each case manager to ensure improvement progression and positive outcomes. Finally, ongoing onsite cross-disciplinary educational programs (e.g., lectures, case conferences, etc.) cover pertinent case management topics.

This chapter does not intend to give the impression that those with more extensive backgrounds in either physical or mental health care cannot or do not have an advantage in providing assistance over those with less experience. Clearly, it is preferable to recruit case managers with greater knowledge and skills in all components of health. It is the supposition of integrated case management, however, that the ability of case managers to *coordinate assistance* in the biological, psychological, social, and health system domains, which create barriers to improvement, trumps greater expertise in any single area, even if it is a primary source of the patient's complexity.

More often than not, it is the interaction of barriers in multiple domains that leads to nonimprovement, rather than failure to recommend the best treatment for a patient's primary illness. For example, it may be that a patient with chronic lung disease has been prescribed a combination of medications that are less effective than those suggested in the most recent studies. A more knowledgeable manager in pulmonary disease may pick this up but fail to realize that the patient is nonadherent to all his medications because he is depressed or has insufficient funds to purchase even the drugs with lower cost.

To provide another example, it may be that a patient with congestive heart failure is having trouble controlling her fluid status. A knowledgeable manager in cardiac disease may realize the need for the patient do daily weights and to see her doctor about changing her water pill but fail to recognize that the patient is too embarrassed to say that she has no scale at home and is functionally illiterate in English and thus does not know which or how many pills to take since she can't read the labels on her medication bottles. In fact, she does not need a change in water pills; she just needs to take the less expensive pills she has more consistently and in the correct dose, based on her weight after the case manager helps her to obtain a scale.

Greater knowledge and assistance in the physical or, for that matter, mental health domain would be less important than addressing issues not commonly uncovered when a disease orientation is the focus of the case manager-patient interaction and assistance paradigm. This is one of the reasons why case management professionals from a variety of disciplines, including nursing and social services, can contribute substantially, especially when management teams with overlapping expertise work together and have the support of nonpsychiatric and psychiatric physician backup.

GENERAL MEDICAL PROFESSIONALS TALK ABOUT UNHEALTHY BEHAVIORS, COPING, AND MENTAL CONDITIONS

We all have personal issues that get in the way of effective functioning, whether they are unhealthy behaviors, such as smoking, dysfunctional eating habits, or sedentary lifestyle; ineffective coping skills; or mental conditions. To a large extent we have been socialized to avoid talking about them, to sweep them under the rug, and to do the best we can with our lives. While it is not the case manager's professional role to personally treat psychological issues, which include all of the preceding examples, it is their job to bring these issues into the open and to initiate activities that have the potential to reverse and/or attenuate barriers to health resulting from them.

Seasoned case managers all know that life circumstances and the way that patients react to them affect their ability to return to health and function. Unless the manager is willing to take the time to include these issues in his or her assessments and intervention, little will be accomplished on behalf of many patients. The first step in becoming effective case managers in the psychological domain is to accept that questions about personal habits and a person's emotional state are as important as knowing about a patient's understanding of his or her physical illnesses and adherence to his or her treatment. For instance, elderly patients often have chronic illnesses with complications that require the use of numerous medications and health-enhancing behaviors. Unless assessment for *cognitive impairment* (e.g., dementia, decreasing the ability to remember to take medications), *emotional state* (e.g., depression, leading to nonadherence with treatment recommendations), and *coping skills* (e.g., not asking for help when help is needed) is a part of the case manager's recognized role, important components related to the patient's return to health will be missed and improvement will not occur.

Interactions with adult patients using integrated case management INTERMED-Complexity Assessment Grid (IM-CAG) technology are based on a series of open-ended questions designed to allow a relationship between the patient and the manager to develop. **Exhibit 5.2** illustrates examples of questions related to main topic areas in the assessment interview of a complex patient. Each of these questions is followed by other exploratory queries that when completed allow anchor point scoring for each of the IM-CAG grid items through a dialogue with the patient. While the initial assessment can often be completed in one interview, divided interviews are occasionally necessary since the time needed to uncover barriers to improvement in patients with health complexity frequently taxes the stamina of those with compromised health. More will be said about this in Chapter 10.

Similar questions are used in pediatric complexity assessments with children/youth and their caregivers/parents as a part of the pediatric IM-CAG (PIM-CAG). Using open-ended questions facilitates the ability to ask personal questions of the patient and their family/caregivers, which are beyond the usual physical health approach prevalent in today's case management environment. For instance, it is a natural consequence when talking with a patient about a poorly controlled, functionally impairing chronic medical illness to include questions about discouragement (depression) due to poor control, behavioral changes, life concerns (anxiety) due to the effect of impairment on extracurricular activities, school, and peer and family relationships, and how they and their parents obtain and/or seek help (coping skills) for the things that they need.

Based on the information gleaned, the case manager can take steps to educate (e.g., smoking cessation or weight loss literature/programs), support (e.g., listening and reflecting with the patient on intervention options, using motivational interviewing techniques), and talk with the patient and providers about referral for relevant services (e.g., coping skill training,

psychiatric treatment). To the extent that health behaviors, coping skills, and emotional conditions interfere with return to health, it is the responsibility of the case manager to assist patients in obtaining help for them.

Case managers with physical health backgrounds who have had little experience in dealing with psychological issues may be hesitant to open Pandora's box and address the flood that might ensue, especially since they do not have experience in addressing problems in this area of health. Their comfort level in addressing psychological issues can be enhanced by recognizing that:

- The population they are working with has been pre-screened as a group to be at high risk for psychological barriers (i.e., many need mental health help)
- The case manager may be the only one available to uncover and assist with the psychological barriers
- Psychological barriers lead to prescribed assistance measures, based on IM-CAG findings, very similar to measures that are taken for physical illnesses
- Overcoming psychological barriers in patients with physical illness may be more important than making sure that the correct general medical interventions have been chosen
- Patients often experience a sense of relief when these issues are addressed by a professional in an open, nonjudgmental fashion

Some suggest that it is better to assign assessment and intervention duties for psychological issues to case managers with backgrounds or experience in mental health fields. While there is truth to the fact that those with mental health training will have a greater appreciation for options, *at least initially,* failure to link mental condition assessment and intervention with other factors retarding improvement, such as impairment caused by a medical condition (biological domain), poor access to needed providers (health system domain), or marginal support in following through on recommendations (social domain), may be more likely

---

EXHIBIT 5.2   Content Areas of Open-Ended IM-CAG Assessment Questions

General Life Situation: "Can you tell me a little about yourself such as where you live, who you live with, how you spend your days, what your hobbies and interests are, and what are the pressures in your life?"

Physical Health: "How is your *(name main medical illness)* affecting you today?"

Emotional Health: "How do you feel emotionally, such as worried, tense, sad, forgetful?"

Interaction With Treating Practitioners: "Can you tell me who you see for your health problems?"

Health System Issues: "Can you tell me whether you have difficulty in getting the health care you need?"

More Sensitive Personal Information: "What kind of person are you, such as outgoing, suspicious, tense, optimistic?"

Additional Information: "What things did I not ask about that you think are important?"

to lead to persistent health problems than the way that a mental health issue is addressed will. Further, many patients with health complexity will have no mental condition per se but will nevertheless need psychological assistance in the form of referral for coping skills training, education, and suggestions about healthy behaviors. In such patients, mental health backgrounds provide little advantage.

MENTAL HEALTH PROFESSIONALS TALK ABOUT GENERAL MEDICAL DISORDERS

While there are geographic and local service area delivery exceptions, for years mental health professionals have assiduously avoided including discussions about general medical health when evaluating and intervening on behalf of mental health patients because the topic area was not included in their training and thus was outside of their expertise. Even psychiatrists, who complete four years of medical school and at least one year of postgraduate experience working in nonpsychiatric settings, are reluctant to include review of nonbehavioral signs and symptoms as a part of their mental health evaluations.

For the most part, mental health clinicians have been taught that the workings of the mind have little to do with those of the body. Some have even been discouraged from discussing medical topics in regard to patients with psychiatric conditions to avoid creating transference and counter-transference problems. For the remainder, who bear none of this misinformation, discussions about medical comorbidity are avoided because many mental health practitioners just do not feel competent to include such questions in their evaluations.

In integrated case management, it is the case manager's professional role to personally bring general medical issues uncovered during patient assessments into the open and initiate activities that have the potential to reverse or attenuate barriers to health resulting from them. For this reason, it is critical for integrated case managers coming from behavioral health backgrounds to develop a sufficient knowledge base about issues in the general medical domain so that they can:

- Comfortably discuss them,
- Ensure that appropriate assistance for them is being given, and
- Connect them with barriers to health in other domains.

Seasoned case managers with mental health backgrounds all know that assistance in overcoming barriers to improvement related to medical illnesses is essential for return to health and function whether related to comorbid mental health problems or not.

Unless an integrated case manager includes physical health issues in his or her assessments and intervention, little will be accomplished on behalf of many, if not most, complex patients, even when the primary problem might be in the mental condition domain.

The first step for mental health professionals in becoming effective case managers in the general medical domain, therefore, is to accept the notion that questions about medical illnesses, their treatment, and their complications are a core part of integrated case management evaluations and to learn what is necessary to routinely address them. For instance, a patient may have major cognitive difficulties and a limited support system. Such a patient is an obvious candidate for significant psychosocial intervention. However, if the case manager fails to uncover, either from the patient himself or from a second source, that the patient, with a history of heart attacks and hypertensive crises, has not been taking his antihypertensive medications, medical complications may far outweigh psychosocial needs.

Based on the information gleaned from a multidisciplinary assessment, case managers with mental health backgrounds can take steps to: (a) educate (e.g., kidney failure diets, weight control), (b) support (e.g., listening and reflecting with the patient on approach alternatives, using motivational interviewing techniques, or connecting the patient with disease advocacy groups), and (c) talk with the patient and providers about referral (e.g., specialist care, employee assistance). To the extent that ineffectively treated general medical problems interfere with return to health, it is the responsibility of the case manager to assist patients in finding appropriate care. Case managers with mental health expertise must overcome their discomfort in asking and assisting with cross-disciplinary problems since they may be the only line of access that complex patients have in getting the physical health treatment that they need.

Similar to what is seen on the general medical side (i.e., a tendency to refer cross-disciplinary patients to other case management specialists), some suggest that it is better to assign assessment and intervention duties for physical health issues only to case managers with backgrounds or experience in general medical fields. While there is truth to the fact that those with physical health training will have a greater appreciation for options, *at least initially,* failure to link general medical assessment and intervention with other factors retarding improvement, such as nonadherence to treatment recommendations or nontreatment for mental conditions (psychological domain), poor coordination of care among providers (health service domain), or the lack of a permanent address and no financial resources (social domain), may lead to persistent health problems

TABLE 5.1	Independent Versus Integrated General Medical and Mental Health Care Delivery and Payment Practices for Discrete Patients		
		INDEPENDENT	**INTEGRATED**
HEALTH SYSTEM			
Interaction of systems		Rare	Uniform
INSURERS			
Patient identifiers		Separate	Single
Payment pool		*Two buckets*	*Single bucket*
Contract benefit descriptions		Disparate	Unified
Network of providers		Medical vs. mental health	All in one
Member and provider support		Separate call-in numbers	One call-in number
Approval process		Disparate	Uniform
Case management support		Discipline specific	Cross-disciplinary
Coding and billing		Separate payment rules	Consistent process
Claims adjudication		Separate processes	Unified single server
Data warehousing and actuarial analysis		Segregated	Consolidated
CLINICAL CARE			
Practice location		Separate	Combined
Service delivery		Segregated	Coordinated
Clinician collaboration and communication		Rare	Routine

more than the way that a physical health issue is addressed will.

The bottom line is that mental health personnel wishing to do integrated case management need to be willing to nurture a new skill set, which will allow them to use a more holistic approach to support for care of the patients that they manage. Importantly, they have to know enough about the general medical conditions and the health system to give sound advice that leads to health improvement. It is a bit like a husband making sure that his wife with breast cancer gets good and appropriate health care. Common sense helps him know when provider support and intervention is doing little to improve her situation. It is this common sense, with a background in or growing knowledge of medical illnesses and the medical system that ultimately helps an integrated case manager bring value to his or her managed patients.

HEALTH SYSTEM HANDLING OF PHYSICAL AND MENTAL CONDITIONS

Since the 1980s, when managed behavioral health administration came into existence, psychiatry holds the distinction of being the only allopathic medical specialty to be segregated from the rest of medicine

(Table 5.1). It can rightly be stated in today's health care environment that this separation itself creates significant barriers to outcome changing care for patients with complex and/or chronic health problems (Exhibit 5.3), most of whom have concurrent physical and mental conditions (Institute of Medicine, Committee on Crossing the Quality Chasm: Adaptation to Mental Health and Addictive Disorders, 2006; Institute of Medicine, Committee on Quality of Health Care in America, 2001). For this reason, part of the training for case managers coming from general medical backgrounds requires that they develop an understanding of behavioral health business practices, the special administrative needs of patients with mental conditions, and an appreciation for the capabilities, based on training and experience, of those who deliver mental health services. Likewise, case managers coming from mental health backgrounds require training that allows them to understand general medical business practices and differences in administrative approaches to patients with physical disorders. Understanding these health system-related issues makes it possible to create a context in which patients with concurrent physical and mental conditions can receive coordinated care and treatment with the potential to improve their composite clinical conditions.

EXHIBIT 5.3   Negative Effects of Segregated Physical and Mental Condition Business Practices

Practice Location

Geographically and/or functionally disparate

Communication

Disincentive to integrate care (time, hassle, lack of clinical/financial accountability)

Mental Health Provider Access

Multiple mental health provider networks serving each physical health provider network leads to a 1-800 call, not a provider referral

Reimbursement

Inequitable discipline-based payment (e.g., primary care physicians are paid better than mental health providers for mental condition treatment despite 36% fewer patients getting minimally effective care)

Inpatient care (e.g., no transfers, patients are discharged and readmitted)

Payment

Benefit-based cost shifting from mental health benefits to general medical benefits through increased and often unnecessary general medical service use

---

INDEPENDENT GENERAL MEDICAL AND MENTAL HEALTH BUSINESS PRACTICES AND THEIR NATURAL CONSEQUENCES

Most reimbursement systems worldwide pay for mental and physical health services from segregated pools of money, even when a discrete country or company administers the total health budget. For those who wish to understand the cascading effect of this business decision, readers are directed to the book *Healing Body and Mind: A Critical Issue for Health Care Reform* (Kathol & Gatteau, 2007). The end result of separate payment pools is that it is virtually impossible for mental and physical health clinicians to practice in the same setting, for treatment to be coordinated, and for communication between general medical and mental condition professionals to allow collaborative care.

Patients with concurrent physical and mental conditions have a challenge getting consistent and timely care since independent payment has led to discriminatory practices in terms of what is covered (benefit restrictions, e.g., chemical dependence exclusions), where treatment can be delivered (the physical vs. mental health setting), who can deliver the care and under which benefits (mental health or general medical professionals; medical or behavioral benefits), how much is paid for the services delivered (lower reimbursement to mental health providers and facilities for the same or often more effective services), and for what duration (annual and lifetime coverage limits). The natural consequences of this for patients are summarized in **Exhibit 5.4**. Unless payment for mental condition services becomes a part of general medical

benefits, the most important barrier (i.e., recognition and accountability for cross-disciplinary physical and mental health treatment and outcomes by the all health practitioners) will not change.

The importance of understanding the effect of the current independent reimbursement environment on care is so that integrated case managers can work with their patients as they overcome the barriers to improvement that are created by a fragmented system. To date, case managers have avoided this thorny area of assistance, focusing rather on issues in either the medical or mental health domains, but not both. With integrated case management, it is just as important to help the managed patient find mental health assistance and to link it to general medical treatment as it is to ensure that proper physical health treatment is being provided.

For instance, it is within the domain of responsibility for the integrated case manager to help a patient with multiple sclerosis find a psychiatrist or psychotherapist for interferon-induced depression, ensure access to and coordination of neurological and mental health services, and document adherence and response to multiple sclerosis and depression treatment. No longer can the manager concentrate on treatment and outcome for multiple sclerosis alone. In fact, responsibility does not end as assistance is given for the disorders experienced by the patient. The patient's social support system, insurance coverage, relationship and communication with providers, and other issues constitute potential barriers to improvement and thus are within the integrated case manager's accountability.

EXHIBIT 5.4   Consequences of an Independent Physical and Mental Condition Payment System

- Nonaccountability for mental health outcomes by non-mental health professionals
  - Few mental health and chemical dependence programs available in the primary care settings (e.g., integrated clinics, screening and brief intervention, buprenorphine programs)
  - Limited use of evidence-based mental health practice or personnel who can provide it
  - Little clinical outcome concern or measurement
- Reduced access to psychiatrists and other mental health professionals
  - Mental health professionals not listed among medical health plan network providers
  - Common nonparticipation in behavioral health plan networks by mental health clinicians (i.e., cash-only practices, thus the sickest patients with mental conditions cannot afford or access care even with insurance coverage)
- Frustration by primary care physicians and other medical specialists related to 4- and 8-week appointment delays for off-site mental condition appointments
- No payment for same-day physical and mental health appointments in medical settings
- Care discontinuity with geographically separate physical and mental health treatment locations
- Noncommunicating health records
- Untimely or no mental health follow-up appointments due to scheduling constraints
- No mental condition treatment in 70% of general medical patients with disorders
- Only a third of the 30% of general medical patients who are treated get evidence-based care
- General medical tests and interventions not paid for in inpatient psychiatric settings leading to financial insolvency for integrated services in complex patients
- Limited interdisciplinary checking about adherence and/or response to treatment

---

PRACTICE ISSUES OF IMPORTANCE IN PHYSICAL AND MENTAL CONDITION CARE

There are differences in practice needs for virtually all disciplines within medicine. Surgeons need operating rooms. Radiologists need imaging equipment. Gerontologists need nursing homes. Pathologists need laboratories. Mental health specialists need commitment laws, special procedures for suicidal or homicidal patients, and long-term care facilities for the serious and persistently mentally ill. Since most case managers coming from general medical backgrounds and some with mental health backgrounds will not be familiar with special mental condition needs, core issues related to the need to provide treatment against a patient's will (competence and commitment) and in dealing with suicidal and homicidal patients or other psychiatric emergencies will be reviewed here.

Likewise, most case managers coming from mental health backgrounds and some from physical health backgrounds will have few, if any, experiences in dealing with medical emergencies. This will also be summarized. Finally, while general pediatric and child psychiatry emergencies are addressed in much the same way that adult emergencies are, there are special considerations in dealing with child/youth emergencies since there are laws relating to decision making that need to be understood. These will also be discussed.

Competence and Commitment

There are situations in which forced treatment is necessary. Even in the non-mental health arena, it is possible to *require* treatment for tuberculosis, HIV, or other communicable diseases in non-psychiatrically ill individuals for public health reasons. While in patients with mental conditions, the reason for mandated detention and treatment is due to adjudicated impairment of decision-making capabilities, the principle is the same. If treatment is not given, danger is introduced to the patient or to a member of the public.

For virtually all clinicians, it is uncomfortable to initiate or be a part of proceedings in which a person may be held against his or her will. Nonetheless, it is a part of quality health care for a segment of the population. In the general medical sector, such activity commonly occurs, albeit without the involvement of the court, on behalf of vulnerable patients with medical causes for incapacity. For instance, many patients with dementia are subtly forced by family and/or their care providers to give up personal autonomy in the name of safety (e.g., driver's licenses, independent living arrangements, etc.). In more acute settings, hospitalized patients with delirium can be restrained and treatment given against their will even at times when there is no imminent danger.

In the mental health setting, forced detention and treatment in most jurisdictions can only be given when: (a) a mental illness is present that impairs judgment, such as dementia, substance dependence, severe eating disorder, mania, or depression and (b) the impaired judgment puts someone in danger. When these criteria are thought to be present, a series of clinical and legal procedures are taken to detain the patient and systematically establish decision-making capacity, based on illness, and dangerousness. Only then can nonemergent treatment be given. Health professionals (medical or mental health) or law enforcement officers typically initiate these adjudication procedures.

In most situations, case managers are only peripherally involved in such matters since they do not themselves provide care. On the other hand, it is important for them to understand the procedures necessary for forced detention and treatment so that they remain objective in working with the patient, the patient's guardian, and the patient's clinicians. Importantly, the manager must remember that they are advocates for the patient's health within the law. In some situations, this means that they support forced treatment despite the patient's objections. Case managers, however, may find themselves helpful arbiters of collaboration between the patient, the patient's family, and the patient's providers since they may be the only impartial bystanders to contentious clinical intervention.

This manual does not go into detail related to competence and commitment since specific laws regulating their administration vary from state to state and country to country. For this reason, those reading this manual should plan on talking with mental health personnel in their local jurisdiction, reading about, or going to a lecture on this topic after training in integrated case management is complete. Details about how incompetence is determined and how commitment proceedings are initiated are not within the scope of action by the case manager. It can, however, be helpful to have this knowledge or know where to find it when working with family members or physicians who are dealing with a patient receiving poor care due to mental health-related nonadherence.

Suicidal or Homicidal Concerns

Nothing is more uncomfortable than having a patient tell you that he or she is thinking about killing himself or herself or another, especially when this is something that you have not dealt with in the past. While such situations are necessarily emergent in nature, depending on the level of intent, when a case manager has an understanding of the steps that need to be taken, it takes some, but not all, of the sting from the situation.

Unlike issues related to forced detention and treatment for incompetent and committed patients, integrated case managers will likely, at some time during their work with patients, encounter situations *legally requiring* action. For this reason, in all settings in which integrated case management is provided, part of the early onsite training for case managers coming from general medical backgrounds (and some with mental health backgrounds who have dealt only with less severely ill patients) should include how to respond to suicidal or homicidal ideation or behavior in their patients. General guidelines for handling concerns about suicidal behavior can be found in **Exhibit 5.5** and for homicidal behavior in **Exhibit 5.6**. Additional onsite training about these topics can be given at the same time that emergency medical procedures are reviewed for case managers coming from behavioral health backgrounds (e.g., what to do for a patient describing cardiac-type chest pain or a person who has suddenly become nonresponsive while talking on the phone). The reason for doing this as an onsite procedure is that specifics about what is to be done are determined by the setting in which the circumstance arises (i.e., in a clinic, over the phone, at a patient's home, etc.) and also the laws in the region in which the case management services are delivered.

Suicidality and homocidality constitute a special clinical situation, which, in most jurisdictions, requires action (e.g., emergency response activation, if needed, or notification of life threat to named individual) by any health professional who encounters it. This is a personal responsibility for the case manager, requiring swift and decisive attention. Lack of informed consent to speak to mental health professionals or law enforcement when suicidality is present or when there is a threatened individual in the case of homocidality is superseded by the potential danger associated with the situation. When possible, it is helpful to involve the patient's health professionals, but accountability for action rests with the case manager.

It is thus imperative for case managers when first initiating health privacy parameters with a new patient to indicate that confidentiality will be maintained in all situations except when the patient describes potential danger to self or others. Thus, patients know that dangerousness legally obliges the case manager to protect the patient or a threatened individual. It is much better to explain this up front than to do so in the heat of the situation.

Medical Emergencies

In many ways, it is easier for professionals with mental health backgrounds to adapt to and deal with medical emergencies than it is for those coming from general medical backgrounds to learn how to deal with forced treatment (competence and commitment) and

---

EXHIBIT 5.5   **Procedures for Handling Patients With Suicidal Concerns**

Expression of Suicidality or Self-Harm

- Listen to the patient to clarify for level of intent
  Level 1. Not want to live; would not resist death
  Level 2. Active thoughts of harming self
  Level 3. Thought of method to do it without plan
  Level 4. Plan for harming self
- Identify risk factors
  - Depression
  - Drug or alcohol intoxication/dependence
  - Acute crisis
  - Prior attempts
  - Worsening life circumstances
  - Other risk factors
- Action for Level 1 without risk factors *(occurs often in complex patients)*
  - Explain you are not a mental health therapist and will try to connect them with help
- Action for Level 1 with risk factors of concern or Levels 2 through 4
  - Direct transfer to crisis line; suicide hot line *(better than to personal doctor or mental health professional)*
  - If direct transfer refused or patient hangs up and serious concern remains, call 911 to send law enforcement
  - Discuss with medical director and/or supervisor for further suggestions/involvement

Suicide Attempt

- Call 911 to have ambulance/law enforcement sent to location

With Levels 2 Through 4:

- Do not try to talk them down
- Do not tell them to go to their doctor or to the emergency room
- Do not try to do something personally such as go to their house, call them back later, etc.

EXHIBIT 5.6   **Procedures for Handling Patients With Homicidal Thoughts**

General Threat to Others

- Listen to the patient and clarify circumstances
- Refer to a mental health specialist or encourage the patient to talk with his or her mental health provider *(this is usually something that requires a psychiatrist)*
- Inform mental health specialist if patient is seeing one
- Maintain relationship if possible but do not become involved in the dispute/difficulty
- Discuss with medical director and/or supervisor for further suggestions/involvement
- Remain neutral; if neutrality not possible, discuss with medical director/supervisor or drop case

Threat to an Identifiable Person

- Do as with a general threat as previously noted
- Based on local protocol, notify the identified person about the threat in a timely fashion *(legally required by Tarasoff rule in the United States)*

---

dangerous behavior (suicidal and/or homicidal ideation). In patients with medical illness, less contentious interventions are usually required. Since case managers are not involved in the direct treatment of patients with whom they work, in emergency situations, they merely need to know how to activate the emergency medical response system or how to direct the patient to an appropriate provider.

Perhaps a greater challenge for case managers with non-medical backgrounds will be to know when an emergency situation exists rather than what to do when one is identified. Again, it is not the case manager's responsibility to know about all medical emergencies or how to treat them. Instead, he or she should use common sense and be proactive when potential emergency situations arise. Unlike the patient, case managers will usually have colleagues or a medical director to draw on for assistance. Thus, they can more easily obtain further information and advice about what to do. If no one is available, then directly transferring the patient to their primary physician's office or to a 24-hour nurse line may be in order. If it is obviously an emergency situation, a direct transfer or call to the local emergency response number may be the appropriate course of action.

In all circumstances, the case manager should act with the safety of the patient in mind. Often this involves getting immediate acute medical assistance onsite. For this action, few will fault the case manager. After the crisis is over, it is a good idea to review the course of events with a supervisor to ensure that appropriate steps were taken on behalf of the patient. Finally, follow up with the patient to find out how things turned out.

Special Pediatric and Child Psychiatry Circumstances

Both a child/youth and a parent/caregiver are affected by decisions concerning the health of a child/youth; however, as children mature they increasingly develop the capacity to understand and consent to their medical care and to have control about who has access to information about their personal health care. Although rare, occasions do arise when there are disagreements between children and their parents about the proper course of action. Further, there are domains where parents may intervene in their children's care (e.g., by asking for information from the youth's physician without consideration of whether they have their youth's consent to do so). Therefore, it is important for pediatric case managers to be aware of relevant legislation in the jurisdiction in which they work with regard to issues of consent and confidentiality. In most countries, the age at which a youth can make independent health decisions is 18 years. In isolated locations, the age of majority can be as high as 21 (e.g., Mississippi, Egypt) or as low as 14 (e.g., Samoa and Puerto Rico). The age of majority in specific locales can be easily found on the Internet.

While the age of majority is the most common arbiter of who makes health-related decisions, there are some situations in which younger individuals can become their own decision makers. For instance, in some states and countries, youth aged 14 can become emancipated minors and thus make their own decisions by declaration, by legal petition, by marriage, or by joining the armed services. Factors concerning decision making become even more complicated in relation to sexual activity (e.g., the age of consent for sexual activity is most often 16 to 18 years

but can be as low as 14 years or as high as 21 years in some countries). Another common area of early health decision making, again generally related to early sexual activity, relates to a youth's right to initiate birth control, to have an abortion, or to be treated for a sexually transmitted disease without parental notification/consent. Legal authorities and the Internet can usually clarify local laws, but it is preferable for the case manager to be familiar with them through educational activities at his or her location of practice.

Pediatric case managers must be informed of local legislation guiding decisions about who is able to give health consent in various situations, who requires notification and at what ages, and whether there are exceptions. Without having a firm understanding of these rules, case managers are at risk of acting based on information from the wrong decision maker, providing personal health information without proper consent, or alienating one or the other party because of lack of information about regional laws.

Having provided these cautionary notes, it should be noted that pediatric case managers are most effective when they can facilitate child/youth and parent/caregiver communication as assistance related to barriers to health is given. In most situations, the child/youth and the parent/caregiver have the same goals and work together to maximize health. Information provided to them by the case manager about what constitutes the age of majority, can often obviate a dispute that would otherwise arise about who makes the final health-related decision.

Case managers also need to be well versed in the legislation governing mandatory reporting of child abuse or neglect in the jurisdictions in which they practice. Typically, when there is reasonable suspicion that child abuse or neglect is occurring, any health professional, teacher, or law enforcement officer is *required* to report it. Child abuse and neglect is generally defined as any type of cruelty inflicted on a child, including emotional abuse, physical harm, neglect, and sexual abuse or exploitation. For most types of abuse, mandatory reporting is required under the age of 18, although there may be different age requirements in different jurisdictions. Since this is an area in which case managers, virtually all of whom are health professionals, can be criminally prosecuted for not reporting to child protective agencies, it is important for them to understand laws on mandatory reporting in locations where they provide case management services. This is the case manager's responsibility, though he or she may collaborate with other clinicians involved in the care of the child/youth in providing information.

PRACTITIONERS FOR MENTAL HEALTH DISORDERS

All practitioners do not have the same intervention capabilities—for example, a physical therapist does not prescribe medication but is an expert in rehabilitation procedures. A chiropractor can treat back pain but not pneumonia. A psychologist can perform evidence-based psychotherapy and complete psychodiagnostic assessments but does not know how to administer psychotropic medications. This seems self-evident; however, there has been a tendency in the past 25 years to assume that exposure to any mental health professional can be expected to result in the same outcome. Nothing could be further from the truth.

Exhibit 5.7 summarizes the training and skill sets commonly used by mental health and substance use disorder practitioners. While it provides general guidelines for the type of services that can be expected when a patient participating in case management is being assisted by the professional involved, it does not guarantee that outcome-changing care will be given. For instance, it is unreasonable to expect that a patient with schizophrenia or bipolar affective disorder will have a good outcome if treated by a general practitioner coupled with a psychologist or social worker. Certainly, psychological and social interventions are important in such patients; however, a core principle of treatment for patients with these diagnoses requires specialists versed in the nuances of psychopharmacology. This is particularly true for patients with health complexity, for whom comorbid medical conditions are also present and multiple medications are being used.

In these situations, diplomacy is critical as attempts are made to guide a patient to the set of clinicians most likely to be of benefit. It is for this reason that outcome monitoring is so important. For instance, if a patient with unipolar major depression has persistent Patient Health Questionnaire-9 (PHQ-9) depression scale scores fluctuating around 20 (a high score suggesting serious depression) while on medication prescribed by her primary care physician in adequate doses and for adequate duration, then assisting with involvement by a psychologist who has expertise in interpersonal or another efficacy-based form of psychotherapy or a psychiatrist who might try an alternative antidepressant may turn nonresponse into response. Not infrequently, using the assistance of the case manager's medical director can facilitate such an adjustment to care.

Even after such an adjustment is made, it remains within the purview of the case manager to follow continued intervention and outcomes. Other factors may play a role in nonresponse, such as poor coordination of interventions among practitioners, workplace conflicts that have not been dealt with, no-shows for appointments, and so forth. It may be the relationship between the patient and case manager that allows the issues retarding improvement to come to light. In these situations, the case manager can truly tip the scale toward recovery.

ASSISTING PATIENTS WITH MENTAL CONDITIONS

The integrated case management approach is built on the principles of communimetrics (**Exhibit 5.8**), developed prior to the creation of the IM-CAG complexity assessment tool (Lyons, 2006). Of particular importance in relation to the discussion of mental conditions is principle four—that is, that psychological items are agnostic to etiology. It is not the job of the case manager to explore or try to understand the *cause* of distressing psychological symptoms. Rather, the case manager is responsible for identifying the presence or concern about the presence of symptoms and for assisting the patient in finding treatments most likely to quickly reverse symptoms. Just as in patients with physical illnesses, symptoms of psychiatric illnesses are associated with suffering, impaired function, and increased need for health services. Reversing symptoms is the best way to alter these consequences.

Some people consider mental conditions untreatable. In fact, in today's world nothing could be further from the truth. Granted, some illnesses and patients are harder to treat than others, but this is true for both physical and mental illnesses (Table 2.2).

GENERAL PHYSICAL AND MENTAL HEALTH ASSISTANCE

The first step for any case manager is to help patients understand their illnesses and the things that they can do to get better. This most often means that the patient is provided with information about his or her illnesses and is given an opportunity to have questions about them answered. The case manager should recognize that the majority of the literature sent to patients about their illnesses finds its way into the wastebasket, most often without being read. For this reason, the case manager must have a discussion with the patient about his or her illness to ensure that there is a basic understanding of symptoms, treatments, anticipated time to improvement, and parameters that document outcomes. During this discussion, it is helpful to find out about the patient's or a family member's reluctance for the patient to enter treatment. This is common with mental conditions because of misinformation about the value of treatment or the patient's feeling that he or she can use his or her will power or prayer to overcome symptoms. This is one area in which motivational interviewing skills come in handy.

EXHIBIT 5.7   Behavioral Health Personnel Skill Sets

Psychiatrists: medical doctors (MDs, DOs) specializing in mental and substance use disorders

Knowledge base

Physiological and psychological basis of the behavioral manifestations of physical illness and medications; major and minor behavioral, emotional, and cognitive disturbances; research

Interventions

Psychotherapy, medications for mental and substance use disorders, light therapy, electroconvulsive therapy, vagal stimulation, all other available therapies for mental illness and substance use disorders

Subspecialties

Child and adolescent, substance use disorders, geriatrics, psychosomatic medicine, forensic, or physicians with dual training in psychiatry *and* in family practice, pediatrics, internal medicine, or neurology

Psychologists: non-medically trained specialists in mental and substance use disorders

Knowledge base

Psychological aspects of mental and substance use disorders; neurocognitive and neuropsychological testing; psychological, organizational, and developmental assessments; research

Educational levels

Doctoral (PhD, EdD, PsyD), master's or bachelor's (special license or supervision for clinical practices in most states)

Interventions

Psychotherapy, biofeedback, hypnosis, behavior change techniques

Subspecialties

Clinical (health, neuropsychology, geropsychology, counseling), school, industrial-organizational, developmental, social, research

Psychiatric Nurses: medically trained nurses specializing in mental and substance use disorders

Knowledge base

Medical and psychological problem resolution for psychiatric disturbances whether related to medical or psychiatric disease (APNs: advanced training in physiology, psychology, and psychopharmacology of mental illness and substance use disorders)

Educational levels

Advanced practice nurses (APNs), clinical nurse specialists (CNSs), registered nurses (RNs)

Interventions

Variable up to level of APN that can have prescribing and independent decision-making privileges

Subspecialties

Adult, child and adolescent, family, public health

Social Workers: non-medically trained specialist (MSW, other) who assist clients through socially difficult situations

Knowledge base

Social and environmental problems and system issues that affect a person's life

Interventions

Assisting with supportive counseling and crisis intervention, discharge planning, community and health

Subspecialties

Family and school, medical and public health, mental and substance use disorders

Other Behavioral Health Personnel: substance use disorder counselor, marriage and family therapist, counselor, practical nurse, etc.

From *Healing Body and Mind: A Critical Issue for Health Care Reform* (p. 34), by R. Kathol and S. Gatteau, 2007, Westport, CT: Praeger. Copyright ©2007 by Roger G. Kathol & Suzanne Gatteau.

EXHIBIT 5.8	**Principles of Communimetrics Used With the IM-CAG**

- Each item is relevant to the service plan
- Complexity levels of the items translate into actions
- A patient's outcome is more important than the service recommended
- Psychological items are agnostic as to etiology
- Items are designed to allow communication about potential barriers to health among key stakeholders, including the patient

---

The second step is to ensure that the patient is getting treatments that are likely to lead to the quickest and most effective improvement. In Chapter 6, case managers will become familiar with several common mental and physical health conditions and with how to document symptom improvement. For instance, in patients with depression and anxiety, both medication and psychotherapy can be effectively used alone or in combination. What frequently occurs in the primary care setting, however, is that a patient is given a prescription, which is not filled, or is referred to a counselor, who gives support but not evidence-based therapy for the underlying condition. Neither of these situations would portend improvement for the patient. Thus, it may be necessary to educate the primary care physician about depression or anxiety treatment adherence problems or efficacy-based psychotherapies so patient-physician collaboration can be enhanced to the benefit of the patient.

In patients with general medical disorders—such as those with diabetes—medication, diet, and exercise play an interacting role in symptom improvement and blood sugar control. What frequently occurs, however, is that a patient is given a prescription for oral hypoglycemics, which is either not filled or taken in lower than prescribed doses to save on cost; a diet, which is too difficult to follow or not understood; and an exercise program, for which there is no time or interest. Unless each of these barriers to improvement is discussed and reasonable alternatives are uncovered, the situation heralds a low likelihood of improvement for the patient. Thus, it may be necessary to educate the primary care physician about the patient's treatment adherence problems and/or to discuss compromises that might be more acceptable to the patient. Again, the challenge is in creating a therapeutic win for the patient in concert with the suggestions for care by his or her doctor.

Finally, the case manager needs to connect mental health symptoms and treatment with general medical illness treatment and its adherence. Worse outcomes for medical conditions, documented in patients with concurrent physical and mental disorders, will not improve unless equal attention is given to the administration of and follow-through for the patient's combined health conditions. Part of this connection process will likely include either having the patient tell his or her general medical clinicians about the coexisting mental condition or making sure that descriptions of it are included in the reports that the patient's clinician receives about progress through case management.

In order to effectively complete the three tasks just described, the case manager must learn basic information about:

- The symptoms experienced by the patient when he or she has conditions of note.
- Complications that can occur because of the conditions and steps to prevent them
- First-line and to some extent second-line treatments (since case managers will be working with complex patients).
- The measures used to follow whether the diseases are under control and whether progressive improvement is occurring (physical, laboratory, imaging, and other findings). For this, case managers need to know how to interpret common follow-up tests or examinations. This is one of the areas of great value that staffing active cases with a physician (medical director) brings. Such supervision can be the difference between case management success and failure.
- A general timeline for when outcomes should be expected if effective treatment is being given.

Case managers cannot be expected to have the same level of understanding about illnesses as the clinicians treating the patients or even, to some extent, the patients themselves. They, however, should have sufficient understanding to be able to identify common sense barriers to improvement, how to try to support the patient and clinician in reversing them, and what measures to use to document that the changes are effective.

In patients with physical and mental conditions not included in Chapter 6, case managers will likely be less familiar with symptoms and treatments. This is perhaps a greater challenge and concern for case managers who come from mental health backgrounds but who have little or no training in medical illnesses (e.g., psychologists, substance abuse counselors, etc.).

Clearly, additional and systematic training is necessary for these individuals if they are to be considered for roles as case managers. Even for case managers with nursing or social work training, however, many patients will have illnesses about which they are unfamiliar. When this is the case, they should elicit suggestions from their medical director (physician) during supervisory sessions, present the case at an internal case conference, and/or ask for suggestions from colleagues (or their supervisor) who may have a better understanding of the illnesses and the type of help that can be provided.

As case managers work with their patients, they should continue to learn about new physical and mental conditions. Luckily, we live in the information age. It is easy to Google medical topics at reputable websites (e.g., WebMD, Medscape, Mayo Clinics, the National Institutes of Health). Through quick, focused searches, case managers should have sufficient understanding of the basics of most medical conditions, whether common or rare, to be able to help their patients ask questions of their providers so that they can better understand their illnesses, the treatments, and the steps needed to get better. It may be as simple as translating what the doctor told them to do into understandable language.

For instance, one provider could not understand why a patient was having so much trouble with fluid balance since the patient insisted that she was strictly adhering to a liter and a half 24-hour water restriction. It was only after the case manager uncovered that the patient did not include coffee, tea, and soft drinks as water that it became clear that the patient was literally only limiting herself to six cups of H_2O. Recognition of this fact led to appropriate fluid restriction, fewer water pills, and better control.

REFERENCES

Institute of Medicine, Committee on Crossing the Quality Chasm: Adaptation to Mental Health and Addictive Disorders. (2006). *Improving the quality of health care for mental and substance-use conditions.* Washington, DC: National Academies Press.

Institute of Medicine, Committee on Quality of Health Care in America. (2001). *Crossing the quality chasm: A new health system for the 21st century.* Washington, DC: National Academies Press.

Kathol, R., & Gatteau, S. (2007). *Healing body and mind: A critical issue for health care reform.* Westport, CT: Praeger.

Lyons, J. S. (2006). The complexity of communication in an environment with multiple disciplines and professionals: Communimetrics and decision support. *Medical Clinics North America, 90*(4), 693–701.

CHAPTER 6

Examples of Basic Information on Common Physical and Mental Conditions

OBJECTIVES

- To put into context the role of cross-disciplinary illness understanding for use in integrated case management
- To share basic information about the assessment and treatment of several common mental conditions: depression, anxiety, psychotic disorders, substance use disorders, and attention deficit and hyperactivity disorder
- To share basic information about the assessment and treatment of several common chronic general medical disorders/presentations: diabetes, chronic obstructive pulmonary disease, chronic renal disease, unexplained somatic complaints, and asthma

INTRODUCTION

Many clinicians think that the most important component in becoming an integrated case manager relates to the need to learn about illnesses in the specialty domain to which the manager has had little exposure. While it is true that basic information about the illnesses of the patients with whom the case manager is working is necessary, it is, in fact, a small part of all the special knowledge and skills that integrated case managers require. Case managers bring their greatest value to patients as they synthesize disease-specific management with other areas in patients' lives that prevent return to health. Integrated case managers focus their activities on specific risks and needs, some of which will be disease related, but with the global picture in mind.

This chapter discusses several frequently seen general medical and mental health disorders in adults and children/youth. The primary purpose of this chapter is to give case managers an idea about the depth of basic knowledge about an illness condition that is necessary to provide sound case management to patients experiencing such conditions. It does not, however, prepare case managers to assist with a myriad of other common and uncommon medical and mental health conditions to which they will be exposed. Specifically, it is intended to break the ice for historically medical case managers as they choose to venture into the world of behavior and mental health and for historically mental health case managers as they open the door to assisting with general medical conditions. Included among the conditions are two that are commonly seen in children/youth: asthma and attention deficit hyperactivity disorder. In a sense, this chapter is intended to demystify

illnesses typically seen outside the professional's chosen discipline and to share the message that general medical and mental conditions are more similar than dissimilar when it comes to assisting patients regain health.

What is more important than in-depth knowledge of diseases and their specific interventions is an understanding of the level of information necessary to connect them to other factors in patients' lives as a coherent integrated case management plan is created and executed. Such an integrated care plan provides the best guarantee of rapid stabilization and health improvement as discussed in Chapter 2.

As important as the specific content about the illnesses summarized is the framework provided (see the subheadings under each condition) with regard to the type of information about a condition that case managers should obtain as they start to work with new managed patients. With access to the Internet, support from case management colleagues, and access to assistance/supervision from medical directors and physician clinician colleagues, who are part of the case management team, there is little reason that basic information about virtually any illness cannot be quickly assimilated and understood by health-savvy case managers. This is a necessary skill for case managers working with complex patients. An initial place to access needed information about many common medical conditions is MedlinePlus (http://medlineplus.gov/), a service of the U.S. National Library of Medicine and the National Institutes of Health. Additional information may come from proprietary medical education vendors, published guidelines, or other reputable sources.

In the context of integrated case management, disease-specific actions are certainly appropriate but should be connected with barriers to improvement in other complexity domains that contribute to poor health outcomes. How case managers systematically approach the use of disease- and non-disease-related material as they help patients regain or stabilize health will be discussed in Chapters 7 through 11.

SUMMARY OF MAJOR DEPRESSIVE DISORDER

Major depression is the condition most commonly included among disease management programs if an insurance company or disease management vendor chooses to include management assistance for a mental health condition. The reason for this is that it is present in about 10% of the general population at any given time but can reach levels of 30% to 50% in patients with concurrent chronic medical conditions, such as diabetes, congestive heart failure, or chronic renal disease (Ciechanowski, Katon, Russo, & Hirsch, 2003; Druss, Rosenheck, & Sledge, 2000; Hunkeler et al., 2006; Katon, Unutzer, et al., 2006; Kessler et al., 2003; Stewart, Ricci, Chee, Hahn, & Morganstein, 2003; Von Korff & Goldberg, 2001). Supplementary information about depression can be found at:

- http://www.nimh.nih.gov/health/topics/depression/index.shtml
- http://www.impact-uw.org/

Pathophysiology: low mood with impairment of function and an unknown cause. The major current hypothesis includes the presence of neurotransmitter dysregulation in the limbic system (vulnerability). Unfortunate life circumstances can also produce similar symptoms in nonvulnerable individuals, such as in association with the death of a family member. Since sadness is a normal reaction to life circumstances, the diagnosis of major depression should not be purely related to the number of depressive symptoms. It should also reflect their duration and the context in which symptoms of depression occur.

Predisposition: family propensity (genetics); associated medical illnesses (e.g., Cushing's syndrome, Alzheimer's disease, Parkinson's disease, asthma, diabetes, obesity); substance abuse; certain medications (e.g., steroids, beta interferon, and chronic use of benzodiazepines); stressful life experiences may precipitate an episode in vulnerable individuals.

Major Subclasses: subsyndromal, also known as sadness or minor depression; unipolar major depressive disorder (low mood only); bipolar affective disorder (includes periods of mania or hypomania). All of the preceding can be related to general medical conditions, other psychiatric illnesses, or medications.

Core Symptoms: (a and b) dysphoria and/or lack of interest (one of these two is required for a diagnosis),

(c) difficulty concentrating, (d) low energy, (e) agitation or retardation, (f) appetite change, (g) sleep disturbance, (h) feelings of guilt or worthlessness, (i) suicidal thoughts. Mania and/or hypomania are core symptoms that distinguish bipolar from unipolar depression. The Patient Health Questionnaire-9 (PHQ-9) is now used as a standard for symptom documentation and follow-up in medical and mental health settings (Lowe, Unutzer, Callahan, Perkins, & Kroenke, 2004). It is not a diagnostic tool but is convenient to establish baseline symptoms and follow illness progression.

Complications: personal, home, and work impairment; greater morbidity and mortality associated with concurrent general medical illnesses, tests, and procedures; higher cost of health care, especially medical; suicidal risk.

Treatments for Depression: the following lists include the primary approaches to depression treatment with evidence of value for patients. Other interventions can be used as adjuncts to these treatments but are not considered primary treatments, such as supportive psychotherapy, crisis intervention, exercise, healthy diet, good sleep habits, healthy foods, acupuncture, and massage. Outcome measurement will further guide the treatment strategy.

- Education about the illness
- Personal support
- Antidepressant and/or mood stabilizing (for bipolar) medication (benzodiazepines, sedative hypnotics, and alcohol should be avoided since they make depression worse.)
- Selected forms of psychotherapy (e.g., cognitive behavioral therapy, interpersonal psychotherapy, problem-solving therapy)
- Family treatment/support
- Electroconvulsive therapy (ECT)

Interventions for Factors Associated With Depression

- Suicide prevention
- Assistance with return to normal function (home, work, social, etc.)
- Coordination of depression treatment with medical illness treatment; special emphasis on adherence to all recommended interventions

Impact: higher health care service use, functional impairment, medical and psychiatric morbidity, earlier medical and psychiatric mortality.

SUMMARY OF DIABETES MELLITUS

Diabetes mellitus (Ciechanowski, Katon, & Russo, 2000; Egede, 2006; Katon, Unutzer, et al., 2006) is a disorder in which insulin, the hormone that transfers sugar from the blood to cells during food digestion, is either not produced (10% for type 1 autoimmune diabetes) or fails to have its expected action (90% for type 2 insulin-resistant diabetes). As a result, sugar excessively accumulates in the blood, causing symptoms and even diseases in other parts of the body.

About 7% of the population suffers from diabetes, and that number is growing, especially in the United States, since more people are overweight and fewer participate in healthy exercise. It is perhaps the most important of the chronic conditions covered in this chapter since it affects such a large percentage of the population and it is eminently treatable. When left ineffectively treated, diabetes predictably leads to other health complications, disability, morbidity, and early mortality. For this reason, case managers can have a substantial effect on patient outcomes if they can alter behaviors that perpetuate poor control.

Supplementary information on diabetes can be found at:

- http://diabetes.niddk.nih.gov/intro/index.htm
- http://www.nlm.nih.gov/medlineplus/diabetes.html

Pathophysiology: type 1 autoimmune reaction causing death of pancreatic islet cells (insulin producing); type 2 unknown mechanism in which insulin resistance develops, making higher levels of insulin necessary to control blood sugar levels; gestational, which occurs in approximately 5% of pregnant women and is associated with later type 2 diabetes in many individuals.

Predisposition: type 1 diabetes occurs earlier in life (often in childhood) and usually requires insulin for sugar control. Type 2 diabetes occurs later in life, particularly in those with a family history or those who are overweight. Certain ethnic groups, such as American Indians, Hispanics, Pacific Islanders, and those of African descent, are at greater risk for the development of diabetes, as are those on medications associated with weight gain, such as corticosteroids and a number of antidepressant and antipsychotic medications. The prevalence of diabetes in the United States has increased substantially in the last 25 years, probably because of a combination of increased obesity, less exercise, an aging population, and growth in ethnic subgroups (**Figure 6.1**) (Centers for Disease Control and Prevention, http://www.cdc.gov/diabetes/statistics/prev/national/figraceethsex.htm).

Major Subclasses: prediabetes (elevated blood sugar without signs or symptoms of clinical diabetes), often treatable with diet and exercise; non-insulin-dependent diabetes (usually type 2, adult onset treated with diet, exercise, and oral hypoglycemics); insulin-dependent diabetes (type 1 and advanced type 2, requires insulin for blood sugar control and complication prevention); brittle diabetes (any diabetes that is hard to control despite treatment adherence).

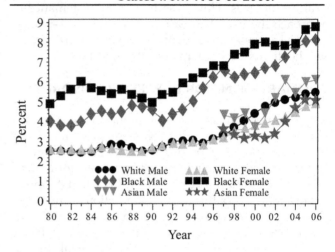

FIGURE 6.1   Diabetes prevalence in the United States from 1980 to 2006.

Core Symptoms: (a) excessive thirst and urinating, (b) fatigue, (c) hunger, (d) symptoms of diabetic complications (see "Complications").

Laboratory Findings: fasting blood sugar: > 125 mg/dl; HbA1c ([estimates long-term control] 4% to 6%: normal; 7%: average blood sugar = 150 mg/dl; 8%: average blood sugar = 180 mg/dl; 9%: average blood sugar = 210 mg/dl).

Complications (Usually Occur After a Long History of Poor Control)

- Obesity
  - □ Preventive measures: weight control, education about diet and exercise
  - □ Symptoms: fatigue, other illnesses
  - □ Treatment: diet, exercise, weight loss medications, surgery
- Hyperlipidemia
  - □ Preventive measures: monitoring lipid levels
  - □ Symptoms: none
  - □ Treatment: diet, weight loss, lipid-lowering medications
- Hypertension
  - □ Preventive measures: monitoring blood pressure control
  - □ Symptoms: none
  - □ Treatment: low salt diet, weight loss, antihypertensive medications
- Depression
  - □ Preventive measures: screening for early symptoms with PHQ-9
  - □ Symptoms: sadness, low energy, nonadherence, disability, and so forth
  - □ Treatment: antidepressant medications, mood stabilizers, psychotherapy, referral

- Coronary heart disease
  - Preventive measures: education about graded exercise, diet
  - Symptoms: chest pain
  - Treatment: weight loss, anti-anginal cardiac strengthening medications, stint, surgery
- Stroke
  - Preventive measures: weight and blood pressure control
  - Symptoms: focal neurological symptoms
  - Treatment: acute intervention, blood thinners, rehabilitation
- Peripheral neuropathy
  - Preventive measures: monitoring neurological examinations
  - Symptoms: numbness, pain, cold extremities
  - Treatment: pain medications, local trauma protection
- Kidney disease/failure
  - Preventive measures: use of angiotensin-converting enzyme (ACE) inhibitors, monitoring creatinine levels
  - Symptoms: fatigue, low urine output
  - Treatment: dialysis, transplantation
- Retinal hemorrhage
  - Preventive measures: monitoring annual eye examinations
  - Symptoms: blurred vision, lost eyesight
  - Treatment: laser treatment
- Poor circulation
  - Preventive measures: weight control
  - Symptoms: claudication
  - Treatment: vasodilating medications, revascularization
- Skin ulcers
  - Preventive measures: protective footwear, safe nail care, good hygiene
  - Symptoms: pain, infection
  - Treatment: skin and nail care, antibiotics, amputation
- Infections
  - Preventive measures: good hygiene, vaccinations
  - Symptoms: fever, pain, swelling
  - Treatment: antibiotics, focal infection care, amputation

Treatments: diet, exercise, insulin, oral hypoglycemics, and treatment of complications.

Intervention for Factors Associated With Diabetes Mellitus

- Assistance with return to work
- Close attention to mental health symptoms and their treatment
- Assistance with diabetes monitoring and preventive measures

Impact: higher health care service use, functional impairment, disability, medical morbidity, and earlier medical mortality.

SUMMARY OF ANXIETY DISORDERS

Anxiety, concern, or worry is a normal emotional reaction to stress. In fact, in most individuals it is a helpful adaptive mechanism since it can sharpen focus and enhance concentration. It becomes an illness only when it occurs in the absence of provocation, endures for prolonged periods of time, or creates symptoms in excess of those expected from precipitating circumstances. Anxiety related to life events occurs frequently. It is not an illness.

Anxiety, as a disorder, can manifest as continuous unprovoked excessive worry (generalized anxiety disorder), spontaneous discrete attacks lasting 5 to 15 minutes (panic disorder), situation-related anxiety (social phobia), intrusive thoughts or actions (obsessive-compulsive disorder), or persistent reflection about prior traumatic events (posttraumatic stress disorder [PTSD]). One or more of these forms of anxiety affect about a fifth of the population each year and are associated with depressive symptoms and/or substance abuse in about a half of those cases.

Perhaps the greatest challenge for providers in assisting patients with anxiety is separating out what is normal anxiety from that which is pathological since the former responds well to support, reassurance, and time for stressful events to pass, whereas the latter requires treatment. This is particularly important in patients with chronic medical conditions since the presence of anxiety is associated with a high degree of disability and cost (Katon, Russo, et al., 2006; Roy-Byrne et al., 2005; Roy-Byrne et al., 2008; Salvador-Carulla, Segui, Fernandez-Cano, & Canet, 1995; Sherbourne, Jackson, Meredith, Camp, & Wells, 1996).

Supplementary information about anxiety disorders can be found at:

- http://www.nimh.nih.gov/health/topics/anxiety-disorders/index.shtml

Pathophysiology: nervousness/tension, phobias, obsessions, compulsions causing impairment of function with unknown cause. The major current hypothesis includes the presence of neurotransmitter dysregulation in the limbic system.

Predisposition: genetics/familial predisposition; medications (e.g., caffeine, stimulants); medical illnesses (e.g., chest pain, irritable bowel); substance abuse and withdrawal; major trauma (PTSD).

Core Symptoms: nervousness/tension, anxiety (panic) attacks, phobias, obsessions, compulsions that persist and impair the individual's ability to function. Generalized anxiety and panic are the two most commonly seen and treated anxiety problems, though simple phobias have a higher prevalence. The Generalized Anxiety Disorder-7 (GAD-7), not considered a diagnostic tool, is now being used as a standard for symptom documentation and follow-up (Spitzer, Kroenke, Williams, & Lowe, 2006).

Complications: functional impairment, increased health care service use, poor medical illness outcomes, increased mortality from cardiovascular disease, higher rates of depression and suicide attempts, substance abuse.

Treatment for Anxiety: the following list includes the primary approaches to anxiety treatment with evidence of value for patients. Other interventions can be used as adjuncts to the treatments listed but are not considered primary treatments for those with anxiety disorders—supportive psychotherapy, crisis intervention, exercise, healthy diet, good sleep habits, healthy foods, acupuncture, massage, breathing into a paper bag. They can, however, be primary treatments for anxiety that is related to common life stresses.

- Anti-anxiety medications (higher doses of selective serotonin reuptake inhibitors [SSRIs] are usually needed for symptom control than those used for depression; benzodiazepines are less commonly used for treatment of chronic anxiety since they increase depressive symptoms [depression comorbidity] and are potentially addicting or habit forming)
- Cognitive behavioral therapy with exposure to phobic- and/or panic-producing stimuli (exposure is of significant importance, especially in those with panic-producing stimuli)
- Coping skills training and progressive relaxation
- Reversal of hyperventilation
- Avoidance of anxiety-producing substances (e.g., caffeine, stimulants, alcohol in excess or withdrawal from alcohol)

Intervention for Factors Associated With Anxiety

- Assistance with return to normal function (home, work, social, etc.)
- Coordination of anxiety treatment with medical illness treatment; special emphasis on adherence to all recommended interventions

Impact: higher health care service use, functional impairment, medical and psychiatric morbidity, and earlier medical mortality

SUMMARY OF CHRONIC OBSTRUCTIVE PULMONARY DISEASE

Chronic obstructive pulmonary disease (COPD; Peytremann-Bridevaux, Staeger, Bridevaux, Ghali, & Burnand, 2008; Wilper et al., 2008) is a disorder in which the walls of small air sacs in the lungs break down so that they lose their elasticity and oxygen exchange

capacity. COPD, also called emphysema and chronic bronchitis, affects 1 in 10 individuals between the ages for 18 and 64. Prevalence increases with age, though many younger patients will also have early stages of COPD without seeing a physician or receiving treatment. As the disease progresses, mucous forms in the damaged airways, putting patients with this condition at risk for pneumonia. COPD is of significant concern to case managers because those who become symptomatic with advancing illness are progressively disabled, require constant oxygen supplementation, and are often hospitalized with acute exacerbations of their condition.

Supplementary information on COPD can be found at:

- http://www.nhlbi.nih.gov/health/dci/Diseases/Copd/Copd_WhatIs.html
- http://www.mayoclinic.com/health/copd/DS00916

Pathophysiology: obstruction of airways due to mucous plugging; collapse of bronchi associated with alveolar airways damage and loss of elasticity

Predisposition: genetics (alpha 1 antitrypsin deficiency), cigarette smoke (primary and secondary), female gender

Major Subclasses: emphysema (primarily due to damage to the walls of the small air sacs, leading to less oxygen exchange surface area but little in the way of inflammation and mucous); chronic bronchitis (primarily due to chronic inflammation and irritation of the small lung passageways with mucous production, clogging of the air passages, and ultimately damage to the small air sacs). Both lead to inability to get enough oxygen into the blood.

Core Symptoms: shortness of breath (air hunger), wheezing, sputum production, and rapid heart rate.

Laboratory and Other Findings: spirometry (forced expiration volume in 1 second [FEV1]; peak expiratory flow rates [PEFRs]: mild disease if between 65% and 85% of predicted; moderate disease if 50% to 65% of predicted; severe if less than 50% of predicted); pulse oximetry (95% to 100%); chest X-ray (evidence of emphysema/chronic bronchitis).

Complications

- Respiratory insufficiency and failure
  - Preventive measures: stop smoking, influenza and pneumococcal vaccine, flu shots
  - Symptoms: inability to get breath without assistance
  - Treatment: refer to doctor/emergency room
- Damage to the heart due to low oxygen levels
  - Preventive measures: continuous oxygen replacement by nose or mouth at appropriate levels; monitoring pulse oximetry readings

- □ Symptoms: signs of heart failure
- □ Treatment: chronic oxygen, treatment of heart failure
- Pneumonia
  - □ Preventive measures: influenza and pneumococcal vaccine, warm clothing
  - □ Symptoms: fever, cough, sputum production, worsening shortness of breath
  - □ Treatment: antibiotics, antiviral agents
- Depression/anxiety
  - □ Preventive measures: monitoring for early symptoms using PHQ-9 and GAD-7 screening
  - □ Symptoms: symptoms of anxiety or depression
  - □ Treatment: medication and/or psychotherapy

Treatments: oxygen, reducing or stopping smoking or exposure to smoke/allergens; bronchodilators; steroids; respiratory therapy, antidepressants, adherence checks

Intervention for Factors Associated With COPD

- Assistance with obtaining appliances and home oxygen
- Review of allergen/smoke exposure and assistance with avoidance
- Smoking cessation help
- Development of a plan for early treatment when exacerbation is starting but before emergency room is needed

Impact: high health care service use, especially inpatient care; functional impairment; disability; medical morbidity; earlier medical mortality

SUMMARY OF PSYCHOTIC DISORDERS

Psychotic disorders are a group of serious illnesses that alter a person's ability to think clearly, make good judgments, respond emotionally, communicate effectively, understand reality, and behave appropriately. When symptoms are severe, people with psychotic disorders have difficulty staying in touch with reality and often are unable to meet the ordinary demands of daily life. However, even the most severe psychotic disorders are usually treatable. Included among these disorders are schizophrenia, brief psychotic episodes, severe affective disorders, delusional disorders, medication-induced psychosis, delirium, and other medical illness-related psychoses. The disorders are typified by hallucinations and delusions but also include behaviors that prevent people from interacting effectively with others (e.g., mania, catatonia).

The reason that these disorders are included in this chapter has less to do with the frequency with which they occur and more to do with the impact that they have on personal health and future problems, both physical and mental. While many of these patients can be symptomatically controlled with medications, they remain at high risk for:

- Continued intermittent psychiatric symptoms and complications
- Lack of adherence to treatment
- Poor outcomes of concurrent physical illness
- Side effects from their antipsychotic medications
- High service use
- Insurability challenges
- Functional impairment

Over half of all health care service use in patients with psychotic disorders is for general medical, not psychiatric, intervention. Morbidity and mortality are high.

Supplementary information on psychosis can be found at:

- http://www.nlm.nih.gov/medlineplus/psychoticdisorders.html
- http://www.webmd.com/schizophrenia/guide/mental-health-psychotic-disorders

Pathophysiology: major current hypotheses include imbalance of dopamine and neuronal and/or neurotransmitter abnormalities; idiopathic.

Predisposition: positive family history (small but definite contributor); substance abuse or use of medications known to cause psychotic symptoms (e.g., levodopa; corticosteroids; chronic marijuana use, especially in adolescents).

Symptoms: hallucinations; delusions; disorganized or incoherent speech; confused thinking; strange, possibly dangerous behavior; slowed or unusual movements; loss of interest in personal hygiene; loss of interest in activities; problems at school or work and with relationships; cold, detached manner with the inability to express emotion; mood swings or other mood symptoms, such as depression or mania.

Complications: persistent decline with some suicidality; other psychiatric disorders (e.g., depression, chemical dependence); side effects of medications (e.g., obesity, diabetes); emphasema; nonadherence to treatment of medical and mental conditions; nontreatment of concurrent medical conditions with complications

Treatment for Psychotic Symptoms: medication (necessary for virtually all); electroconvulsive therapy (ECT) (especially for mania and catatonia); supportive psychotherapy, cognitive behavioral therapy, and crisis intervention; close monitoring and follow-up; sometimes forced hospitalization and treatment is necessary.

Intervention for Factors Associated With Psychosis

- Monitor for adverse medication effects and medical illnesses
- Assist with social support connections
- Assist with getting medical care

- Try to prevent incarceration due to aberrant behaviors
- Ensure insurance support for antipsychotic and other medications, clinical care

Impact: high medical and psychiatric health care service use, especially when symptoms persist and/or the illness progresses despite treatment; functional and economic impairment; medical morbidity; premature death by 15 to 25 years; increased criminal arrest risk.

SUMMARY OF CHRONIC KIDNEY DISEASE

The kidneys filter waste products from the blood, maintain salt and water balance, and perform a number of homeostatic bodily functions through the endocrine system. While all functions are important, it is the first two that create the greatest challenge when kidney reserves fail and dialysis is either being considered or is already being used. At or around the time that a patient's creatinine clearance level reaches 30% of normal, it becomes predictable when total kidney function failure can be expected to lead to hemodialysis, peritoneal dialysis, organ transplantation, or death.

In many patients, kidney disease is one of several organ system problems for which care is needed. Further, kidney failure necessarily ties the patient to a complicated medical procedure either performed at home or in a dialysis center. If, alternatively, the patient has a kidney transplant, then he or she requires close follow-up to catch and reverse rejection episodes. Transplant patients also must be watched for infection since the immunosuppressive drugs administered after the transplant can compromise the body's infection-fighting capabilities. In short, patients with chronic renal disease can be very complex and have challenging lifestyles.

Supplementary information on kidney disease can be found at:

- http://kidney.niddk.nih.gov/
- http://www.nlm.nih.gov/medlineplus/kidneydiseases.html

Pathophysiology: impairment of kidney filtering capacity from any cause (e.g., diabetes, chronic hypertension, polycystic kidneys, medication abuse/overuse, primary kidney disease).

Predisposition: genetics; many illnesses (e.g., diabetes, rheumatic fever, hypertension, long-term analgesic use, other).

Major Subclasses: Alport syndrome (genetic), analgesic nephropathy, glomerulonephritis of any type (one of the most common causes), kidney stones and infection, obstructive uropathy, polycystic kidney disease (genetic), reflux nephropathy.

Core Signs and Symptoms: poor appetite, nausea and vomiting, tiredness, fluid retention (swollen ankles or shortness of breath), itching, cramps, restless legs, hypertension, sallow appearance, anemia, electrolyte disturbances.

Laboratory and Other Findings: renal function tests (creatinine, blood urea nitrogen [BUN], creatinine clearance)

Complications (Other Than Renal Diet and Fluid Control)

- Hypertension
  - Preventive measures: monitoring blood pressure
  - Symptoms: none
  - Treatment: antihypertensive medications, salt restriction
- Pericarditis
  - Preventive measures: monitoring for symptoms on chest examinations
  - Symptoms: exercise intolerance
  - Treatment: diet, drainage
- Anemia
  - Preventive measures: monitoring blood counts
  - Symptoms: fatigue
  - Treatment: medication, transfusion (rare)
- Depression/anxiety
  - Preventive measures: monitoring for early symptoms using PHQ-9 and GAD-7 screening
  - Symptoms: symptoms of anxiety or depression
  - Treatment: medication or psychotherapy
- Bone disease
  - Preventive measures: monitoring calcium and parathyroid hormone levels, bone density measures
  - Symptoms: aches and pains in bones
  - Treatment: medication, diet
- Dialysis and transplantation
  - Case managers need to read about problems related to these treatments

Treatments: treat underlying kidney disease cause, such as diabetes and hypertension; renal failure diet; fluid balance; ACE inhibitors; dialysis; transplantation; antidepressants.

Intervention for Factors Associated With Kidney Disease/Failure

- Assist with social support connections/equipment needs for at home or center dialysis
- Lifestyle adjustments to functional needs

Impact: high health care service use; lifelong dialysis or renal transplantation sequelae; functional impairment and disability; medical morbidity; earlier medical mortality.

SUMMARY OF ALCOHOL ABUSE AND DEPENDENCE

During the last decade, there have been many advances in the way that assistance can be brought to those at risk for or those currently experiencing alcohol abuse and dependence (Anton et al., 2006; Kane et al., 2004; Mundt, French, Roebuck, Manwell, & Barry, 2005; Parthasarathy, Mertens, Moore, & Weisner, 2003). For those case managers who work with populations in which other forms of substance use disorders are common, they should take time to learn about assistance to those individuals as well.

Supplementary information on alcohol abuse and dependence can be found at:

- http://www.nlm.nih.gov/medlineplus/alcohol.html
- http://www.niaaa.nih.gov/FAQs/General-English/default.htm

At these educational/informational Web sites, case managers will come to realize that alcohol abuse and dependence are being viewed differently than in years past. It used to be that the target for treatment was almost exclusively directed to patients with end-stage alcohol-related problems. Current recommendations include strategies for early intervention.

Pathophysiology: change in alcohol metabolism and physiologic response to alcohol.

Predisposition: genetics; familial; environmental; selected psychiatric illnesses (e.g., depression, antisocial personality disorder, anxiety).

Signs and Symptoms

- *At-risk drinking*: for females < 65 years old, more than 3 drinks per day or 7 drinks per week; for males < 65 years old, more than 4 drinks per day and 14 drinks per week
- *Alcohol abuse*: during the last 12 months repeatedly at risk of bodily harm (auto accidents), relationship trouble, role failure, or run-ins with the law due to at-risk drinking
- *Alcohol dependence*: three or more in the last 12 months of
  - ☐ Not being able to stick to drinking limits
  - ☐ Not been able to cut down or stop
  - ☐ Shown tolerance
  - ☐ Shown signs of withdrawal
  - ☐ Kept drinking despite problems
  - ☐ Spent a lot of time drinking
  - ☐ Spent less time on other matters

Complications From Alcohol Abuse and Dependence: physical illnesses (alcohol-related and failure to adhere to treatment of existing medical conditions); auto accidents and other trauma; worsening of other existing psychiatric conditions (e.g., depression); personal, social, and economic loss.

Prevention: screening and brief intervention (**Exhibit 6.1**) was specifically designed for the 10% to 16% of patients with at-risk drinking before they become part of the 4% to 8% who develop abuse and/or dependence.

Treatment of Alcohol Abuse: screening and brief intervention in primary care setting (for at-risk drinking); medical management of intoxication/withdrawal; discuss group support, such as alcoholics anonymous (AA); treat associated psychiatric illness (e.g., depression, anxiety).

Treatment of Alcohol Dependence: support efforts to cut down and/or abstain (substance use disorder treatment programs); pharmacologic (e.g., naltrexone, acamprosate, topiramate); treatment of concurrent psychiatric illness (e.g., depression, anxiety).

Conceptualization: when addressing the needs of patients with alcohol abuse problems, liken their abuse to abuse of cigarettes in a lung cancer patient or food in an obese diabetic with complications (i.e., take the need for health care assistance at face value and provide it). It is not necessary to condone the alcohol abuse/dependence, but it is necessary to include

---

EXHIBIT 6.1   Screening and Brief Intervention for At-Risk Drinking and Alcohol Abuse

- Two primary care physicians visits 1 month apart; extra support calls after each physician visit for those with alcohol abuse
- Intervention
  - ○ Discuss the fact that a potential drinking problem exists
  - ○ Review prevalence of drinking and willingness to consider change
  - ○ If the answer is "yes to change," set up goals; if the answer is "no to change," follow and revisit
  - ○ Workbook on healthy behaviors and adverse effects of alcohol
  - ○ Goal review and adjustment at follow-up
  - ○ Review need for visit with addiction specialist

treatment of the abuse/dependence as a part of treatment for its medical complications, just like helping a smoker with chronic lung disease stop smoking and an obese patient with coronary artery disease control weight. Regardless of the primary cause of illness or complications, both the physical health conditions and the alcohol abuse/dependence require attention. Further, treatment of the patient should often involve participation by the patient's family.

Intervention for Factors Associated With Alcohol Abuse/Dependence

- Search for and treat medical complications
- Provide family support/treatment for impact on family functioning
- Work with employee assistance programs to facilitate sobriety maintenance and persistent employment
- Adjust social environment (e.g., help patient remove him or herself from a substance abuse culture)

Impact: higher health care service use, especially when concurrent medical or psychiatric illness present; functional impairment; medical morbidity; earlier mortality (little documented effect of at-risk drinking on health care service use but progression leads to significant problems).

SUMMARY OF UNEXPLAINED SOMATIC COMPLAINTS

Eighty-five percent of the most common patient complaints in the medical setting have no objective relationship to a medical condition (Kroenke & Mangelsdorff, 1989). These unexplained symptoms fall into the category of somatoform disorders in the psychiatric nomenclature. The vast majority of these resolve without complication and typically do not resurface. In 1% to 2% of patients with unexplained somatic complaints, however, they come to the attention of case managers (i.e., those patients with frequent, pervasive, recurrent, and high cost complaints). These individuals are at significant risk for diagnostic test and/or treatment-related (iatrogenic) illness (e.g., adverse drug reactions, medication dependence, cancer resulting from excess X-ray testing, or for inappropriate consumption of very high levels of costly medical services and medications without health benefit; Rost, Kashner, & Smith, 1994; Smith, Monson, & Ray, 1986). With these patients, case managers become involved and thus should have a general understanding about what constitutes excessive unexplained somatic complaints, also called somatization disorder (Kroenke & Rosmalen, 2006), and how such patients can be conservatively treated by their doctors at reasonable cost and without intervention-related complications.

Supplementary information on unexplained somatic complaints can be found at:

- http://emedicine.medscape.com/article/918628-overview
- http://www.nlm.nih.gov/medlineplus/ency/article/000955.htm

Pathophysiology: idiopathic

Predisposition: hypersuggestibility (pithiatism); illness preoccupation (health anxiety); untreated or ineffectively treated mental health condition (e.g., depression, anxiety)

Symptoms: focused or multifocal protean symptoms and complaints leading to multiple visits to general or specialty medical physicians, numerous tests and medications, and repeated escalating procedures, including surgeries

Complications: adverse medication reactions, complications from tests and procedures, prescribed medication dependence

Treatment for Unexplained Somatic Symptoms: tests, procedures, medications, and consultations only when objective findings on examination can be documented; single primary physician follows patient; cognitive behavioral therapy with symptom reframing (Fink, Rosendal, & Toft, 2002); letter to general medical physician about conservative intervention by psychiatry consultant (Fink et al., 2002; Rost et al., 1994; Smith et al., 1986); reassurance by primary care physicians (**Exhibit 6.2**; Kathol, 1997).

Intervention for Factors Associated With Unexplained Somatic Symptoms

- Treat mental health condition if present (about 50% of patients)
- Assistance with return to employment
- Work with practitioner to help limit the number of medications, tests, and consultations
- Open communication among practitioners
- Send educational material to treating physicians about unexplained somatic complaints (Kroenke, 2007)

Impact: high incidence of iatrogenic illness with associated morbidity and cost; high and unnecessary medical expenditures; disability and impaired function; job loss and health-related financial stress.

SUMMARY OF ATTENTION DEFICIT AND HYPERACTIVITY DISORDER

Attention deficit hyperactivity disorder (ADHD) is a neurobehavioral disorder typified by difficulty staying focused and paying attention, difficulty controlling behavior, and hyperactivity (overactivity).

EXHIBIT 6.2   **Critical Steps for Primary Care Professionals in Reassurance Therapy**

1. Question and examine the patient (a real examination)
2. Acknowledge presence of symptom(s); empathize but be forward thinking (i.e., live with/through the symptom)
3. Assure the patient that serious medical illness in not causing symptom(s) (e.g., "It is not cancer")
4. Specifically suggest that symptom(s) will resolve (give time frame for improvement)
5. Help the patient to return to normal activity; confirm it will not hurt him or her
6. Consider nonspecific treatment; give the patient an excuse to get better
7. Follow the patient; confirm improvement and that nothing is missed

From "Reassurance Therapy: What to Say to Symptomatic Patients With Benign or Non-Existent Medical Disease," by R. G. Kathol, 1997, *International Journal of Psychiatry in Medicine, 27(2)*, p. 175. Copyright ©1997 by Roger Kathol.

About 3% to 5% of children are affected. Several types of ADHD have been described, including a predominantly inattentive subtype (attention deficit disorder—ADD), a predominantly hyperactive-impulsive subtype, and a combination of the two (the most common, ADHD). ADHD has its onset in childhood, but can continue into teen years and even adulthood.

This is the most common mental health issue that pediatricians face in a typical practice. Since there are a limited number of child psychiatrists and restricted payment for child psychologists and child psychiatrists in the medical setting, many children with this condition do not have access to specialty mental health services despite ADHD's prevalence. As a result, many children/youth with this disorder are treated with medication (e.g., psychostimulants), with little input by mental health professionals. No one knows whether children/youth are being overmedicated or undermedicated by pediatricians who have limited background and understanding about how to evaluate for the presence of ADHD, how to implement treatment, and how to follow progress.

Supplementary information on ADHD can be found at:

- http://www.nimh.nih.gov/health/publications/attention-deficit-hyperactivity-disorder/complete-index.shtml
- http://www.webmd.com/add-adhd/default.htm

Pathophysiology: genetics; presumed neurotransmitter imbalance.

Predisposition: low birth weight; head injury; childhood toxic exposures (e.g., lead).

Symptoms: inattention, hyperactivity, impulsivity, commonly associated with oppositional defiant disorder (ODD—tantrums, arguing, and angry or disruptive behaviors toward authority figures).

Complications: poor school performance, truancy, social isolation; parent-child conflict; more trouble with mental health and substance use problems as youth and adults; increased rates of criminal behavior in adulthood.

Treatment for Attention Deficit Hyperactivity Disorder

- Medications—stimulants (e.g., methylphenidate, amphetamine, atomoxetine, bupropion and other antidepressants as secondary interventions)
- Psychotherapy—behaviorally oriented parent training: long-term use of goal setting and rewards and consequences (no data or poor response to other forms of psychotherapy)

Intervention for Factors Associated With ADHD

- Support to parents and teachers

Impact: trouble at school; poor school performance; difficulty in developing peer relationships; disciplinary difficulties; parents miss work to assist child (job loss and/or difficulties).

SUMMARY OF ASTHMA

Asthma is a chronic lung disease that inflames and narrows the airways. It typically starts in childhood with about a third of those experiencing asthma symptoms being children. Also called "reactive airway disease," it is exacerbated when an asthmatic is exposed to various precipitants, such as allergens, especially cats, but also molds, dusts, smoke, perfumes, industrial chemicals, and the like; exercise; or cold weather. While there are currently very effective treatments for asthma, it remains a significant health problem resulting in millions of emergency room visits annually in the United States alone.

Bronchospasm (narrowing of the bronchial tubes) is caused by the inflammation of the muscles surrounding the air passageways. The inflammation makes the airways smaller and therefore makes it more difficult for air to move in and out of the lung. In some cases, breathing may be so labored that an asthma attack becomes life-threatening.

Supplementary information on asthma can be found at:

- http://www.lungusa.org/lung-disease/asthma/
- http://www.webmd.com/asthma/default.htm

Pathophysiology: immune hypersensitivity to triggers causing bronchospasm and airway closure.

Predisposition: genetics; reactive airways early in life; obesity.

Symptoms: shortness of breath, wheezing, tight chest, coughing (especially at night).

Complications: airway remodeling due to long-term inflammation; status asthmaticus (nonresponsive bouts of asthma, which are potentially life threatening); short stature; hospitalization and death.

Treatment for Asthma

- Avoid triggers
- Medications: anti-inflammatory agents, steroids, inhalers (bronchodilators, steroids, cromolyn, other), antibiotics, oxygen, fluids

Intervention for Factors Associated With Asthma

- Treatment of concurrent mental health problems, such as depression or anxiety

Impact: death in 2 of 10,000 annually; hospitalization in 3 of 100 annually

CLOSING COMMENTS

In this chapter, five mental health and five general medical conditions were reviewed to illustrate basic information that would help an integrated case manager to effectively assist patients experiencing these conditions. The depth of information is sufficient to allow a case manager to have a general idea about whether the patient's current exposure to clinical care would be likely to lead to outcome improvement. Importantly, a good case manager would not stop at the level of information described in the preceding sections if additional information was necessary to stabilize a patient's health. When needed, case managers would tap case management colleagues, their supervisor, or the supervising physician for expanded information about a topic and suggestions about assistance measures that may be useful.

REFERENCES

Anton, R. F., O'Malley, S. S., Ciraulo, D. A., Cisler, R. A., Couper, D., Donovan, D. M., et al. (2006). Combined pharmacotherapies and behavioral interventions for alcohol dependence: The COMBINE study: A randomized controlled trial. *Journal of the American Medical Association, 295*(17), 2003–2017.

Centers for Disease Control and Prevention. Retrieved April 21, 2010 from http://www.cdc.gov/diabetes/statistics/prev/national/figraceethsex.htm.

Ciechanowski, P. S., Katon, W. J., & Russo, J. E. (2000). Depression and diabetes: Impact of depressive symptoms on adherence, function, and costs. *Archives Internal Medicine, 160*(21), 3278–3285.

Ciechanowski, P. S., Katon, W. J., Russo, J. E., & Hirsch, I. B. (2003). The relationship of depressive symptoms to symptom reporting, self-care and glucose control in diabetes. *General Hospital Psychiatry, 25*(4), 246–252.

Druss, B. G., Rosenheck, R. A., & Sledge, W. H. (2000). Health and disability costs of depressive illness in a major U.S. corporation. *American Journal Psychiatry, 157*(8), 1274–1278.

Egede, L. E. (2006). Disease-focused or integrated treatment: Diabetes and depression. *Medical Clinics North America, 90*(4), 627–646.

Fink, P., Rosendal, M., & Toft, T. (2002). Assessment and treatment of functional disorders in general practice: The extended reattribution and management model—an advanced educational program for nonpsychiatric doctors. *Psychosomatics, 43*(2), 93–131.

Hunkeler, E. M., Katon, W., Tang, L., Williams, J. W., Jr., Kroenke, K., Lin, E. H., et al. (2006). Long term outcomes from the IMPACT randomised trial for depressed elderly patients in primary care. *British Medical Journal, 332*(7536), 259–263.

Kane, R. L., Wall, M., Potthoff, S., Stromberg, K., Dai, Y., & Meyer, Z. J. (2004). The effect of alcoholism treatment on medical care use. *Medical Care, 42*(4), 395–402.

Kathol, R. G. (1997). Reassurance therapy: What to say to symptomatic patients with benign or non-existent medical disease. *International Journal Psychiatry Medicine, 27*(2), 173–180.

Katon, W., Russo, J., Sherbourne, C., Stein M. B., Craske, M., Fan, M. Y., et al. (2006). Incremental cost-effectiveness of a collaborative care intervention for panic disorder. *Psychological Medicine, 1*–11.

Katon, W., Unutzer, J., Fan, M. Y., Williams, J. W., Jr., Schoenbaum, M., Lin, E. H., et al. (2006). Cost-effectiveness and net benefit of enhanced treatment of depression for older adults with diabetes and depression. *Diabetes Care, 29*(2), 265–270.

Kessler, R. C., Berglund, P., Demler, O., Jin, R., Koretz, D., Merikangas, K. R., et al. (2003). The epidemiology of major depressive disorder: Results from the National Comorbidity Survey Replication (NCS-R). *Journal of the American Medical Association, 289*(23), 3095–3105.

Kroenke, K. (2007). Efficacy of treatment for somatoform disorders: a review of randomized controlled trials. *Psychosomatic Medicine, 69*(9), 881–888.

Kroenke, K., & Mangelsdorff, A. D. (1989). Common symptoms in ambulatory care: Incidence, evaluation, therapy, and outcome. *American Journal Medicine, 86*(3), 262–266.

Kroenke, K., & Rosmalen, J. G. (2006). Symptoms, syndromes, and the value of psychiatric diagnostics in patients who have functional somatic disorders. *Medical Clinics North America, 90*(4), 603–626.

Lowe, B., Unutzer, J., Callahan, C. M., Perkins, A. J., & Kroenke, K. (2004). Monitoring depression treatment outcomes with the patient health questionnaire-9. *Medical Care, 42*(12), 1194–1201.

Mundt, M. P., French, M. T., Roebuck, M. C., Manwell, L. B., & Barry, K. L. (2005). Brief physician advice for problem drinking among older adults: An economic analysis of costs and benefits. *Journal Studies Alcohol, 66*(3), 389–394.

Parthasarathy, S., Mertens, J., Moore, C., & Weisner, C. (2003). Utilization and cost impact of integrating substance abuse treatment and primary care. *Medical Care, 41*(3), 357–367.

Peytremann-Bridevaux, I., Staeger, P., Bridevaux, P. O., Ghali, W. A., & Burnand, B. (2008). Effectiveness of chronic obstructive pulmonary disease-management programs: Systematic review and meta-analysis. *American Journal Medicine, 121*(5), 433–443.

Rost, K., Kashner, T. M., & Smith, R. G., Jr. (1994). Effectiveness of psychiatric intervention with somatization disorder patients: Improved outcomes at reduced costs. *General Hospital Psychiatry, 16*(6), 381–387.

Roy-Byrne, P., Stein, M. B., Russo, J., Craske, M., Katon, W., Sullivan, G., et al. (2005). Medical illness and response to treatment in primary care panic disorder. *General Hospital Psychiatry, 27*(4), 237–243.

Roy-Byrne, P. P., Davidson, K. W., Kessler, R. C., Asmundson, G. J., Goodwin, R. D., Kubzansky, L., et al. (2008). Anxiety disorders and comorbid medical illness. *General Hospital Psychiatry, 30*(3), 208–225.

Salvador-Carulla, L., Segui, J., Fernandez-Cano, P., & Canet, J. (1995). Costs and offset effect in panic disorders. *British Journal Psychiatry Suppl*(27), 23–28.

Sherbourne, C. D., Jackson, C. A., Meredith, L. S., Camp, P., & Wells, K. B. (1996). Prevalence of comorbid anxiety disorders in primary care outpatients. *Archives Family Medicine, 5*(1), 27–34; discussion 35.

Smith, G. R., Jr., Monson, R. A., & Ray, D. C. (1986). Psychiatric consultation in somatization disorder. A randomized controlled study. *New England Journal Medicine, 314*(22), 1407–1413.

Spitzer, R. L., Kroenke, K., Williams, J. B., & Lowe, B. (2006). A brief measure for assessing generalized anxiety disorder: The GAD-7. *Archives Internal Medicine, 166*(10), 1092–1097.

Stewart, W. F., Ricci, J. A., Chee, E., Hahn, S. R., & Morganstein, D. (2003). Cost of lost productive work time among US workers with depression. *Journal of the American Medical Association, 289*(23), 3135–3144.

Von Korff, M., & Goldberg, D. (2001). Improving outcomes in depression. *British Medical Journal, 323*(7319), 948–949.

Wilper, A. P., Woolhandler, S., Lasser, K. E., McCormick, D., Bor, D. H., & Himmelstein, D. U. (2008). A national study of chronic disease prevalence and access to care in uninsured U.S. adults. *Annals Internal Medicine, 149*(3), 170–176.

CHAPTER 7

Adult Integrated Case Management Using INTERMED-Complexity Assessment Grid Methodology

- To provide an overview of the INTERMED-Complexity Assessment Grid (IM-CAG) and its administration in adult integrated case management programs
- To describe anchor point scoring for each item in the IM-CAG
- To connect case manager actions with IM-CAG anchor point scores for each item
- To delineate barriers to improvement uncovered by each IM-CAG item, the goals for health change related to them, and how success is measured and documented

BASICS OF THE ADULT INTERMED-COMPLEXITY ASSESSMENT GRID

The adult INTERMED-Complexity Assessment Grid (IM-CAG), adapted from the European version (see Appendix 15; Stiefel et al., 2006), is at the heart of this manual because it is a method through which illness and life situation (health) complexity can be codified, documented, quantified, and acted upon (**Table 7.1**, see page i2 for color version; also see Appendixes 4, 6, 8). In this chapter, the student will systematically review anchor point scoring and potential actionable steps for each cell score in each domain. The chapter will clarify the barriers to improvement addressed by each item, the goals desired when barriers for an item are identified, and the success metrics that can be used to document that the barrier has been addressed by the patient-case manager team and whether improvement has occurred.

This chapter and Chapter 9 are the chapters of the manual on which readers performing only adult case management should devote considerable time since they will allow consistent scoring of IM-CAG items from case manager to case manager, connect problems with actions, lead to efficient use of case manager time, and improve outcomes for patients assisted through the integrated case management process. They form the basis for care plan development and working with patients through health-related barrier resolution, stabilization of health, and case graduation.

HEALTH COMPLEXITY ASSESSMENT USING THE IM-CAG

As discussed in Chapter 2 (see the section "Health Complexity"), individualized care is the approach used by case managers to help patients with health complexity as they bring their illnesses back under control. Whenever an item in the IM-CAG is scored, in addition to the clinical anchor points for each cell, as defined in this chapter, the case manager should keep the following question in mind: "Will the situation recorded for this cell interfere with clinical outcomes if standard medical care is given?" Another important consideration, particularly when there is debate between two anchor point levels for an individual item (e.g., scoring a 0 vs. a 1 or a 2 vs. a 3), is to consider the immediacy of need for action on behalf of the patient. The time frame for action can inform the final decision.

Each of the domains is subdivided into two historical content cells, two current content cells, and one vulnerability cell. By dividing the domains in this way, it is possible for the case manager to develop an appreciation for and a perspective about how the patient's prior life experiences relate to his or her present clinical and personal situation and to anticipated vulnerabilities.

For consistency in scoring, all historical complexity items refer to the last 5 years. The two exceptions are the cells labeled "Mental Health History" and "Access to Care." Mental Health History (HP2) relates to the patient's entire life, and Access to Care (HHS1) relates to the last 6 months. All current complexity items

TABLE 7.1   INTERMED-Complexity Assessment Grid Scoring Sheet

Date	HEALTH RISKS AND HEALTH NEEDS					
Name	**HISTORICAL**		**CURRENT STATE**		**VULNERABILITY**	
Total Score =	Complexity Item	Score	Complexity Item	Score	Complexity Item	Score
Biological Domain	Chronicity **HB1**		Symptom Severity/Impairment **CB1**		Complications and Life Threat **VB**	
	Diagnostic Dilemma **HB2**		Diagnostic/Therapeutic Challenge **CB2**			
Psychological Domain	Barriers to Coping **HP1**		Resistance to Treatment **CP1**		Mental Health Threat **VP**	
	Mental Health History **HP2**		Mental Health Symptoms **CP2**			
Social Domain	Job and Leisure **HS1**		Residential Stability **CS1**		Social Vulnerability **VS**	
	Relationships **HS2**		Social Support **CS2**			
Health System Domain	Access to Care **HHS1**		Getting Needed Services **CHS1**		Health System Impediments **VHS**	
	Treatment Experience **HHS2**		Coordination of Care **CHS2**			

Comments

(Enter pertinent information about the reason for the score of each complexity item here. For example, poor patient adherence, death in family with stress to patient, non-evidence-based treatment of migraine, etc.)

Scoring System

Green	0	= no vulnerability or need to act
Yellow	1	= mild vulnerability and need for monitoring or prevention
Orange	2	= moderate vulnerability and need for action or development of intervention plan
Red	3	= severe vulnerability and need for immediate action or immediate intervention plan

Biological Domain Items		**Psychological Domain Items**	
HB1	*Physical illness chronicity*	HP1	*Problems handling stress and/or problem solving*
HB2	*Historic problems in diagnosing the physical illness*	HP2	*Prior mental condition difficulties*
CB1	*Physical illness symptom severity and impairment*	CP1	*Resistance to treatment; nonadherence*
CB2	*Current difficulties in diagnosis and/or treatment*	CP2	*Current mental condition symptom severity*
VB	*Risk of physical complications and life threat if case management is stopped*	VP	*Risk of persistent personal barriers or poor mental condition care if case management is stopped*
Social Domain Items		**Health System Domain Items**	
HS1	*Personal productivity and leisure activities*	HHS1	*Health system-related access to appropriate care*
HS2	*Relationship difficulties*	HHS2	*Experiences with doctors or the health system*
CS1	*Residential stability or suitability*	CHS1	*Logistical ability to get needed care at service delivery level*
CS2	*Availability of social support*	CHS2	*Communication among providers and coordination of care*
VS	*Risk of work, home, and relational support needs if case management is stopped*	VHS	*Risk of persistent poor access to and/or coordination of services if case management is stopped*

This scoring sheet is an example of what is used for adult patients. In practice, it is often easier to use the acronym IM-CAG instead of the full, more explanatory name as it is discussed. Scoring usually is completed using documentation software.

refer to the 30-day period prior to the date that the IM-CAG assessment is completed. All vulnerability complexity items refer to the 3- to 6-month period after the date that the IM-CAG assessment is completed.

The IM-CAG assesses health complexity using a four-point Likert-type scoring system. Unlike other Likert scales, however, each item score on the IM-CAG suggests actions to be taken by the case manager working on behalf of the patient or by the patient on his or her own behalf within a time frame (Appendix 8). A score of 0 (green) indicates that the patient needs no assistance in the item content area. A score of 1 (yellow) suggests that observation and/or prevention is needed; 2 (orange) indicates the need to do something soon (i.e., intervention/plan development); and 3 (red) indicates that an immediate intervention/plan is required. (In the manual text, grayscale scoring progresses from lightest [0] to darkest [3].) To the extent possible, activities by the case manager and the patient should be a part of a patient-manager developed care plan with goals and objectives.

While each item in the IM-CAG will generate an individual score and have an associated set of actions, of equal and perhaps greater importance is that the items themselves are often linked to each other. As readers will come to realize, the IM-CAG does more than just identify and address each item that creates barriers to improvement. It also helps case managers connect barriers and to develop plans to counteract those barriers as a unit. In fact, it is the integration of items and scores that will become the most important component of the IM-CAG approach used by the case manager-patient unit to quickly and effectively return the patient to health and productivity.

For instance, the case manager may be working with an employee of an appliance assembly plant who is being treated for back pain. During the IM-CAG evaluation, the patient is also found to have depression, which is often seen in patients with back pain. Obviously, it would be important to concurrently document adherence to treatment for both depression and the back pain. The IM-CAG allows the connection and resulting action. Use of the IM-CAG also allows assessment of social issues (e.g., work-related disability) that could have a bearing on improvement. In fact, discussion with the patient, using IM-CAG methodology, may reveal that there are performance problems or conflicts at work decreasing the incentive for the patient to get better. Thus, work-related intervention would take an equal place with depression and back pain treatment as addressing three linked barriers to improvement in the care plan. This will be covered in greater detail after each domain and item is better understood.

All care plans include education of the patient and, when appropriate, significant others about the patient's illnesses, the interaction of illnesses, and the treatments. Often the case manager will provide information about diseases or help the patient formulate questions for their physicians, who will serve as the primary arbiter of information and treatment. As discussed in Chapter 4 (see the section "Motivational Interviewing: A Patient-Centered Process"), this case management educational role should always be approached through discussion, rather than a didactic format, so that the patient can internalize the message and connect it to a rationale and desire to change.

In the context of IM-CAG use, case managers support approaches to care that are likely to improve outcomes, breakdown barriers, and assist with health system navigation. In essence, they serve as coaches and direction finders for patients with health complexity. They must, therefore, have knowledge about the patients' conditions, as reviewed in Chapter 6 (see the "Introduction" section), to have an appreciation about whether the interventions patients are receiving are likely to lead to symptom control and potential resolution. Focus is not just on the type of treatment that the patients are getting but also on important factors that affect treatment response, such as having questions answered by their practitioners, the frequency of visits to their doctors, the coordination of care by different practitioners, the ability to pay out-of-pocket expenses for medications, and so forth.

Since clinicians are the focal point of effective treatment, it is important for case managers to form alliances with the patient's treatment team as they work with a patient. This can be facilitated by sending a flier to practitioners (Appendix C, www.springerpub.com/kathol) on case management and the role it can play in assisting them with complex patient care and a letter stating that their patient has been entered into a case management program (Appendix D, www.springer pub.com/kathol). In the correspondence, the patient's clinicians should learn that the case manager:

1. Is not treating his or her patient but is assisting the patient in adhering to the clinician's treatment suggestions,
2. Works with his or her patient on both clinical and nonclinical barriers to improvement,
3. Will be involved with the patient for only a limited duration (i.e., during health stabilization), and
4. Wishes to collaborate and communicate with the clinician in achieving the greatest benefit for the patient.

It is also helpful to send updates of case manager-patient activities and to seek suggestions about how the case manager can help the patient's care team get better results. A scored IM-CAG grid and the notes summary are ideal and automatic communication tools to facilitate this through the CMSA software capability.

Many of the cells on the IM-CAG are associated with barriers to treatment adherence. Though stubborn unwillingness to be treated (CP1) could be the reason for nonadherence, it is by no means the only, nor necessarily the main, reason. Other examples include, but are not limited to, insufficient funds to pay for treatment, memory deficits, language barriers, contrary advice from family members, and cultural factors (**Exhibit 7.1**). Since nonadherence is clearly associated with worse clinical outcomes (Katon, Cantrell, Sokol, Chiao, & Gdovin, 2005; Sokol, McGuigan, Verbrugge, & Epstein, 2005), the case manager and patient should work together collaboratively to reverse barriers to treatment adherence identified within and across domains.

IM-CAG DOMAINS

Each domain in the IM-CAG has five items: two historical, two current, and one vulnerability. These correspond to recognized barriers to improvement for which specific actions can be taken. In order for them to be used consistently and effectively, it is necessary for case managers utilizing IM-CAG methodology to learn how to apply the standardized anchor points associated with each item and the potential actions that case managers could take in association to each score. Understanding the anchor points occurs through studying this manual. The actions listed in the exhibits in this chapter are intended only to provide illustrations to case managers about what could be considered when items are scored at specific levels. When other actions would be appropriate related to individual item scores in given patients, they should be included in care plan development.

Face-to-face training through the Case Management Society of America (CMSA) or in an established, university-based academic program after the completion of manual-based knowledge acquisition ensures proper application of anchor point scores through the use of relationship-building, scripted, open-ended questions. Finally, actual use of the questions and then scoring cells in the IM-CAG during supervised mock interviews solidifies the connection of anchor points to actions and linkages among actions.

BIOLOGICAL DOMAIN

Cells in the biological domain address how the patient's physical illness duration and severity, diagnostic/therapeutic complexity, and the interaction of illnesses create barriers to improvement. The biological domain is composed of: (a) chronicity (HB1), (b) diagnostic dilemma (HB2), (c) symptom severity/impairment (CB1), (d) diagnostic/therapeutic challenge (CB2), and (e) complications and life threat (VB). Each of these constitutes independent yet interacting physical complexity items that affect health.

The ultimate goal associated with the biological complexity items is to help patients understand and

EXHIBIT 7.1 Barriers to Treatment Adherence

- **Language,** for example, Spanish speaking only
- **Culture,** for example, resistance to medication
- **Religion,** for example, Scientologist's hostility toward psychiatric treatment
- **Health and treatment orientation,** for example, nonbelief in the allopathic approach to care (Western medicine)
- **Education,** for example, does not read or does not understand about his or her illness (health literacy)
- **Cognitive impairment,** for example, impairment secondary to medical or behavioral illness
- **Technology,** for example, no telephone
- **Geography,** for example, no transportation, remote living
- **Coverage issues,** for example, benefit exclusions
- **Dependency issues,** for example, caregiver/guardian refusal
- **Provider,** for example, no providers in patient's location or needed specialist availability
- **Parental consent,** for example, parent does not agree with treatment approach
- **Finances,** for example, no money for copayments
- **Lack of interest in change,** for example, disability-related disincentive
- **Social,** for example, protective resistant husband, family sees no need
- **Psychological,** for example, active paranoia about health care system
- **Stigma of having a mental illness and seeking treatment,** for example, job in jeopardy
- **Prior adverse health care experience,** for example, having been told "It's all in your head"
- **Denial of illness,** for example, personal view of just having a tough time rather than depression

overcome obstacles related to their general medical conditions that interfere with health stability. Resolution of illnesses is not central to integrated case management work processes since many patients with health complexity have chronic, noncurable conditions. Rather, the goal is to assist patients with achieving maximum control of their physical illnesses so that they can stabilize health, regain function, and decrease their total cost of their care.

Most patients with IM-CAG scores high enough to warrant case management will have more than one illness. In many patients, physical illness will also be mixed with psychological problems and/or somatization (Kroenke, 2007). Thus, sorting out which illness is associated with which symptom, in itself, can create a diagnostic and therapeutic challenge. For instance, depression is associated with symptoms of fatigue, weight loss, low energy, and sleep disturbance, and it can magnify other physical complaints, such as headaches, back pain, and so forth. By rights, these symptoms should show up in scores for psychological items—that is, mental health history (HP2), mental health symptoms (CP2). However, they can create scoring confusion since, taken at face value by a primary care or specialty medical clinician, they could

contribute to biological items, raising scores for diagnostic dilemma (HB2) and diagnostic/therapeutic challenge (CB2). This will be covered in greater detail in the Chapter 9 section "Biological Domain."

Complexity item: Chronicity (**Exhibit 7.2** and **Exhibit 7.3**).

Barriers to improvement. Old understanding of illnesses and treatments, burnout, frustration with lack of control, complicated needs.

Goals. Sufficient understanding of illnesses to participate in treatments; control of frustration with motivation to participate in care; identified outcome targets and a method to achieve them; communication among providers and coordination of services.

Success metrics. Patient understands illnesses and participates in treatments; patient personally engages in illness stabilization.

Complexity item: Diagnostic dilemma (**Exhibit 7.4** and **Exhibit 7.5**).

Barriers to improvement. Poor historical understanding of illnesses and their interactions by clinicians or patients leads to ineffective, inefficient, inconsistent, and costly evaluations and interventions.

Goals. Clarity about the patient's illnesses and their treatments; patient, caregiver, and practitioner

---

EXHIBIT 7.2   HB1 Chronicity Anchor Points

0. Less than 3 months of physical symptoms/dysfunction; acute health condition
1. More than 3 months physical symptoms/dysfunction or several periods of less than 3 months
2. A chronic disease
3. Several chronic diseases

EXHIBIT 7.3   Actions Related to HB1 Chronicity Scores

1. **More than 3 months physical dysfunction or several periods of less than 3 months:**
   - Review patient's understanding of persistent dysfunction
   - Observe to see if condition turns chronic with physical limitations
   - Assure primary care or specialist follow-up
2. **A chronic disease:**
   - Review patient's understanding of the chronic illness and treatment
   - Simplify and assist with a systematic approach to illness control
   - Ensure active involvement and collaboration by primary care physician and medical specialists, if needed
   - Assess and ensure treatment of co-occurring mental condition
   - Confirm assessments of patient symptoms and/or measure clinical outcomes over time (e.g., diabetic neuropathy, HbA1c, etc.)
   - Enable unfettered access to physical health and mental health records by all treating clinicians
3. **Several chronic diseases:**
   - *Immediately* perform actions under #2
   - Include customized actions based on interview
   - Review understanding of illnesses and treatments
   - Confirm communication and coordination of care among practitioners

---

EXHIBIT 7.4   **HB2 Diagnostic Dilemma Anchor Points**

0. No period of diagnostic complexity
1. Diagnosis was clarified quickly
2. Diagnostic dilemma solved but only with considerable diagnostic effort
3. Diagnostic dilemma not solved despite considerable diagnostic effort

---

EXHIBIT 7.5   **Actions Related to HB2 Diagnostic Dilemma Scores**

1. **Easy diagnoses:**
   - Observe for changes in clinical status
2. **Diagnostic dilemma with single or multiple conditions:**
   - Review diagnoses, interventions, and treatments for fidelity with the patient's course and improvement with treatment
   - Assess attitude of patient about diagnosis and workups; educate about process
   - Bring in case management medical director to review if it is outside the case manager's level of expertise to get a big picture assessment of the accuracy of diagnoses and treatment
   - Facilitate doctor-to-doctor communication, if needed
   - Discuss ways that case management can assist the patient in improving outcomes
   - Ensure that assessment for concurrent mental conditions has been done and treatment is being given, if present
   - Diplomatically communicate discordant understanding with patient and clinicians
3. **Diagnostic dilemma not solved despite considerable diagnostic efforts:**
   - *Immediately* perform actions under #2
   - Include customized actions based on interview
   - Seek patient's input about unresolved problems
   - Case manager serves as link among clinicians caring for patient, the case management medical director, and the patient to maintain communication, collaboration, and outcome orientation

---

concordance about the cause of symptoms and their treatment; clarity about the biological/psychological interaction.

Success metrics. Understanding of all contributing illnesses to poor outcomes by patient, clinicians, caregivers, and other health participants; agreement on etiology and future prioritized assessments/interventions to the degree possible.

Complexity item: Symptom severity/impairment (**Exhibit 7.6** and **Exhibit 7.7**).

Barriers to improvement. Difficulty in controlling and/or stabilizing acute/severe physical symptoms; irresolvable and/or aggravating functional impairment.

Goals. Maximal improvement and the least impairment; longitudinal approach to care coordination, intervention, and follow-up; prevention of symptom and impairment progression; rehabilitation and/or living situation matches health needs and impairments.

Success metrics. Stabilized illness parameters with appropriate support for continued treatment in place; activated illness progression prevention measures; rehabilitation for functional impairment and appro-

priate level of personal/equipment support and residential care

Complexity item: Diagnostic/therapeutic challenge (**Exhibit 7.8** and **Exhibit 7.9**).

Barriers to improvement. Inaccurate diagnoses or unshared clinical interpretations among providers or between providers and patients on the importance of contributing illnesses and their interventions; failure to diagnose nonphysical health contributors to poor outcomes or to include them among interventions, such as mental disorders, malingering, poor motivation to improve due to work conflicts, and so forth.

Goals. Clarity about biological and nonbiological contributors to physical health outcomes; prioritized administration and coordination of interventions for physical and mental conditions that lead to health improvement; open communication (e.g., shared IM-CAG and summary comments), among patients, caregivers, and primary and secondary practitioners about diagnostic uncertainty and about the risks and potential benefits of various interventions on outcomes.

EXHIBIT 7.6   CB1 Symptom Severity/Impairment Anchor Points

0. No physical symptoms or symptoms resolve with treatment
1. Mild symptoms, which do not interfere with current functioning
2. Moderate symptoms, which interfere with current functioning
3. Severe symptoms leading to inability to perform many functional activities

---

EXHIBIT 7.7   Actions Related to CB1 Symptom Severity/Impairment Scores

1. **Mild symptoms; no functional impairment:**
   - Observe
   - Review for less invasive, less expensive treatment options
2. **Moderate to severe symptoms; impairment present:**
   - Ensure that treatment and follow-up provided is coordinated through efforts of primary care and specialty medical physicians
   - Confirm active involvement of mental health team for patients with comorbid mental conditions
   - Activate ongoing assessment of patient symptoms over time (e.g., labs, X-rays, complications, etc.)
   - Maximize adherence
   - Enable unfettered access to physical health and mental condition records by all treating clinicians
   - Evaluate patient's understanding of illness and impairment; educate if appropriate
   - Delineate impairments and ensure rehabilitation and support measures
3. **Severe symptoms leading to inability to perform activities of daily living:**
   - *Immediately* perform actions under #1 and #2
   - Include customized actions based on interview
   - Find out what works best for the patient
   - Assist with ongoing communication among practitioners
   - Enlist family assistance when available
   - Consider alternative treatment settings, living arrangements, rehabilitation services
   - Augment home care availability
   - Enlist case management medical director assistance and suggestions when needed

---

EXHIBIT 7.8   CB2 Diagnostic/Therapeutic Challenge Anchor Points

0. Clear diagnoses and/or uncomplicated treatments
1. Clear differential diagnoses and/or diagnosis expected with clear treatments
2. Difficult to diagnose and treat; physical cause/origin and treatment expected
3. Difficult to diagnose or treat; other issues than physical causes interfering with diagnostic and therapeutic process

---

Success metrics. Factors contributing to persistent symptoms and treatment resistance identified; documentable outcome change occurring with appropriate intervention.

Complexity item: Complications and life threat (**Exhibit 7.10** and **Exhibit 7.11**).

Barriers to improvement. Without individualized assistance, general medical support system would not provide ongoing physical health care that limits progression of disease and functional impairment.

Goals. General medical care environment consistent with longitudinal control of illness after case management activities have stopped.

Success metrics. Clinical services available to the patient that control symptoms and prevent disease progression likely to be consistently delivered for the foreseeable future.

PSYCHOLOGICAL DOMAIN

Cells in the psychological domain address patients' ability to adapt to their environment, to follow providers' health recommendations, and to access and receive treatment for psychiatric illnesses that lead to personal suffering and dysfunction. The psychological domain is composed of: (a) barriers to coping (HP1),

EXHIBIT 7.9   Actions Related to CB2 Diagnostic/Therapeutic Challenge Scores

1. **Quick diagnoses expected with easy treatments:**
   - Ensure coordination of services
2. **Difficult to diagnose and treat; physical cause/origin and treatment expected:**
   - Scrupulously ensure that patient is following through on evaluations and treatments
   - Make sure that clinicians know the outcomes of exams and tests done by colleagues
   - Assist in measuring outcomes of interventions
   - Maintain communications with and between patient and clinical team (e.g., using IM-CAG results)
   - Have case management medical director review case for additional ideas and talk to clinicians, if warranted
   - Assist patient in getting answers to questions about health from practitioners
   - Consider setting up a case conference among clinicians
3. **Difficult to diagnose and treat; psychological, social, economic issues cloud picture:**
   - *Immediately* perform actions under #2
   - Include customized actions based on interview
   - Make sure that clinicians know about mental conditions and/or social and health system factors that may be playing a role
   - Confirm that the patient is being seen in a timely fashion by appropriate practitioners
   - Have case management medical director talk with patient's clinician about expanded differential and potential treatments
   - Facilitate mental health referral through primary care physicians if possible
   - Include patient in discussions about roles of nonphysical factors in symptoms/treatment

---

EXHIBIT 7.10   VB Complications and Life Threat Anchor Points

0. Little or no risk of premature physical complications or limitations in activities of daily living
1. Mild risk of premature physical complications or limitations in activities of daily living
2. Moderate risk of premature physical complications or permanent and/or substantial limitations in activities of daily living
3. Severe risk of physical complications associated with serious permanent functional deficits and/or dying

---

EXHIBIT 7.11   Actions Related to VB Complications and Life Threat Scores

1. **Mild risk of premature physical complications or limitations in activities of daily living:**
   - Ensure adherence to treatment and troubleshoot barriers that crop up
   - Consider transfer back to standard care
2. **Moderate risk of premature physical complications or permanent and/or substantial limitations in activities of daily living:**
   - Address issues causing nonadherence to treatment
   - Establish continuity of physical and mental condition services
   - Stabilize communication and collaboration among providers and patient
   - Establish methodology to follow clinically relevant outcomes with patient and clinicians (e.g., HbA1c, visits to emergency room, missed work/disability, etc.)
   - Monitor with case management medical director through case conferences
   - Consider intermittent long-term contact with patient
3. **Severe risk of physical complications and serious functional deficits and/or dying:**
   - Perform actions under #2
   - Include customized actions based on interview
   - Consider exploring alternative providers with patient after discussion with medical director
   - Ensure physical health condition assessment and treatment follow through
   - Intermittent long-term contact with patient until risks change
   - Assist with hospice and long-term care, if appropriate

(b) mental health history (HP2), (c) resistance to treatment (CP1), (d) mental health symptoms (CP2), and (e) mental health threat (VP). Unlike in the biological domain, the psychological domain relates not just to those with mental health and substance use disorders (i.e., mental conditions) as potential barriers to health; it also includes health behaviors exhibited by patients with and without mental conditions. Thus a patient with asthma but no psychiatric illness may score in the 2 to 3 range in sections of the psychological domain because of his or her personal belief system, understanding of his or her illness, and so forth. For instance, poor coping mechanisms in individuals with asthma who are encountering stress can reduce their ability to adhere to treatment recommendations. Other patients may require blood after auto accidents but may be resistant to infusions (treatment) based on their religious beliefs. Neither of these constitutes the presence of a mental condition; rather, they represent nonpathologic variances in behaviors that affect outcomes for physical and mental health disorders and for maintenance of health.

The ultimate goal for case management assistance associated with psychological complexity items is to help patients understand and overcome obstacles related to health behaviors and mental conditions that interfere with health stability. The integrated case manager's objective is mental condition symptom resolution or maximum improvement (HP2 and CP2) and reversal of interfering health behaviors (HP1 and CP1). Importantly, in many complex patients, this should be done in coordination with assistance for their physical illnesses since reversal of some psychological barriers to improvement is the lynchpin of physical health improvement.

Complexity item: Barriers to coping (**Exhibit 7.12** and **Exhibit 7.13**).

Barriers to improvement. Personality traits or nonproductive coping mechanisms lead to problems in following through on health-related recommendations.

Goals. Development of coping skills that lead to improved health-related activities; substance usage

---

EXHIBIT 7.12   HP1 Barriers to Coping Anchor Points

0. Ability to manage stresses/life and health circumstances, such as through seeking support or hobbies
1. Restricted coping skills, such as a need for control, illness denial, or irritability
2. Impaired coping skills, such as nonproductive complaining or substance abuse but without serious impact on medical condition, mental health, or social situation
3. Minimal coping skills manifested by destructive behaviors, such as substance dependence, psychiatric illness, self-mutilation, or attempted suicide

---

EXHIBIT 7.13   Actions Related to HP1 Barriers to Coping Scores

1. **Restricted coping skills:**
   - Provide active listening and patient education
   - Ensure/encourage counseling on coping mechanisms
   - Consider training in stress-reduction techniques (one to three sessions, often with a counselor)
2. **Impaired coping skills with frequent conflicts and/or substance abuse:**
   - Identify support for stressful situations
   - Encourage counseling on coping mechanisms
   - Enable training in stress-reduction and conflict-resolution techniques (one to five sessions, often with a counselor)
   - Involve employee assistance program (EAP) to address worksite-related stressors
   - Suggest adjustments in living/work location/activities, if possible
   - Endorse screening and brief intervention for alcohol abuse
   - Consider talking with primary care physician about substance abuse counseling and/or mental health referral for assessment
3. **Minimal coping skills with dangerous behaviors:**
   - *Immediately* perform actions under #2
   - Include customized actions based on interview
   - Assist in support system or crisis management for patient through collaboration with providers
   - Encourage providers to refer for mental health assessment and intervention (e.g. cognitive behavior therapy [CBT], dialectic behavior therapy [DBT], or medication)
   - Facilitate referral for substance abuse/dependence treatment

and psychiatric symptoms under sufficient control that they do not impair coping ability.

Success metrics. Stress reduction and problem-solving capabilities; reduction in substance misuse/abuse/dependence; treatment that controls psychiatric symptoms.

Complexity item: Mental health history (**Exhibit 7.14** and **Exhibit 7.15**).

Barriers to improvement. Historical psychiatric symptoms that are associated with maladaptive or ineffective function.

Goals. Residual psychiatric symptom control and monitoring; ready mental health practitioner access if needed.

Success metrics. Screening and follow-up for potential recurrent psychiatric symptoms in place; support structure for mental condition treatment and follow-up by appropriate providers in place.

Complexity item: Resistance to treatment (**Exhibit 7.16** and **Exhibit 7.17**).

Barriers to improvement. Nonadherence to outcome-changing treatment leads to persistent symptoms or illness complications and high health care service use.

Goals. Adherence to acceptable treatments; knowledge of therapeutic objectives.

Success metrics. Documented adherence associated with health stabilization or outcome improvement.

EXHIBIT 7.14   HP2 Mental Health History Anchor Points

0. No history of mental health problems or conditions
1. Mental health problems or conditions, but resolved or without clear effects on daily function
2. Mental health conditions with clear effects on daily function, needing therapy, medication, day treatment, partial program, and so forth
3. Psychiatric admissions and/or persistent effects on daily function

---

EXHIBIT 7.15   Actions Related to HP2 Mental Health History Scores

1. **Mental conditions resolved or without effect on life activities:**
   - Encourage regular primary care screenings for mental conditions with intervention, if appropriate
   - Check for access to support from mental health professionals
2. **Mental conditions that interfered with life activities or required treatment:**
   - Ensure the patient's understanding of potential for recurrence of mental health conditions by using lay language
   - Link potential for medical and physical condition interactions, if indicated
   - Ensure potential for active involvement by psychiatrist and mental health team (psychologists, social workers, nurses, substance use disorder and other counselors, etc.) support when conditions destabilize
   - Confirm maintenance and continuation treatment provided by primary care professionals (medical home) with mental health specialist assistance
   - Facilitate ongoing monitoring of patient symptoms over time (e.g. PHQ-9, GAD-7, etc.)
   - Activate communication and unfettered access to physical and mental health records by all treating clinicians
3. **Psychiatric admissions and/or persistent effects on daily function:**
   - *Immediately* perform actions under #2
   - Include customized actions based on interview
   - Encourage primary involvement and treatment by a mental health team for mental conditions working in close collaboration with primary care physicians who care for concurrent physical illness
   - When possible, facilitate colocation of the patient's physical and mental health clinicians who actively interact in an integrated clinic setting

---

EXHIBIT 7.16   CP1 Resistance to Treatment Anchor Points

0. Interested in receiving treatment and willing to cooperate actively
1. Some ambivalence though willing to cooperate with treatment
2. Considerable resistance and nonadherence; hostility or indifference toward health care professionals and/or treatments
3. Active resistance to important medical care

EXHIBIT 7.17   Actions Related to CP1 Resistance to Treatment Scores

1. **Ambivalence:**
   - Educate patient/family about illnesses
   - Initiate discussions with patient about resistant behaviors using motivational interviewing and problem-solving techniques to reduce resistance
   - Explore other barriers to treatment adherence (**Exhibit 7.1**)
   - Inform providers of adherence problems and work with them to consider alternative interventions, if needed
2. **Resistance, hostility, indifference:**
   - Perform actions under #1
   - Review need for other health professional or clinic to provide care with case manager's medical director
   - Actively explore and attempt to reverse other sources of resistance (e.g., family member's negativism, religious objections, cultural influences, relationships with treating physician)
3. **Active resistance:**
   - *Immediately* perform actions under #1 and #2
   - Include customized actions based on interview
   - Work with treating clinicians in considering and instituting alternative interventions
   - If needed, work with case management medical director to find second opinion practitioners
   - If irresolvable and pervasive, consider discontinuation of case management

EXHIBIT 7.18   CP2 Mental Health Symptoms Anchor Points

0. No mental health symptoms
1. Mild mental health symptoms, such as problems with concentration or feeling tense, which do not interfere with current functioning
2. Moderate mental health symptoms, such as anxiety, depression, or mild cognitive impairment, which interfere with current functioning
3. Severe psychiatric symptoms and/or behavioral disturbances, such as violence, self-inflicted harm, delirium, criminal behavior, psychosis, or mania

EXHIBIT 7.19   Actions Related to CP2 Mental Health Symptoms Scores

1. **Mild mental health symptoms:**
   - Ensure primary care treatment with access to support from mental health professionals
   - Facilitate unfettered access to physical and mental health records by all treating clinicians
2. **Moderate mental health symptoms:**
   - Perform actions under #1
   - Ensure that acute, maintenance, and continuation of treatment is being provided by primary care physicians with mental health support and backup
   - Facilitate primary maintenance and continuation treatment provided by primary care physician (medical home) with mental health specialist assistance—that is, a psychiatrist and mental health team (psychologists, social workers, nurses, substance abuse counselors, etc.)—when condition destabilizes, becomes complicated, or demonstrates treatment resistance
   - Assist with instituting symptom documentation recording system, such as PHQ-9, GAD-7, and so forth
   - Ensure crisis plan is available
3. **Severe psychiatric symptoms and/or behavioral disturbances:**
   - *Immediately* perform actions under #1 and #2
   - Include customized actions based on interview
   - Support active and aggressive treatment for mental conditions by a mental health team working in close collaboration with primary care physicians, who care for concurrent physical illness
   - When possible, encourage geographically collocated physical and mental health personnel to facilitate ease of coordinating treatment
   - Confirm persistent symptom documentation recording system, such as PHQ-9, GAD-7, and so forth
   - Ensure physical and mental health treatment adherence

Complexity item: Mental health symptoms (Exhibit 7.18 and **Exhibit 7.19**).

Barriers to improvement. Difficulty in controlling disruptive emotions, cognitions, and behaviors related to mental health and substance use disorders, leading to personal suffering and impairment.

Goals. Mental condition symptom improvement or stabilization; adherence to ongoing active treatment.

Success metrics. Mental health symptom improvement/stabilization; appropriate mental health professional involvement; social/environmental support in place; mental health symptoms do not interfere with general medical treatment and outcomes.

Complexity item: Mental health threat (**Exhibit 7.20** and **Exhibit 7.21**).

Barriers to improvement. Without individualized assistance, general medical and mental health system would provide inadequate support to maintain coping strategies, treatment adherence, and psychiatric symptom control, leading to return of unhealthy and potentially destructive behaviors.

Goals. Patient-based accessible coping skills and strategies; comfort with and adherence to recommended interventions; consistent psychiatric and mental health team access and outcome-changing mental health treatment when needed.

Success metrics. Stabilized mental conditions; ready access to and availability of mental health services; health improvement associated with consistent treatment adherence; reduction in patient crises (personal, health, social).

SOCIAL DOMAIN

Cells in the social domain address the patient's financial and residential stability, interpersonal relationships, ability to interact with others effectively, and the level of support available when difficulties or crises occur. The social domain is composed of: (a) job and leisure (HS1), (b) relationships (HS2),

---

EXHIBIT 7.20 **VP Mental Health Threat Anchor Points**

0. No mental health concerns
1. Risk of mild worsening of mental health *symptoms*, such as stress, anxiety, feeling blue, substance abuse, or cognitive disturbance with limited impact on function; mild risk of treatment resistance (ambivalence)
2. Moderate risk of mental health *disorder* requiring additional mental health care; moderate risk of treatment resistance
3. Severe risk of psychiatric disorder requiring frequent emergency room visits and/or hospital admissions; risk of treatment refusal for serious disorder

---

EXHIBIT 7.21 **Actions Related to VP Mental Health Threat Scores**

1. **Mild risk of worsening mental health symptoms:**
   - Ensure access to support
   - Ensure/encourage continuous follow-up care with intermittent mental health assessments, when appropriate
   - Suggest booster sessions for coping and stress reduction, when needed
   - Consider transfer back to standard care
2. **Moderate risk of worsening mental health symptoms:**
   - Perform actions under #1
   - Set up maintenance and continuity program that involves the treating primary care physicians, clinical nurse specialists, and mental health specialists
   - Assist in establishing a regular symptom documentation system, such as PHQ-9, GAD-7, and so forth
   - Facilitate guideline development for mental health team involvement with patient in the primary care clinic to assist with treatment adjustments (best provided in an integrated primary care clinic)
   - Address adherence and patient-provider relationship issues
   - Involve caregivers in all activities after informed consent obtained
   - Institute verbal, paper, and electronic communication capabilities for all clinical professionals working with the patient
3. **Severe and persistent risk of psychiatric disorder with frequent health service use:**
   - Perform actions under #1 and #2
   - Include customized actions based on interview
   - Confirm care continuity with both general medical and mental health specialists
   - Work with the patient's clinicians in establishing collaborative clinical goals with the patient
   - Consider long-term involvement

(c) residential stability (CS1), (d) social support (CS2), and (e) social vulnerability (VS). Each of these constitutes independent yet interacting social complexity items that affect health and may create barriers to improvement.

The social domain addresses patients' social connectedness and how their living situations may influence health issues. For instance, a person living on the street is unlikely to be able to adhere to even short-term treatment suggestions unless a shelter is found in the proximity to where health care is provided. In a less dramatic, yet equally impairing, example, a person with memory deficits and limited supervisory support is likely to inappropriately use prescribed medications, leading to poor illness control, complications, and even hospitalization.

The goal related to social complexity items is to help patients with limited resources or support systems maximize their living situation so that they are better able to participate in their personal health. As in other domains, integrated case managers cannot be expected to correct many adverse social situations contributing to health instability. They can, however, initiate many simple interventions, such as connecting the patients to drug company-sponsored medication support programs or community housing projects that can make a significant impact on health and function.

Complexity item: Job and leisure (**Exhibit 7.22** and **Exhibit 7.23**).

Barriers to improvement. Not having a job can lead to loss of insurance, to limited money needed for out-of-pocket health expenses, and to an unstable living situation. Little leisure activity or a recognized daytime role (such as homemaker, retiree, etc.) suggests impaired socializing skills, personal impairment, or limited financial resources, which decrease the likelihood of mobilizing support when help with health care is needed.

Goals. Economic stability and social activities.

Success metrics. Return to employment, school, and leisure activities.

Complexity item: Relationships (**Exhibit 7.24** and **Exhibit 7.25**).

Barriers to improvement. Impaired interpersonal skills lead to destructive relationships and a worsening health care support system.

Goals. Social skills that will lead to personal relationships; connectedness that is useful during times of need.

Success metrics. Improved interactions with family, friends, colleagues, and significant others.

Complexity item: Residential stability (**Exhibit 7.26** and **Exhibit 7.27**).

Barriers to improvement. Unstable, unsafe, or inadequate living situations may prevent access to consistent health providers, health care services, or effective treatment or create an inherent risk for health deterioration.

Goals. A safe and consistent living situation.

Success metrics. A safe and stable living environment that leads to consistent and appropriate health access and care.

EXHIBIT 7.22   HSI Job and Leisure Anchor Points

0. A job (including housekeeping, retirement, studying) and having leisure activities
1. A job (including housekeeping, retirement, studying) without leisure activities
2. Unemployed now and for at least 6 months with leisure activities
3. Unemployed now and for at least 6 months without leisure activities

---

EXHIBIT 7.23   Actions Related to HSI Job and Leisure Scores

1. A job; few leisure activities:
- Explore interests/hobbies with the patient and encourage rekindling activity

2. At least 6 months unemployed (but employable); leisure activities:
- Assist patient in getting disability assistance, exploring schooling opportunities, and so forth
- Educate patient on how to get public assistance for living and health care needs
- Set up with social service, job finding services, vocational rehabilitation, or other community resources if a new job is a possibility
- Follow up; continue encouraging patient-initiated activities

3. At least 6 months unemployed (but employable); few leisure activities:
- *Immediately* perform actions under #1 and #2
- Include customized actions based on interview
- Explore impact of no job and few activities on health access
- Explore community resources with patient

EXHIBIT 7.24   HS2 Relationships Anchor Points

0. No social disruption
1. Mild social dysfunction; interpersonal problems
2. Moderate social dysfunction, such as inability to initiate or maintain social relations
3. Severe social dysfunction, such as involvement in disruptive social relations or social isolation

---

EXHIBIT 7.25   Actions Related to HS2 Relationships Scores

1. **Mild social dysfunction; interpersonal problems:**
   - Observe interpersonal difficulties during patient interviews and adjust recommendations to accommodate for limitations (i.e., introversion, family discord, etc.)
2. **Moderate social dysfunction:**
   - Encourage social skills training (one to six sessions, often with a counselor)
   - Foster involvement of family, significant others, or social service
   - Assess impact of social problems on patient's health issues, address if present
   - Explore alternative socialization opportunities
3. **Severe social dysfunction:**
   - *Immediately* perform actions under #1 and #2
   - Include customized actions based on interview
   - Encourage mental health assessment and treatment if appropriate and/or needed through primary care physician

---

EXHIBIT 7.26   CS1 Residential Stability Anchor Points

0. Stable housing; fully capable of independent living
1. Stable housing with support of others (e.g., family, home care, or an institutional setting)
2. Unstable housing (e.g., no support at home or living in a shelter; change of current living situation is required)
3. No current satisfactory housing (e.g., transient housing or dangerous environment; immediate change is necessary)

EXHIBIT 7.27   Actions Related to CS1 Residential Stability Scores

1. **Stable housing situation with support of others:**
   - Make sure vulnerability needs match support
2. **Unstable housing:**
   - Initiate contact with social service or other community resources to look into housing options
   - Get assistance to help correct the cause of the residential instability, such as financial limitations, family conflict, natural disaster, and so forth
   - Follow up on results of suggestions
   - Use knowledge of community resources to push the system
3. **Unsafe or transient housing:**
   - *Immediately* connect the patient with social service to find a shelter, such as for battered women, or other suitable housing
   - Perform actions under #2
   - Include customized actions based on interview

EXHIBIT 7.28   **CS2 Social Support Anchor Points**

0. Assistance readily available from family, friends, and/or acquaintances, such as work colleagues, at all times
1. Assistance generally available from family, friends, and/or acquaintances, such as work colleagues, but possible delays
2. Limited assistance available from family, friends, and/or acquaintances, such as work colleagues
3. No assistance readily available from family, friends, and/or acquaintances, such as work colleagues, at any time

---

EXHIBIT 7.29   **Actions Related to CS2 Social Support Scores**

1. Assistance generally available but possible delays:
   - Initiate assistance mechanism, if needed
2. Limited assistance readily available:
   - Talk with patient's available personal contacts about what they can do along with the patient
   - Set up with social services or other agency to assist patient with finding needed community resources
   - Follow up on recommendation outcome
   - Use knowledge of community resources to push the system
   - Get ideas about options from other health professionals familiar with patient's social setting
3. No assistance readily available:
   - *Immediately* perform actions under #2
   - Include customized actions based on interview
   - Consider helping to transfer patient to a location with a higher level of care (e.g., group home, assisted living facility)

Complexity item: Social support (**Exhibit 7.28** and **Exhibit 7.29**).

Barriers to improvement. Lack of personal support system, which is required for return to health stabilization, overwhelms the patient's ability to follow through on needed care.

Goals. Social and living situation that allows access to support for chronic and acute health needs that are in excess of the patient's personal resources.

Success metrics. Assistance for health needs available through accessible support system chronically and in times of crisis.

Complexity item: Social vulnerability (**Exhibit 7.30** and **Exhibit 7.31**).

Barriers to improvement. Without individualized assistance, an inconsistent or inadequate social support system, unstable living situation, poor social skills, or lack of financial resources could lead to poor health care access, worsening illness control, physical and mental condition complications, and high health care service use.

Goals. Consistent and appropriate social support and residential living after case management ends; financial stabilization.

Success metrics. Financial resource access covering basic needs; appropriate and consistent living arrangements; personal support with optimized relationships for the foreseeable future.

HEALTH SYSTEM DOMAIN

There is more to maintaining or improving health than getting the right diagnosis and receiving the right treatment recommendations. It is also necessary for the patient: (a) to have access to care, including insurance for payment, providers that speak the patient's language, and geographic access to needed specialists; (b) to have sufficient trust in practitioners to follow their advice; (c) to have needed physical and mental condition services temporally and geographically available; (d) to have clinicians who communicate with each other so that treatment recommendations are coordinated; and (e) to have support for needed services throughout an illness episode.

The health system domain is composed of: (a) access to care (HHS1), (b) treatment experience (HHS2), (c) getting needed services (CHS1), (d) coordination of care (CHS2), and (e) health system impediments (VHS). Each of these constitutes independent yet interacting health system complexity items that can lead to barriers to improvement. The health system domain addresses the patients' experiences in trying to get health services and their ability to navigate an increasingly complicated delivery and reimbursement environment as they do so. This is the area of health care that has a great impact on disease outcomes and yet is the least addressed in most case management programs.

EXHIBIT 7.30 **VS Social Vulnerability Anchor Points**

---

0. No risk of need for changes in the living situation, social relationships and support, or employment
1. Mild risk of need for changes in the living situation (e.g., home health care), social relationships and support, or employment
2. Risk of need for social augmentation/support, financial/employment assistance, or living situation change in the foreseeable future
3. Risk of need for social augmentation/support, financial/employment assistance, or living situation change now

---

EXHIBIT 7.31 **Actions Related to VS Social Vulnerability Scores**

---

1. Some health assistance needs:
   • See if current location can accommodate potential need
   • Consider transfer back to standard care
2. Risk of need for alteration in social situation in the foreseeable future:
   • Continue to work with family
   • Assist, engage, and push social service to find resources and make ready the procedures for help and/or placement
   • Follow outcomes of recommendations
   • Use knowledge of community resources to push the system
3. Risk of need for alteration in social situation now:
   • Perform actions under #2
   • Include customized actions based on interview
   • Attempt to set up long-term living arrangements

Examples abound relating to how the health system influences health outcomes:

■ Patients who cannot find a mental health provider to see them for severe depression because of provider network inadequacies
■ Patients with concurrent chest pain and anxiety, in whom the heart specialist and psychologist do not even know that they are working with the same individual, presenting to both with identical symptoms
■ Patients with young children and no car who have appointments with doctors on the same day yet in offices miles apart

Health system domain items not only address how support for health care is organized and coordinated but also how patients experience the system. Since the relationship between patients and their clinicians predicts adherence and outcomes, it is also important for the case manager to uncover mistrust and provider relationship issues that alter patients' participation in their own care.

The ultimate goal associated with the health system complexity items is to help patients establish trusting therapeutic relationships with clinicians that are appropriate for their illnesses, to confirm that providers are communicating with each other, and to assist patients with overcoming system-level and logistical access barriers to receiving outcome-changing treatment.

Complexity item: Access to care (**Exhibit 7.32** and **Exhibit 7.33**).

Barriers to improvement. (System level) Lack of or insufficient health care coverage or payment mechanism for needed services, living in a rural setting, lack of translators, psychiatric bed shortages, long wait lists, among other system-level factors can make it difficult to access practitioners who can give outcome-changing treatment.

Goals. Medical and mental health insurance coverage, geographic clinician accessibility, translation services, and culturally sensitive services; practitioners willing to accept patients who have the resources needed to provide effective treatment.

Success metrics. Timely, affordable, and appropriate health care pertinent to the patient's health conditions unencumbered by payment, language, cultural, or geographic issues; no barriers to integrated medical and mental health care.

EXHIBIT 7.32   HHSI Access to Care Anchor Points

0. Adequate access to care
1. Some limitations in access to care due to financial/insurance problems, geographic reasons, family issues, language, or cultural barriers
2. Difficulties in accessing care due to financial/insurance problems, geographic reasons, family issues, language, or cultural barriers
3. No adequate access to care due to financial/insurance problems, geographic reasons, family issues, language, or cultural barriers

---

EXHIBIT 7.33   Actions Related to HHSI Access to Care Scores

1. Some limitation in accessing care:
- Assist in identifying culturally sensitive willing providers, interpretation services, and ensuring access to timely appointments

2. Difficulties in accessing care:
- Work with patient in finding health insurance and in identifying willing providers
- Ensure timely culturally sensitive appointments and translation services (use conference calls or telephonic access if necessary)
- Assist in flexing benefits (with health plan) when possible to get appropriate care (go up the supervisory ladder)
- Push the system to shorten wait list priority
- Connect physical and mental health financial/administrative support for services
- Assist with appeals of inappropriately denied care (use case management medical director, if necessary)

3. No adequate access to care:
- *Immediately* perform actions under #2
- Include customized actions based on interview
- Enlist social service to assist with actions in #2 and in finding insurance product or general assistance clinic
- Assist with post-emergency room and post-hospitalization follow-up locations
- Advocate for patient

Complexity item: Treatment experience (**Exhibit 7.34** and **Exhibit 7.35**).

Barriers to improvement. Biases against allopathic medical services, an inconsistent patient-provider relationship, or prior provider experiences that engendered mistrust and negative regard predicts future nonadherence and nontreatment for existing health problems or the use of the emergency health system.

Goals. Adherence to care from consistent and trusted providers; resolution of doctor mistrust and negative experiences to the extent possible; open communication between clinicians and patients; reconciled biases against allopathic medicine.

Success metrics. Collaborative and mutually acceptable doctor-patient relationships; satisfaction with care; adherence to illness appropriate treating practitioner's interventions.

Complexity item: Getting needed services (**Exhibit 7.36** and **Exhibit 7.37**).

Barriers to improvement. (Care delivery level) Logistical lack of availability of or referral to specialists, poorly coordinated appointments, and/or inadequate transportation make it difficult for the patient to get the type of care that is needed; money is not available to cover out-of-pocket costs of medications, equipment, or needed services.

Goals. Transportation available and scheduled appointments with the patient's providers are coordinated using telemedicine access or other means if needed; referral to needed providers for targeted illnesses and outcomes (e.g., psychologist or psychiatrist); funds to pay for out-of-pocket expenses related to needed medications, equipment, and services.

Success metrics. Full capability to attend appointments; minimized appointment conflicts and numbers of visits; able to buy medications, equipment, and needed services (e.g., rehabilitation); appropriate referrals to clinical providers or for medical services that are needed to reverse symptoms and impairment.

Complexity item: Coordination of care (**Exhibit 7.38** and **Exhibit 7.39**).

Barriers to improvement. If providers do not know what each other are doing, duplication or missed services can occur; this increases chance for nontreatment, conflicting treatment, and drug interactions.

Goals. Established communication between and among providers; primary provider coordinates services (medical home); unified medical and mental health record systems accessible to all clinicians involved in patient's care.

Success metrics. All health personnel involved in patient's care are aware of and coordinating the services they are providing with others who work with the patient; record system interconnectivity.

Complexity item: Health system impediments (**Exhibit 7.40** and **Exhibit 7.41**).

Barriers to improvement. Without individualized support, loss of persistent and consistent access to coordinated services from preferred and trusted

---

EXHIBIT 7.34   HHS2 Treatment Experience Anchor Points

0. No problems with health care professionals
1. Negative experience with health care professionals (patient or relatives)
2. Dissatisfaction with or distrust of doctors; multiple providers for the same health problem; trouble keeping consistent and/or preferred provider(s)
3. Repeated major conflicts with or distrust of doctors, frequent emergency room visits or involuntary admissions; forced to stay with undesirable provider because of cost, provider network options, or other reasons

---

EXHIBIT 7.35   Actions Related to HHS2 Treatment Experience Scores

1. **Negative experience with health care providers:**
   - Assess for adherence to assessment and treatment recommendations
   - Periodically ask about current relationship with clinical practitioners
   - Help patient to ask questions of or to challenge practitioners
2. **Changes doctors more than once because of dissatisfaction; multiple providers:**
   - Assess types of conflicts with practitioners
   - Adjudicate conflict when possible (directly or indirectly)
   - Ensure treatment adherence
   - Foster communication between patient and practitioner about conflicts
   - Assist patient in getting to a different provider if needed, where outcomes would be better
   - Involve case management medical director for assistance
3. **Repeated major conflicts with doctors, frequent emergency room visits, or involuntary admissions:**
   - *Immediately* perform actions under #2
   - Include customized actions based on interview
   - Assist in finding someone to work with patient on conflict resolution techniques
   - Involve the case management medical director to talk with practitioners about relationship
   - Consider assisting patient with finding another professional or location of care
   - Mental health consultation to assess for personality or chemical dependence issues contributing to conflict
   - Look at insurance alternatives with patient

EXHIBIT 7.36   CHS1 Getting Needed Services Anchor Points

0. Easily available treating practitioners and health care settings (general medical or mental health care); money for medications and medical equipment
1. Some difficulties in getting to appointments or needed services
2. Routine difficulties in coordinating and/or getting to appointments or needed services
3. Inability to coordinate and/or get to appointments or needed services

EXHIBIT 7.37   **Actions Related to CHS1 Getting Needed Services Scores**

1. **Some difficulties in getting to appointments or needed services:**
   - Review correlation of disorders with treatment being given
   - Check for barriers
   - Assist with finding money for medications, equipment, and needed services
2. **Routine difficulties in coordinating and/or getting to appointments or needed services:**
   - Assess alternative care locations and practitioner availability
   - Review options with the patient and ensure timely access
   - Consider accessing services through telemedicine
   - Assist with finding money for medications, equipment, and needed services
   - Check for appointment flexibility in current clinic system
   - Help patient find needed medical and/or mental health specialists and set up appointments (out of region/network if necessary)
   - Review difficulties with primary care physician (medical home)
3. **Inability to coordinate and/or get to appointments or needed services:**
   - *Immediately* perform actions under #2
   - Include customized actions based on interview
   - Establish medical home
   - Work with primary care (or specialty) physician (medical home) to coordinate appointments (e.g., diabetologist and psychiatrist)
   - Assist with transportation for patient and coordination of assessments/follow-ups
   - Enlist assistance of community agencies and social services

---

EXHIBIT 7.38   **CHS2 Coordination of Care Anchor Points**

0. Complete practitioner communication with good coordination of care
1. Limited practitioner communication and coordination of care; primary care physician coordinates medical and mental health services
2. Poor communication and coordination of care among practitioners; no routine primary care physician
3. No communication and coordination of care among practitioners; primary emergency room use to meet nonemergent health needs

---

EXHIBIT 7.39   **Actions Related to CHS2 Coordination of Care Scores**

1. **Limited practitioner communication and coordination of care:**
   - Encourage record sharing and communication among clinicians, including mental health and complementary medicine
   - Open links for important communication
2. **Poor communication and coordination of care among practitioners:**
   - Determine and augment communication links between physical and mental health practitioners
   - Ensure note sharing, preferably common record system, among clinicians working with patient
   - Assist in coordinating appointments and transportation
   - Help patient get same-day appointments for different problems
   - Investigate availability of integrated clinics
   - Identify reasons for missed appointments to overcome barriers
3. **No communication and coordination of care among practitioners:**
   - *Immediately* perform actions under #1 and #2
   - Include customized actions based on interview
   - Serve as link for patient with various practitioners (e.g., with informed consent (see Appendix 3 if needed), obtain and fax notes for distribution to various clinic sites)
   - Talk with treating practitioners on behalf of patient but also educate patient on how to do so
   - Create alternatives to emergency room use
   - Enlist assistance from case management medical director to try to establish a medical home

---

EXHIBIT 7.40 **VHS Health System Impediments Anchor Points**

0. No risk of impediments to coordinated physical and mental health care
1. Mild risk of impediments to care, such as insurance restrictions, distant service access, and limited provider communication and/or care coordination
2. Moderate risk of impediments to care, such as potential insurance loss, inconsistent practitioners, communication barriers, poor care coordination
3. Severe risk of impediments to care, such as little or no insurance, resistance to communication, and/or disruptive work processes that lead to poor coordination

---

EXHIBIT 7.41 **Actions Related to VHS Health System Impediments Scores**

1. **Mild risk of impediments to care:**
   - Ensure that insurance benefits cover health needs
   - Assist in maintaining coverage
   - Review practitioner communication procedures
   - Consider transfer back to standard care
2. **Moderate risk of impediments to care:**
   - Work with patient, practitioner providing medical home, social services, and community agencies to establish the best health setup possible in the region
   - Assist in finding insurance products, needed providers, and communicating clinic systems
   - Pay special attention to physical and mental health links
3. **Severe risk of impediments to care:**
   - Perform actions under #2
   - Include customized actions based on interview
   - Help patient find and establish a medical home that will persist over time
   - Assist in overcoming barriers to practitioner involvement with patient
   - Consider setting up a physical and mental health clinicians' case conference
   - Attempt to enlist assistance of community-based case manager (public health)
   - Ensure that insurance benefits cover health needs
   - Assist in maintaining coverage
   - Review and assist with practitioner communication procedures

---

providers or logistical difficulties in getting needed services would prevent the availability of treatments that restore health.

Goals. Consistent geographically accessible and consistent care by trusted practitioners willing to treat the patient within his or her budget; sustained coordination and communication about care among patient's providers; resolution of language, transportation, or cultural barriers to effective treatment.

Success metrics. Stable access to and support for health needs from trusted providers; widespread communication among providers; positive patient-provider relationship for the foreseeable future.

REFERENCES

Katon, W., Cantrell, C. R., Sokol, M. C., Chiao, E., & Gdovin, J. M. (2005). Impact of antidepressant drug adherence on comorbid medication use and resource utilization. *Archives Intern Medicine, 165*(21), 2497–2503.

Kroenke, K. (2007). Efficacy of treatment for somatoform disorders: A review of randomized controlled trials. *Psychosomogical Medicine, 69*(9), 881–888.

Sokol, M. C., McGuigan, K. A., Verbrugge, R. R., & Epstein, R. S. (2005). Impact of medication adherence on hospitalization risk and healthcare cost. *Medical Care, 43*(6), 521–530.

Stiefel, F. C., Huyse, F. J., Sollner, W., Slaets, J. P., Lyons, J. S., Latour, C. H., et al. (2006). Operationalizing integrated care on a clinical level: The INTERMED project. *Medical Clinics North America, 90*(4), 713–758.

CHAPTER 8

Child/Youth Integrated Case Management Using Pediatric INTERMED-Complexity Assessment Grid Methodology

OBJECTIVES

- To describe the development of integrated case management for children/youth with health complexity
- To depict similarities and differences between the INTERMED-Complexity Assessment Grid (IM-CAG) and the Pediatric INTERMED-Complexity Assessment Grid (PIM-CAG) as a method to document and measure health complexity in children/youth
- To connect case manager actions with PIM-CAG anchor point scores
- To explain how the PIM-CAG assessment leads to the development of an integrated case management care plan

INTRODUCTION

Since integrated case management capabilities for patients with health complexity became available in the adult setting, there has been interest in having a complementary version for use with children and youth. This chapter represents the introduction of pediatric integrated case management, based on the concept that the level of child/youth complexity drives action and thus potential value for the child/youth, his or her family, and the health system. The pediatric version parallels the adult approach to integrated case management, which capitalizes on INTERMED research experience from Europe during the last 15 years (Huyse & Stiefel, 2006). In addition, the integrated case management approach utilizes the expertise and suggestions of the health professionals that introduced, utilize, and now provide training in the Child and Adolescent Needs and Strengths (CANS) approach which is a behavioral health assessment process for children and adolescents being used in more than 30 states or provinces throughout the United States and Canada (Lyons, 2004; Lyons, Baerger, Almeida, & Lyons, 1999). Like the integrated case management program, the CANS is based on communimetrics, a documentation and measurement approach that facilitates communication among professionals and connects clinically relevant information with actions that can be taken on the behalf of children/youth. The primary developer of the CANS approach, John Lyons, PhD, has served as an INTERMED consultant since its inception in the 1990s.

The pediatric version of the INTERMED-Complexity Assessment Grid (PIM-CAG) forms the core of the child/youth complexity assessment process (Appendixes 5 and 7). As the pediatricians, child psychiatrists, child psychologists, pediatric case managers, and creators of the adult IM-CAG contributed to the development of this child/youth tool, it became apparent that there were a number of concept areas (items) in the adult version that needed to be adapted for use with children/youth. Further, the addition of several further concept areas was required to address developmental issues and the fact that both the child/youth and the caregiver/parent would influence outcomes in the integrated case management process. The final PIM-CAG assessment tool was thus developed based on discussion and consensus among contributors with experience and expertise in working with children, review of the literature on psychosocial and health system correlates of pediatric chronic illness, coupled with suggestions by those who had been involved in the development and use of the adult integrated case management approach to health support. This allowed significant overlap of domains, items, and anchor points between the adult and pediatric versions.

The PIM-CAG is specifically developed for use by care managers rather than by treating practitioners, with a special emphasis on case management. Since the role of case managers is to uncover barriers to improvement, but not to provide treatment themselves, it is not considered necessary for the PIM-CAG to contain grid items that delineate all of the discrete areas in which physical or mental health intervention may be helpful. Rather, item anchor points are intended to inform case managers about complexity-based barriers to improvement and the actions that can be taken to overcome them. Through their identification, case managers can assist the child/youth and caregiver/parent with obtaining needed services from appropriate providers. One item could trigger multiple actions by the case manager involving more than one provider. Alternatively, covered content by an item anchor point score could suggest to a single provider contacted for child/youth assistance by the case manager to include multiple areas of intervention. Because the PIM-CAG, like the IM-CAG, is both an assessment and communication tool, it can be used to place the child/youth, the caregivers/parents, and the treating practitioners on common ground regarding the child's/youth's complexity level and treatment needs. On the other hand, it does not reveal specific treatments that are needed nor which type of professional should provide them.

Importantly, the PIM-CAG goes far beyond mere treatment of general medical or mental health conditions. It assesses many other factors potentially influencing the ability of the child/youth to maximize their health status such as cognitive ability, family and peer relationships, school functioning, financial and housing needs, adverse life events, trust of providers, and caregiver/parent health. Like the IM-CAG it is a comprehensive assessment of major factors in the child's/youth's life that can affect health stabilization and return to maximum function.

While the PIM-CAG is an assessment tool through which pediatric integrated case management will be performed, it is the application of the assessment to care planning and subsequent work with the children/youth and their families that results in stabilized health and function. By disentangling and prioritizing those areas in which action can be taken to alter outcomes, it then becomes possible to methodically address the needs of the child/youth and to work toward return to standard care.

SIMILARITIES AND DIFFERENCES BETWEEN THE PIM-CAG AND THE IM-CAG

Like the IM-CAG, the PIM-CAG (**Table 8.1**, see page i3 for color version) is at the heart of the integrated case management assessment since it provides a method through which illness and life situation (health) complexity can be codified, documented, quantified, and acted upon on behalf of the child/youth. Those case managers reading this manual, and especially those who will be case managing children/youth, are encouraged to review Appendixes F (see www.springerpub.com/kathol), 7, and 9. Appendix F (or Exhibit 10.2) outlines the complete list of open-ended questions that can be used to uncover areas of complexity in all domains and for all items while building a relationship with the child/youth and the child's/youth's caregivers/parents. Appendix 7 systematically delineates all of the pediatric items and anchor points in each domain and the rules for their use. Appendix 9 contains a representative compendium of potential actions that might be considered by the case manager, the child/youth, the caregiver/parent, health professionals, and/or educational personnel when item anchor points are triggered.

Rather than reviewing each item in the PIM-CAG in detail, this chapter will provide an overview of how the PIM-CAG relates to the IM-CAG. Since it parallels the IM-CAG in application, with a scoring grid and scoring system that has been adapted to children/youth, the PIM-CAG results will drive the development of a prioritized care plan, the actions taken on behalf of the child/youth, and the integrated case management process through which health stabilization can occur.

Finally, the central task of pediatric integrated case management is to uncover barriers to improvement for a *child/youth* and for the case manager to work with the child/youth and his or her family in reversing those barriers. During the child/youth assessment, caregivers'/parents' needs will also be assessed. In some situations, identified needs will be of equal or greater magnitude than those of the child/youth. Since the child/youth is targeted for help during pediatric integrated case management, this means that the case manager working with the child/youth must decide whether assistance to the caregiver/parent warrants referral of the caregivers/parents for assistance of their own or whether such assistance is within the realm of the child's/youth's case manager.

This can sometimes be a difficult decision since some assistance to caregivers/parents is routine in the application of any child/youth case management. Nonetheless, needs of the parents, caregivers, and/or other family members can overwhelm time available or the ability of the case manager to influence change for the child/youth. In these situations, worksite organizational rules, direction from supervisors, and/or common sense should dictate the direction taken by the case manager.

THE CHILD/YOUTH AND CAREGIVERS/PARENTS INTERVIEW AND ASSESSMENT

Integrated case management is based on the assumption that the relationship between the case manager and the patient is a driving force for change to health stability and reduced impairment. Thus, similar to the adult IM-CAG, the PIM-CAG is scored from a scripted discussion with the child/youth and/or caregivers/parents using open-ended questions. Scripted questions can be found and reviewed in Appendix F and Exhibit 10.2.

TABLE 8.1   Pediatric INTERMED-Complexity Assessment Grid Scoring Sheet

Date	HEALTH RISKS AND HEALTH NEEDS					
Name	**HISTORICAL**		**CURRENT STATE**		**VULNERABILITY**	
Total Score =	Complexity Item	Score	Complexity Item	Score	Complexity Item	Score
Biological Domain	Chronicity **HB1**		Symptom Severity/Impairment **CB1**		Complications and Life Threat **VB**	
	Diagnostic Dilemma **HB2**		Diagnostic/Therapeutic Challenge **CB2**			
Psychological Domain	Barriers to Coping **HP1**		Resistance to Treatment **CP1**		Learning and/or Mental Health Threat **VP**	
	Mental Health History **HP2**		Mental Health Symptoms **CP2**			
	Cognitive Development **HP3**					
	Adverse Developmental Events **HP4**					
Social Domain	School Functioning **HS1**		Residential Stability **CS1**		Family/School/Social System Vulnerability **VS**	
	Family and Social Relationships **HS2**		Child/Youth Support **CS2**			
	Caregiver/Parent Health and Function **HS3**		Caregiver/Family Support **CS3**			
			School and Community Participation **CS4**			
Health System Domain	Access to Care **HHS1**		Getting Needed Services **CHS1**		Health System Impediments **VHS**	
	Treatment Experience **HHS2**		Coordination of Care **CHS2**			

Comments
(Enter pertinent information about reason for score of each complexity item here. For example, poor patient adherence, death in family with stress to child/youth, non-evidence-based treatment of celiac disease, etc.)

Scoring System

Green	0	= no vulnerability or need to act
Yellow	1	= mild vulnerability and need for monitoring or prevention
Orange	2	= moderate vulnerability and need for action or development of intervention plan
Red	3	= severe vulnerability and need for immediate action or immediate intervention plan

Biological Domain Items		**Psychological Domain Items**	
HB1	*Physical illness chronicity*	**HP1**	*Problems handling stress or engaging in problem solving*
		HP2	*Prior mental condition difficulties*
HB2	*Physical health diagnostic dilemma, prenatal exposures*	**HP3**	*Cognitive level and capabilities*
		HP4	*Early adverse physical and mental health events*
CB1	*Physical illness symptom severity and impairment*	**CP1**	*Resistance to treatment; nonadherence*
CB2	*Current difficulties in diagnosis and/or treatment*	**CP2**	*Current mental conditions symptom severity*
VB	*Risk of physical complications and life threat if case management is stopped*	**VP**	*Risk of persistent personal barriers or poor mental condition care if case management is stopped*

(Continued)

TABLE 8.1   **Pediatric INTERMED-Complexity Assessment Grid Scoring Sheet (Continued)**

Social Domain Items		Health System Domain Items	
HS1	Aptitude-correlated academic and social success	**HHS1**	Health system causes for poor access to appropriate care
HS2	Child/youth living environment and interactions		
HS3	Caregiver/parent physical and mental health condition and function	**HHS2**	Mistrust of doctors or the health system
CS1	Food and housing situation	**CHS1**	Ability to get and ease of getting needed services
CS2	Child/youth support system		
CS3	Caregiver/parent support system	**CHS2**	Coordination of and transitioning to age-appropriate care as requested
CS4	Attendance, achievement and behavior at school		
VS	Risk for home/school support or supervision needs if case management is stopped	**VHS**	Risk of persistent poor access to and/or coordination of services if case management is stopped

In practice, it is often easier to use the acronym PIM-CAG Scoring Sheet instead of the full, more explanatory name for this grid.

They have been developed as a guide for the case manager to ensure that all areas of complexity are addressed and that PIM-CAG scoring can be completed. If, however, items on the grid are answered while discussing topics related to other questions, there is no need to repeat questions about that content area unless further clarification is needed.

Before the interview begins, the case manager should review any clinical notes and/or claims information available about the child/youth. When the case manager is assigned to work with the child/youth, it is essential to first determine who the legal guardians are, to define issues of confidentiality and how they will be honored, and to discuss expectations for the child/youth and caregivers/parents. While this is sometimes less complicated with children than youth nearing the age of consent or majority, it remains an issue when the parents are divorced, separated, or in conflict about decisions concerning the child's/youth's health and care.

In the case of young children, the interview will usually be exclusively with a caregiver/parent. Sometimes caregivers/parents will complete the interview together. At other times, each caregiver/parent may wish to converse separately. As the age of the child increases, the child/youth will and should become more involved in the interview. While the caregiver/parent may provide a significant portion of the factual information, it is the child's/youth's health at stake. As early as possible, he or she should become involved in understanding and participating in his or her own care.

During a youth's adolescence, case managers should be sensitive to developing independence. Some youth have no objections to involvement by parents and full sharing of information. With others, privacy is a significant concern. Conversely, parents differ in their level of comfort discussing concerns about their children in the youth's presence. The case manager should be familiar with laws and regulations regarding when and how information between caregiver/parent and youth is to be shared. The youth and caregivers/parents should be informed at the beginning of the case management interview of the privacy standards and confidentiality limits that are relevant. This will prevent breakdown in the case manager-youth relationship when by necessity information obtained from the youth must be shared with the caregiver/parent.

As in the case of adults, children/youth are chosen for case management based on high potential for health complexity. As a result, the case manager should not try to rush through the scripted interview and scoring of the PIM-CAG. In all likelihood, the case manager will be working with the child/youth and caregivers/parents for months or even years as barriers to care are stabilized. While most initial assessments can likely be completed in one interview, if it takes two or three interview sessions to complete the PIM-CAG, it merely means that there has been more time devoted to establishing a relationship with the child/youth and his or her family.

The scripted interview has been primarily designed for use with the child/youth and caregiver/parent, however, the case manager will often seek permission to interface with the child's/youth's practitioners, teachers, relatives, and peers in order to obtain a clearer picture of issues that might be affecting health. It is the job of the case manager to secure appropriate informed consent to talk with stakeholders in the child's/youth's health but then to maximize validity of information through confirmation from multiple sources. When there is conflicting information, attempts should be made to resolve the discrepancy through clarifying conversations with informants having the most reliability.

GENERAL SCORING

The PIM-CAG contains 25 items in four domains, whereas the IM-CAG contains 20 items in four domains. The scoring range for the PIM-CAG, therefore, is from 0 to 75 while the scoring range for the IM-CAG is from 0 to 60. The domains for the adult and pediatric version are the same with the exception that the adult "Social" domain is labeled "Family/Social" in the pediatric version to reflect the importance and involvement of family issues in child/youth complexity. Two new items (concept areas) are added to the psychological domain and three to the family/social domain in the PIM-CAG. Several other items in the IM-CAG have been adapted to reflect child/youth issues.

The same decision point rules about complexity that apply to the IM-CAG also apply to the PIM-CAG—that is, they are based on the level of need for individualized care in order to overcome identified barriers to improvement. When there is debate about anchor point scoring, the immediacy of need for assistance will influence whether a higher or lower anchor point score is chosen. Actions related to anchor point scores are the same for the IM-CAG and PIM-CAG (e.g., 0 equals no action, and 3 equals immediate action).

In the PIM-CAG, "Historical" items refer to the child's/youth's entire life, however, special attention is to be given to the year prior to the assessment. There is one exception: "Access to Care" (HHS1) refers to the last 6 months. "Current" items refer to the 30-day period prior to the date of the PIM-CAG assessment. "Vulnerability" items refer to the 3- to 6-month period after the PIM-CAG assessment. *"Vulnerabilities" in the context of the PIM-CAG specifically relate to the risk of barrier persistence and/or worsening domain-specific problems in the future if individualized care through case management is withdrawn.*

Several items in the complexity grid contain more than one content component that could be creating barriers to improvement—for example, impaired family *or* peer relationships, prior adverse biological (lead exposure) *or* psychological events (sexual abuse), and so forth. When scoring each item, the content component with the *greatest* potential for creating a barrier to improvement should direct the score, rather than the average of the item components. For instance, if the child has little general medical illness severity but has significant impairment related to physical disabilities, the item score would reflect needs related to the impairment.

IM-CAG AND PIM-CAG ITEMS WITH THE SAME ANCHOR POINT WORDING

Of the 25 items in the PIM-CAG, 7 contain the same anchor point wording as in the IM-CAG. These include: "Chronicity" (HB1), "Diagnostic Dilemma" (HB2), "Symptom Severity/Impairment" (CB1), "Complications and Life Threat" (VB), "Mental Health History" (HP2), "Access to Care" (HHS1), and "Getting Needed Services" (CHS1). An additional item in the PIM-CAG, "Caregiver/Family Support" (CS3) is the same as "Social Support" (CS2) in the IM-CAG.

The overlap of these items was considered sufficiently similar for children/youth and adults to retain the same language. Similar anchor point wording also suggests that the actions that would be taken on behalf of children/youth would be similar to those taken on behalf of adults (Appendix 9). Inherent in pediatric case management is the assumption that management activities will involve caregivers/parents (especially in children/youth that have not reached the age of majority), the child/youth, and often the school system. Nevertheless, for items in the IM-CAG and the PIM-CAG with similar anchor point wording, the general approach to altering outcomes will utilize similar care plan principles and approaches.

IM-CAG AND PIM-CAG ITEMS WITH SIMILAR CONSTRUCTS BUT ADAPTED ANCHOR POINT WORDING

Twelve items from the IM-CAG have been adapted to meet the needs of children/youth. Two items, "Barriers to Coping" (HP1) and "Mental Health Symptoms" (CP2), differ only in that they replace child/youth examples of behaviors consistent with anchor point scores for the adult examples. Two additional items, "Resistance to Treatment" (CP1) and "Treatment Experience" (HHS2), merely differ in that the PIM-CAG items reflect the fact that it could be the child/youth or caregiver/parent who creates health barriers related to these concept areas.

Adding these 4 items in which minimal anchor point wording changes occurred to the 8 in which no changes from the adult version were made, totals 12 of 20 adult items that are essentially the same as pediatric items. For 2 items in the PIM-CAG, differences between adults and children/youth led to alteration in item names and anchor point designations: (a) from "Job and Leisure" (adult HS1) to "School and Community Participation" (pediatric CS4) and (b) from "Relationships" (adult HS2) to "Family and Social Relationships" (pediatric HS2). Three items in the PIM-CAG took on adapted anchor points but retained their item names: (a) "Diagnostic/Therapeutic Challenge" (CB2), (b) "Coordination of Care" (CHS2), and (c) "Residential Stability" (CS1).

"Job and Leisure" (adult HS1; Exhibit 7.22) and "School and Community Participation" (pediatric CS4; **Exhibit 8.1**) reflect similar conceptual constructs and thus have similar anchor point wording. Scoring for each addresses *attendance* at the central activity area in the person's life (job versus school) and the level of interaction with others (socialization skills/activities); however, the adult item approaches it from a historical perspective and the pediatric does so from a current state perspective. This is one area of potential confusion; however, it should become less so when a new item, "School Functioning" (pediatric HS1) is described that addresses "Historical" school *performance* and associated behaviors, which were considered to be more important historical complexity indicators for children/youth than were attendance and social interactions.

"Relationships" (adult HS2; Exhibit 7.24) reflects complexity introduced by an adult's inability to form and/or maintain personal relationships. "Family and Social Relationships" (pediatric HS2; **Exhibit 8.2**) addresses the same conceptual construct; however, it delineates in greater detail and with examples the areas

in which troubled relationships for children/youth may create complexity, such as a disturbed family setting or difficulty in developing and sustaining friendships with peers. While other relationships may be important influences in a child's/youth's life that contribute to complexity, such as with a teacher, a religious leader, and so forth, disrupted family and peer groups are most often involved.

"Residential Stability" (adult CS1; Exhibit 7.26) looks at the degree to which housing and support associated with housing stability contribute to health complexity in the adult. While stable housing is also a central need for children/youth, they also require support for child/youth-related activities, such as school attendance and transportation to social events, as well as nutritional sustenance from those in charge of their care. Because of these additional needs, the pediatric item (pediatric CS1; **Exhibit 8.3**) is intended to consolidate child/youth needs affected by the living arrangements of their family/caregivers. Up to this item, actions related to the pediatric complexity cells parallel those of adults adapted for the child/youth situation. The "Residential Stability" item, however, may involve behaviors by caregivers/parents, which create danger for the child/youth. As a result, it may require invoking assistance and/or involvement by child protective services as described in Chapter 5 (**Exhibit 8.4**).

In adults, complexity associated with "Diagnostic/Therapeutic Challenge" (adult CB2; Exhibit 7.8) arises more from the complicated nature of the illnesses and the treatments than from the effect of the treatments on the patient. In children/youth, the level of impact

---

EXHIBIT 8.1   Pediatric CS4 School and Community Participation Anchor Points

0. Attending school regularly, achieving and participating well, and actively engaged in extracurricular school or community activities (e.g., sports, clubs, hobbies, religious groups)
1. Average of one day of school missed/week and/or minor disruptions in achievement and behavior with few extracurricular activities
2. Average of two days or more of school missed/week and/or moderate disruption in achievement or behavior with resistance to extracurricular activities
3. Truant or school nonattendance with no extracurricular activities and no community connections

---

EXHIBIT 8.2   Pediatric HS2 Family and Social Relationships Anchor Points

0. Stable nurturing home, good social and peer relationships
1. Mild family problems, minor problems with social and peer relationships (e.g., parent-child conflict, frequent fights, marital discord, lacking close friends)
2. Moderate level of family problems, inability to initiate and maintain social and peer relationships (e.g., parental neglect, difficult separation/divorce, alcohol abuse, hostile caregiver, difficulties in maintaining same-age peer relationships)
3. Severe family problems with disruptive social and peer relationships (e.g., significant abuse, hostile child custody battles, addiction issues, parental criminality, complete social isolation, little or no association with peers)

EXHIBIT 8.3   Pediatric CS1 Residential Stability Anchor Points

0. Stable housing and financial support for personal growth needs
1. Mild stress with multiple moves, school changes, financial issues
2. Moderate stress with unstable housing and/or living situation support (e.g., living in shelter, poor nutrition); change of current living situation is required
3. Severe stress with no current satisfactory housing (e.g., homelessness, transient housing, child/youth malnourished, or dangerous environment); immediate change is necessary

---

EXHIBIT 8.4   Actions Related to Pediatric CS1 Residential Stability Scores

1. **Inconsistent living situation:**
   - Make sure that child/youth's safety, supervision, and nourishment needs are being met
2. **Unstable housing and/or living situation support:**
   - In collaboration with the parents, if possible, initiate contact with social service or other community resources to look into housing and food services options
   - Get assistance to help correct the cause of the residential instability (e.g., financial limitations, family conflict, natural disaster, etc.)
   - Inquire about outcome
   - Use knowledge of community resources to push the system
3. **Unsafe housing situation for child/youth:**
   - *Immediately* involve protective services to locate a safe living situation for the child/youth (e.g., foster home, youth facility)
   - Perform actions under #2
   - Include customized actions based on interview
   - Report situations requiring legal notification to authorities

---

EXHIBIT 8.5   Pediatric CB2 Diagnostic/Therapeutic Challenge Anchor Points

0. Uncomplicated diagnosis; treatment with few unpleasant side effects or risks
1. Clear differential diagnoses and/or diagnosis expected; noninvasive treatment with multiple components and/or minor but tolerable side effects
2. Difficult to diagnose but physical cause/origin expected; invasive treatment and/or multiple components with some risks and unpleasant side effects
3. Difficult to diagnose with interfering factors other than physical cause/origin; daily complex, invasive, and/or cross-disciplinary treatment; potentially serious risks and toxic side effects

---

that treatments themselves have on the child/youth also introduces its own therapeutic challenge. This is addressed by the change in anchor point wording for the pediatric CB2 (**Exhibit 8.5**) and has implications for how the child/youth and his or her caregivers will be assisted as complicated interventions are given.

The need to transition delivery of health services from health professionals that specialize in the care of children/youth to those who primarily treat adults creates a special problem for the pediatric item labeled "Coordination of Care" (pediatric CHS2; **Exhibit 8.6**) as youth reach the age of majority or consent (see Chapter 5 section "Special Pediatric and Child Psychiatry Circumstances"). Particularly in children/youth with health

complexity, there is reluctance for family practitioners or general internists, or even needed specialists, to take on such patients. Not only do complex youth turning to adults consume much clinical time and effort in getting to know them and becoming acquainted with their health needs, they also fall among patients with limited financial resources and/or insurance. For instance, in the United States, complex children/youth may be covered under a specialized youth-focused insurance product before transition, but may become uninsurable because of so-called preexisting conditions at the age of majority. Transition of care is a common area of case management assistance for these youth and is reflected in action items related to the coordination of care (**Exhibit 8.7**).

EXHIBIT 8.6   **Pediatric CHS2 Coordination of Care Anchor Points**

0. Complete practitioner communication with good coordination and transition of care
1. Limited practitioner communication and coordination of care; pediatrician coordinates medical and mental health services
2. Poor communication and coordination of care among practitioners; no routine pediatrician; difficulty in transitioning to age-appropriate care
3. No communication and coordination of care among practitioners; primary emergency room use to meet non-emergent health needs; systemic barriers to age-appropriate care transition

---

EXHIBIT 8.7   **Actions Related to Pediatric CHS2 Coordination of Care Scores**

1. **Limited practitioner communication and coordination of care:**
   - Encourage record sharing and communication among all clinicians, including mental health and complementary medicine
   - Open links for important communication
2. **Poor communication and coordination of care among practitioners:**
   - Determine and augment communication links between physical and mental health practitioners
   - Ensure note sharing among clinicians working with child/youth
   - Assist in coordinating appointments and transportation
   - Help child/youth get same-day appointments for different problems
   - Investigate availability of integrated clinics (medical home)
   - Determine reason for missed appointment (overcome barriers)
   - Assist with transition from pediatric care to adult practitioner care
3. **No communication and coordination of care among practitioners:**
   - *Immediately* perform actions under #1 and #2
   - Include customized actions based on interview
   - Serve as link for child/youth with various practitioners (i.e. fax accumulated clinical information to practitioners after release of information obtained [see Appendix 3 for universal release example])
   - Talk with treating practitioners on behalf of child/youth but also educate caregivers/parents on how to do so
   - Create alternatives to emergency room use
   - Enlist assistance from case management medical director to try to establish a medical home

---

PIM-CAG ITEMS UNIQUE TO CHILDREN/YOUTH

Five new items have been added to the IM-CAG, which allows the PIM-CAG to complete the assessment of health complexity in children/youth. These include: "Cognitive Development" (pediatric HP3), "Adverse Developmental Events" (pediatric HP4), "School Functioning" (pediatric HS1), "Caregiver/Parent Health and Function" (pediatric HS3), and "Child/Youth Support" (pediatric CS2). These five items recognize and capture complexity related to developmental factors, school, peer interactions, and the dependent role of children/youth.

While cognitive deficits can occur in adults (e.g., various dementias), they have a different connotation and impact on complexity than cognitive difficulties in children/youth. This item encompasses the presence of intellectual disabilities, as well as the spectrum of developmental disorders (Asperger's, pervasive developmental disorders, autism). As a result, a separate item called "Cognitive Development" (pediatric HP3; **Exhibit 8.8**)

has been added under the "Psychological" domain for children/youth, whereas cognitive impairment in adults would be historically documented under the "Mental Health History" (adult HP2). There is no question that some adults with cognitive difficulties may require additional case management assistance; however, in children/youth, as anchor point levels for "Cognitive Development" increase, they raise the potential need for specialized educational settings, support personnel in the home, and assistance with socialization since development delay is not understood and is often handled poorly by uninformed and/or insensitive peers (**Exhibit 8.9**).

Another item, which has been added to the "Psychological" domain, is "Adverse Developmental Events" (pediatric HP4; **Exhibit 8.10**). Its purpose is to expose physical and mental health factors that may influence past and potentially future cognitive ability, emotions, and/or behavior (e.g., toxic exposures, traumatic brain injuries, psychological or sexual abuse, and central nervous system illnesses). While some of the

---

EXHIBIT 8.8   **Pediatric HP3 Cognitive Development Anchor Points**

0. No cognitive impairment
1. Possible developmental delay or immaturity; low IQ
2. Delayed development; mild or moderate cognitive impairment
3. Severe and pervasive developmental delays or profound cognitive impairment

---

EXHIBIT 8.9   **Actions Related to Pediatric HP3 Cognitive Development Scores**

1. **Possible developmental delay or immaturity; low IQ:**
   - Assist in establishing level of impairment, including capacity of child to communicate physical needs and symptoms
   - Discuss level of impairment and needs with caregivers, educator, and the pediatrician to ensure appropriate placement in school system
   - Assess need for remedial educational assistance and home support
   - Observe
2. **Delayed development; mild or moderate mental retardation:**
   - Perform actions under #1
   - Assist caregiver/parent and pediatrician in identifying appropriate educational placement and support
   - Review performance/adjustment issues with school facility; involve social services if needed
   - Assess and assist with home support for child/youth based on functional capabilities and respite for caregivers/parents
   - Assess and share child/youth's ability to communicate
3. **Severe and pervasive developmental delays or profound mental retardation:**
   - *Immediately* perform actions under #1 and #2
   - Include customized action based on interview
   - Work with caregiver, pediatrician, and other clinicians to ensure appropriate support for child/youth special needs
   - Consider and assist with placement options, if necessary

---

EXHIBIT 8.10   **Pediatric HP4 Adverse Developmental Events Anchor Points**

0. No identified developmental traumas or injuries (e.g., physical or sexual abuse, meningitis, lead exposure, etc.)
1. Traumatic prior experiences or injuries with no apparent or stated impact on child/youth
2. Traumatic prior experiences or injuries with potential relationship to impairment in child/youth
3. Traumatic prior experiences with apparent and significant direct relationship to impairment in child/youth

---

adverse events are the result of general medical illness or intoxications, this item is included in the "Psychological" domain since the events typically result in mental health symptoms. When there are residual physical effects of the early life trauma, they may additionally be captured in HB2, CB1, or CB2 depending on whether the physical symptoms create a diagnostic dilemma, contribute to symptoms or impairment, or contribute to uncertainty about current diagnosis or treatment.

As mentioned earlier, "School Functioning" (pediatric HS1; **Exhibit 8.11**) is a historical item intended to document past performance in the school setting. In the context of HS1, performance includes a consolidated look at achievement, attendance, and behavior. These three factors are often related to each other

and suggest the need for tighter involvement with the child/youth as barriers are addressed since past performance is often a predictor of future performance. "School and Community Participation" differs from "School Functioning" in that it focuses on current attendance and community socialization. Current performance can also be a school issue but it will commonly be captured under "Mental Health Symptoms" (pediatric CP2) or "Barriers to Coping" (pediatric HP1).

Unlike adults, virtually all children/youth depend on a parent or caregiver for a place to live, nutritional sustenance, personal and emotional development, support during intellectual and social development, assistance with learning decision-making skills, maintenance of a safe environment, and many

---

EXHIBIT 8.11   **Pediatric HS1 School Functioning Anchor Points**

0. Performing well in school with good achievement, attendance, and behavior
1. Performing adequately in school although there are some achievement, attendance, and behavior problems (e.g., missed classes, pranks)
2. Experiencing moderate problems with school achievement, attendance, and/or behavior (e.g., school disciplinary action, few school-related peer relationships, academic probation)
3. Experiencing severe problems with school achievement, attendance, and/or behavior (e.g., home bound education, school suspension, violence, illegal activities at school, academic failure, school dropout, disruptive peer group activity)

EXHIBIT 8.12   **Pediatric HS3 Caregiver (Parent) Health and Function Anchor Points**

0. All caregivers healthy
1. Physical and/or mental health issues, including poor coping skills, and/or permanent disability, present in one or more caregiver, which do not impact parenting
2. Physical and/or mental health conditions, including disrupted coping resources, and/or permanent disability, present in one or more caregiver, which interfere with parenting
3. Physical and/or mental health conditions, including disrupted coping styles, and/or permanent disability, present in one or more caregiver, which prevent effective parenting and/or create a dangerous situation for the child/youth

---

EXHIBIT 8.13   **Pediatric CS2 Child/Youth Support Anchor Points**

0. Supervision and/or assistance readily available from family/caregiver, friends/peers, teachers, and/or community social networks (e.g., spiritual/religious groups) at all times
1. Supervision and/or assistance generally available from family/caregiver, friends/peers, teachers, and/or community social networks; but possible delays
2. Limited supervision and/or assistance available from family/caregiver, friends/peers, teachers, and/or community social networks
3. No effective supervision and/or assistance available from family/caregiver, friends/peers, teachers, and/or community social networks at any time

---

other parenting activities. If one or more of the child's/youth's caregivers/parents is ill or disabled, it can place a direct and/or indirect burden on the child/youth. If the parent/caregiver has poor coping skills; has potentially destructive behaviors, such as chemical dependence, participates in illegal activities, or just neglect the child/youth, they can inflict both intended and unintended psychological and physical trauma. Conversely, caregivers/parents who provide good supervision and support in a caring household have the ability to overcome complexity barriers with their child/youth much more facilely than those without these traits.

For this reason, an item addressing "Caregiver/Parent Health and Function" (pediatric HS3; **Exhibit 8.12**) has been added to provide a general assessment of the person/people responsible for the child's/youth's development, health, and safety. The broad terms "health" and "function" are intended to encompass a composite of physical and mental health, including substance abuse or dependence, personal traits that allow the caregiver/parent to provide effective parenting, and

health limitations that might interfere with the caregiver's/parent's ability to support a child's/youth's development. At the positive end of the spectrum, the item can indicate strengths within the family that can be used to support correction of a child's/youth's barriers to improvement. At the negative end, it could indicate the need to activate child protective services on behalf of the child/youth.

Technically, the last added item is "Caregiver/Family Support" (pediatric CS3) since the adult and child/youth social support items should be similar if not the same. In fact, the "Caregiver/Family Support" item is essentially the same as the IM-CAG "Social Support" (adult CS2) item since parameters for adult support are similar, whereas "Child/Youth Support" (pediatric CS2; **Exhibit 8.13**) involves not so much backup in crisis as supervision, assistance with personal growth issues, and emotional support. Support for children/youth can come from family, peers, teachers, community networks, and so forth and is usually an ongoing need rather than a need related to crisis.

INTEGRATED CASE MANAGEMENT CARE PLAN DEVELOPMENT USING THE PIM-CAG SCORING SYSTEM

As with the adult IM-CAG, the PIM-CAG allows the case manager to separate areas of complexity in the child/youth and his or her caregiver/parent and to prioritize them during the development of a care plan. While each anchor point (Appendix 7) leads to specific actions (Appendix 9) designed to overcome barriers to improvement, the case manager must pull back and look at the interaction of items as well as the items themselves as is described in Chapter 9. Scores of 2 and 3 will drive initial concerns; however, they may be connected with each other or with items having scores suggesting less need for initial attention. For instance, a child may be significantly late for dialysis sessions several times a month with resultant consequences since his parents are not available to transport him to the dialysis center (CHS1). This may be due to a restricted caregiver/family support system (CS3) and several recent moves by the family due to job changes (CS1). Without connecting these dots and working with the child's family to come up with short- and long-term solutions, the case manager will find it difficult to overcome the therapeutic challenge (CB2) and potential symptom worsening (CB1).

REFERENCES

Huyse, F. J., & Stiefel, F. C. (Eds.). *Integrated care for the complex medically* ill. [Special issue.]. Medical Clinics of North America, 90 (2006).

Lyons, J. S. (2004). *Redressing the emperor: Improving our Children's public mental health system.* Westport, CT: Praeger.

Lyons, J. S., Baerger, D. R., Almeida, M. C., & Lyons, M. B. (1999). *Child and Adolescent Needs and Strengths: An information integration tool for early development—CANS—0 to 3 manual.* Chicago: Praed Foundation.

CHAPTER 9

Interpreting Complexity Assessment Grid Anchor Point Scores

- To provide an overview of the Complexity Assessment Grid (CAG) and its administration in integrated case management programs
- To explain general principles in scoring anchor points for each item in the CAG
- To describe how to link anchor points in the development of an actionable care plan
- To indicate the potential use of CAG methodology for change measurement and case manager caseload estimation

USING CAG METHODOLOGY IN INTEGRATED CASE MANAGEMENT

Chapter 7 provided a description of each individual adult complexity item in the INTERMED-Complexity Assessment Grid (IM-CAG). Chapter 8 compared and contrasted the IM-CAG with the pediatric version, the PIM-CAG, which adapts the same methodology to children/youth. Both chapters discuss the barriers that each item was designed to uncover in adult and pediatric populations, the actions that should be considered depending on the anchor point score for each item, the goals related to the initiation of actions, and what constitutes success when attempts are made to alter outcomes when working with a patient. Without an understanding of these basic components of CAG methodology, it would be difficult to efficiently overcome barriers to improvement using integrated case management. CAG methodology is systematic, goal-directed, and action-oriented.

Once case managers start using the IM-CAG and the PIM-CAG, however, they quickly learn that the use of these tools requires more than an understanding of the items and associated actions. The foils used in each item, as well as how the items themselves interact with each other, must also be understood. For instance, as described in Chapter 7, multiple items can, at the same time, be associated with nonadherence (Exhibit 7.1). All potential contributors, and their interactions, will need to be recognized and, if needed, addressed for patients to become adherent to their clinician's recommendations.

Items interact in other more direct ways as well. One of the most common questions/complaints of new case managers using this methodology is that there can be a diagnostic and/or therapeutic challenge in the biological domain (CB2) that is due to mental health symptoms in the psychological domain (CP2). Should the problem be scored red (3) in the biological domain or should emphasis be located in the psychological? After all, the problem *is* related to a mental condition. Should both be scored high? Which should be tackled first? These are the type of questions that this chapter addresses.

In this chapter, the meaning of each CAG item within each domain will be described first in the historical, current state, and vulnerability/prognosis axes. Then items will be connected to other items commonly linked to them. This will help case managers see patterns of interacting items that can be tackled as a unit with the patient, the patient's family, and/or the patient's providers. Unless case managers recognize these links, the patient will not.

Further, CAG methodology is based on more than just a collection of the scored items on which to act. Case managers cannot mindlessly score and assist with each item and assume that they have utilized integrated case management to help the patient. Integrated case management is a way of seeing the patient as a whole while being able to differentiate and extricate components that make return to health elusive.

GENERAL SCORING PRINCIPLES

ITEMS WITH MULTIPLE COMPONENTS

A number of items in the IM-CAG and the PIM-CAG have multiple components—for example, Symptom Severity/Impairment (adult and pediatric CB1), Job and Leisure Problems (adult HS1), and School and Community Participation (pediatric CS4). For instance, patients can have severe illness but no impairment and vice versa. When scoring each item on the CAG, the intent is to uncover components of illness, illness behavior, or personal situations that lead to barriers to improvement and/or stabilization. Thus, if a patient has no diagnostic challenge but treatment is difficult (adult and pediatric CB2), then the severity level consistent with the component of the item that would lead to poor outcome would be preferentially scored and the actions associated with it initiated. For some case managers this apparent conflict creates dissonance, but once they realize that the intent of each item is to uncover areas in which action can be taken to improve the patient's situation, it becomes easy to interpret and score the item.

SCALED SEVERITY RESPONSES

A number of items in each of the domains are scaled on severity with the qualifiers: "No," "Mild," "Moderate," or "Severe." In some instances, examples are used to clarify what constitutes factors that help indicate whether a patient fits into one of the severity indicators for that item. In others, more clinical judgment is needed to make the determination. Regardless, when scaled qualifiers are used and there is uncertainty about whether the item should be scored 1 or 2 or 2 or 3, the case manager then reverts to the immediacy with which action should be taken and the potential value that will be brought to the patient. In most cases, this resolves scoring decisions. For instance, if problems with relationships (adult and pediatric HS2) are considered a major barrier to improvement and immediate action is needed to effectively correct it, this would be scored 3 rather than 2.

When assessing "Vulnerability," scaled severity indicators are also used; however, scoring for vulnerability is not usually associated with immediate action. Rather, vulnerability is used as an estimator of future risk. For this reason, higher scores on scaled vulnerability items will reflect the degree to which historical and current state barriers to care have been and/or need to be addressed and stabilized before the patient is returned to standard care. They will influence how and when the case manager transitions the patient back to standard care by his or her providers. As patients move to a vulnerability level of 1, it is usually time to begin preparing the patient, the patient's family, and their practitioners for case closure by discussing the successes that now allow transition back to standard care. Patients, patients' families (with permission), and the patients' practitioners should be provided with initial and follow-up CAG assessments, care plan outcomes, and ideas about continued patient needs after graduation (Figure 3.5 and Appendix 1G). Patients considered at greater risk for poor outcomes

without continued case management support—that is, vulnerability levels of 2 and 3—would remain in case management and only transition back to standard care when their prognosis has improved.

There is a caveat in scoring the "Vulnerability" items. Essentially, there is no time at which standard care will have exactly the same outcomes as individualized care. Extra help by a case manager, especially in complex patients, routinely brings added value if properly applied. There is, however, a diminishing return as health stabilizes.

It is the case managers' job, with the assistance of their supervisors, to determine when their valuable services could bring greater assistance to new patients. Case managers are most helpful in those with the greatest complexity as long as the patients are willing to participate in regaining health and have remediable problems. Thus, case managers with their supervisors and overseeing physicians must balance the risks associated with closing a case versus keeping it in their patient panel. This can be challenging, particularly when a strong relationship has been built and there is a reluctance on both the patient's and the case manager's part to move on. Case management, however, is time intensive. Without graduating cases, few can be added.

HEALTH PROBLEMS WITH IMPACT ON SEVERAL ITEMS

In the following discussion, situations will be described in which the same patient circumstances directly influence two or more items in the same or different domains. For instance, a patient may be missing much work because of headaches that do not respond to typical analgesics or alterations in headache-related behaviors. Further exploration suggests that recognized and untreated depression is contributing substantially to the persistence of headache symptoms. This set of clinical circumstances has a direct bearing on scoring for items "Diagnostic/Therapeutic Challenge" (CB2) and "Mental Health Symptoms" (CP2).

For CB2, the correct severity level would be 3 since "other issues than physical causes" are contributing to symptom persistence, patient impairment (CB1), and apparent resistance to treatment (CP1). On the other hand, the depression may be only mild to moderate in intensity (CP2) and warrant a score of 2. This is an area in which linking items is critical to achieve rapid resolution of multifaceted components of complexity need.

For the preceding situation using traditional nonintegrated case management techniques, the focus would be on ensuring the correct diagnostic assessment for the headaches and adherence to analgesic treatment. Even in integrated case management, if the linking of items is not considered, there could be similar exclusive and/or disproportionate attention given to the headaches themselves. If headaches are linked to depression, on the other hand, they remain a focus of attention; however, treatment of depression, which may technically be considered to have less imminent need, becomes a primary intervention as an indirect treatment for the headaches.

While this is a much-simplified view of the way that patient circumstances can be related to more than one item, it illustrates the importance of making these connections. It also reinforces the importance of a complete all-domain CAG assessment for complexity before the care plan is fully developed and discussed with the patient and the patient's clinicians. One of the real values of the CAG is that it forces assessment in most areas that create barriers to improvement but are often missed by clinicians because of lack of time, interest, or recognition of importance.

IM-CAG SCORES VERSUS PIM-CAG SCORES

Virtually all research related to the use of CAG methodology has been performed on patients in adult clinical settings. It is only in this manual and in selected research contexts, such as at the Children's Hospital of Eastern Ontario, that adult IM-CAG methodology has been adapted and introduced for use in children/youth through the development of the PIM-CAG. Despite the fact that the adult and pediatric CAGs contain much overlap, users of the PIM-CAG should be aware that value brought through its implementation has not yet been empirically demonstrated. While lack of evidence does not equate to lack of effectiveness, it is worthwhile to discuss issues related to the rationale for and adoption of PIM-CAG use.

First, the PIM-CAG draws on the communimetric method of assessment used in the Child and Adolescent Needs and Strengths (CANS) tool and has benefited from the input and support of those involved in the development of the CANS, namely Dr. John Lyons. While the PIM-CAG adds biological and health service components to the child/youth assessment and has been created specifically in this manual for use by case managers rather than treating clinicians, it incorporates approaches that have demonstrated value when behavioral health outcomes are targeted for intervention. Specifically, the IM-CAG, PIM-CAG, and CANS all incorporate principles of communimetrics in their organizational structure. On these grounds, there is reason to believe that the PIM-CAG should have performance characteristics similar to the CANS and the IM-CAG.

In addition, a pilot study conducted by one of the coauthors (Cohen, J. S., Mack, D., Lyons, J., Operationalizing biopsychosocial case complexity: an initial examination of the interrater reliability of a clinical decision-making tool for use with children and youth with chronic illness, unpublished raw data, 2009) examined interrater reliability of the items on the PIM-CAG. Health professionals trained in the use of the PIM-CAG rated a series of clinical vignettes developed from case records, representing a variety of complexity levels and presenting with varied medical, psychological, social, and health system concerns and symptoms. The results of this pilot study indicated that individual items on the PIM-CAG could be reliability rated, with interclass correlations for the majority of items across all vignettes falling in the range of 0.65 to 0.90. These initial findings support the viability of adapting the IM-CAG methodology to assess complexity in children and youth.

BIOLOGICAL DOMAIN

HISTORICAL

Chronicity (Table 9.1)

Risk scores for chronicity are based on whether the patient suffered any periods of physical complaints or diseases over the past 5 years. An important factor in scoring this item is to note whether the complaints or diseases:

- Were effectively treated thus allowing symptoms to disappear, such as recovery from pneumonia or a car accident
- Spontaneously remitted and did not return, such as an episode of stomach pain
- Were intermittent but of little consequence other than as minor symptoms and/or inconveniences, such as tension headaches or palpitations
- Were chronic, requiring continuous care, such as diabetes, heart failure, kidney diseases, rheumatoid diseases, or Parkinson's disease

If the patient has a chronic disease (anchor point 2) or several chronic illnesses (anchor point 3), this implies several things about the patient. First, he or she should have or develop a long-term relationship with at least one primary health care professional. Further, the quality of this relationship is very important since

TABLE 9.1	Chronicity (HB1)
Score	**Anchor points**
0	Less than 3 months of physical symptoms/dysfunction; acute health condition
1	More than 3 months of physical symptoms/dysfunction or several periods of less than 3 months
2	A chronic condition
3	Several chronic conditions

it will predict patient adherence and the efforts made to regain health. Thus, a score of 2 or 3 on the chronicity item will automatically inform the case manager that the *health system* item titled "Treatment Experience" (HHS2), which explores the patient-doctor relationship, is of relevance.

Second, if a patient suffers from a chronic illness or an acute but serious illness, it alters that patient's lifestyle and usually requires the adoption of healthy behaviors. For patients to adapt, they must possess an ability to cope with frustration and lifestyle limitations and/or to initiate health-related activities, such as dieting, exercising, or taking medication. This links chronicity to the psychological items "Barriers to Coping" (HP1) and "Resistance to Treatment" (CP1). In the PIM-CAG, this could also be present in the caregivers/parents of the child/youth and would be captured in the item labeled "Caregiver/Parent Health and Function" (pediatric HS3), or lead to stress in the caregiver's/parent's ability to support the child/youth, "Child/Youth Support" (pediatric CS2).

Third, epidemiological evidence indicates that chronic diseases have a tendency to cluster. A third of patients with a chronic disease will have several chronic diseases (Smith, 2009). For instance, a common combination of diseases is diabetes, heart failure, and kidney disease. We call this phenomenon multimorbidity. A crucial aspect in the treatment of patients with multiple diseases is the adjustment and coordination of their individual treatments. This brings into play health system items "Getting Needed Services" (CHS1) and "Coordination of Care" (CHS2). In 2005, an elderly patient with five chronic illnesses was discussed in the *Journal of the American Medical Association* (Boyd et al., 2005). If she had complied with all the treatment recommendations by her different specialists, it would have been a full-time job. In patients with multimorbidity, coordinated care is essential.

Fourth, psychiatric disorders are significantly more frequent in patients with chronic physical disease. While depression occurs in 4% of the general population, the incidence is higher in patients with chronic illness. For instance, it is 12% in patients with diabetes, 15% in patients with heart failure, and up to 30% in patients with kidney disease and HIV (Katon & Seelig, 2008; Melek & Norris, 2008; Seelig & Katon, 2008; Sheehan, 2002). Similar high prevalence rates are also seen for anxiety disorders, substance use disorders, and dementia in the frail elderly (Kathol, Saravay, Lobo, & Ormel, 2006). For this reason, special attention is required to document risks for complexity based on the psychological domain items "Mental Health History" (HP2) and "Mental Health Symptoms" (CP2).

The most important effect of concurrent psychiatric disorders in those with chronic illnesses is their negative impact on adherence to treatment (see Chapter 2 section "Impact of Comorbidity on Health and Cost Outcomes") due to a variety of factors (Exhibit 7.1).

Other consequences, however, can be subtler. For instance, the presence of a psychiatric disorder can make patients more vulnerable to loss of insurance ("Access to Care" [HHS1]); can make coordination of care more difficult since physical and mental condition practitioners typically don't communicate with each other ("Coordination of Care" [CHS2]); and can make the logistics of making and attending appointments more challenging ("Getting Needed Services" [CHS1]). They can also alter patients' perceptions of their medical symptoms and lead to more frequent and/or exaggerated general medical complaints, making the diagnostic process more difficult ("Diagnostic Dilemma" [HB2]) or their current diagnosis and treatment more challenging ("Diagnostic/Therapeutic Challenge" [CB2]).

Therefore, scoring one or several chronic diseases on this risk assessment should automatically trigger the need for an integrated treatment plan, which includes the principles of chronic care as formulated by Wagner (Wagner, 1998; Wagner et al., 2005):

- Longitudinal multidisciplinary care, including psychosocial components
- Focus on adherence to therapy
- Attention to the quality of the relationship between patients and their clinicians

Diagnostic Dilemma (Table 9.2)

Often physical complaints indicate a physical disease. However, the majority of physical complaints—that is, about 70% of those seen in primary care patients—gradually disappear and cannot be attributed by doctors to a specific disease (Kroenke & Mangelsdorff, 1989; Kroenke & Rosmalen, 2006). This can be related to several factors. Some patients have waxing and waning physical complaints without any sign of a disease because certain individuals have a tendency to augment normal bodily

TABLE 9.2   **Diagnostic Dilemma (HB2)**

Score	Anchor points
0	No period of diagnostic complexity
1	Diagnosis was clarified quickly
2	Diagnostic dilemma solved but only with considerable diagnostic effort
3	Diagnostic dilemma not solved despite considerable diagnostic efforts

sensations. Other patients may have physical complaints that cannot be linked to a disease because the physical disease is too early in its expression to be detected or cannot be easily identified through existing diagnostic tests. Examples include slowly developing conditions and/or those with diverse symptoms patterns, such as systemic lupus erythematosis and multiple sclerosis.

Alternatively, physical symptoms can be a manifestation of a psychiatric disorder. For instance, patients with panic disorder experience physical symptoms during panic attacks, including pain in the chest, dizziness, a dry mouth, or tingling sensations in their extremities. Patients with depression describe fatigue, low energy, and insomnia but can also have augmentation of symptoms associated with coexisting and objective physical disorders, such as lumbar disc herniation, hypothyroidism, emphysema, and so forth. About 50% of patients with more than four complaints of pain, whether or not these complaints are caused by a physical illness, such as cancer, will suffer from depression. In fact, about 70% of the patients with depressive disorder present in primary care with physical, not psychological, complaints (Kroenke, Jackson, & Chamberlin, 1997).

Illnesses that have created a diagnostic dilemma often can predict future diagnostic and therapeutic challenges ("Diagnostic/Therapeutic Challenge" [CB2]) or could be an indication that there is risk of longer lasting or current psychiatric contributors to symptom development and persistence ("Mental Health History and/or Symptoms" [HP2 and CP2]). They can also influence patients' interactions with or perceptions of health care personnel and trust in the health care delivery system ("Treatment Experience" [HHS2]). Unresolved symptoms frustrate both patients and doctors and lead to unspoken hostility, noncooperation, unnecessary tests and treatments, fruitless referral, and/or neglect. For this reason, clarification of what caused the diagnostic dilemma and how it might be contributing to current treatment resistance is an important activity.

Finally, a diagnostic dilemma can occur in children/youth as a result of limited history taking by treating practitioners or poor records about prenatal toxic exposures, such as to alcohol, cocaine, or heavy metals; in utero infections, such as meningitis or encephalitis; or childhood head trauma. For children/youth falling into this category, it will be important to assess "Cognitive Development" (HP3); to review school performance ("School Functioning" [HS1]) and current school participation ("School and Community Participation" [CS4]); and to make sure that the family has the appropriate support and resources required ("Caregiver/Family Support" [CS3]).

CURRENT STATE

Symptom Severity/Impairment (Table 9.3)

The seriousness of patients' physical complaints is an important determinant of their capacity to function independently. In the case of most acute illnesses, symptoms will disappear or diminish; however, when associated with a new or existing chronic disease, symptoms can disappear, occur intermittently, persist, or increase. Thus, the level of symptom severity or impairment can raise concerns about vulnerabilities in the future ("Complications and Life Threat" [VB]). More serious physical complaints and related impairment may require greater attention to rehabilitation planning or follow-up to prevent the risk of the patient becoming persistently symptomatic or dependent on help from family and friends.

If the level of symptom severity or impairment is significant with a likelihood of the need for future assistance, then social factors require additional attention (e.g., "Social Support" [adult CS2], "Child/Youth Support" [pediatric CS2] "Residential Stability" [adult and pediatric CS1], and "Family/School/Social Vulnerability" [adult and pediatric VS]). Concerns about livelihood may also arise ("Job and Leisure" [adult HS1]) and school attendance in children/youth ("School and Community Participation" [pediatric CS4]). Seemingly nonassociated factors in the health system domain may also come into play. For instance, impaired individuals may lose their insurance (HHS1). Severely ill patients may have difficulty getting out of the house to attend appointments (CHS1). These factors can create multiple vulnerabilities (VB, VS, VHS) or lead to the development of "Mental Health Symptoms" (CP2). In youth, near the age of majority, such factors can lead to difficulties in identifying adult clinicians willing to accept youth with health complexity as they transition to adult care ("Coordination of Care" [pediatric CHS2]).

TABLE 9.3	Symptom Severity/Impairment (CB1)

Score	Anchor points
0	No physical symptoms or symptoms resolve with treatment
1	Mild symptoms, which do not interfere with current functioning
2	Moderate symptoms, which interfere with current functioning
3	Severe symptoms leading to inability to perform many functional activities

Diagnostic/Therapeutic Challenge (Tables 9.4 and 9.5)

Patients may have physical symptoms in which the relation of illness to its treatment is clear and unequivocal (e.g., typical symptoms of an upper respiratory infection or a broken arm). In other patients, new or existing physical complaints may be obscure or treatment resistant (e.g., chronic pelvic pain, dizziness). Symptoms become difficult to diagnose when they are caused by:

- A rare (uncommon) disease (e.g., celiac disease [gluten intolerance])
- A condition early in its development (e.g., pancreatic cancer)
- An atypical presentation of a common illness (e.g., weakness in a patient with cardiac ischemia)
- An augmentation of normal bodily sensations (e.g., ascribing acute joint pain to rheumatoid disease)
- A manifestation of psychiatric illness (e.g., concern about occult cancer in a patient with depression, somatoform disorder, or psychotic somatic delusions)

Unexplained treatment resistance or not knowing which treatment to use, on the other hand, could relate to:

- Diagnostic uncertainty or an incorrect diagnosis
- Nonadherence
- Poor or incorrect treatment instructions (e.g., misplaced decimal in a medication prescription)
- Delayed response
- Treatment-resistant illness (e.g., brittle diabetes)
- Use of ineffective treatments (e.g., joint space debridement in osteoarthritis of the knee)
- Need for a combination of treatments (e.g., diet, exercise, oral hypoglycemics, and an antidepressant for a diabetic patient)

- Treatment for an illness when no physical condition is present, (e.g., somatization disorder, malingering)

The case manager is not responsible for diagnosis or treatment, however, coming to some understanding about the barriers to improvement can make a major difference in the future clinical and functional state of the patient, use of health care resources, and the risk for iatrogenic illness. Thus, it is an area in which careful review of clinical information, discussions with care providers, and questions to the case manager's physician supervisor can be particularly helpful. For instance, when a patient has a condition such as back pain and is not responding to evidence-based therapeutic interventions or is falling outside of disability duration guidelines (Denniston, 2009), then further testing or referral may be in order (HB2). Alternatively, treatment nonresponse could be related to the existence of unconsidered psychiatric illness, such as depression (CP2) or poor coping mechanisms (HP1).

An important subgroup of patients who often score high on this item are those who have a psychiatric condition known as somatization disorder (see Chapter 6 section "Summary of Unexplained Somatic Complaints"). An easy way to conceptualize patients with this type of health disturbance is that they are on the far end of the spectrum of those who augment normal bodily sensations or physical characteristics. For them, a grumbling stomach can raise concerns about an ulcer; a simple benign fatty deposit (lipoma) can raise concerns about terminal cancer. While these patients will often have one or more objectively diagnosed medical

TABLE 9.4	Diagnostic/Therapeutic Challenge (Adult CB2)
Score	**Anchor points**
0	Clear diagnoses and/or uncomplicated treatments
1	Clear differential diagnoses and/or diagnosis expected with clear treatments
2	Difficult to diagnose and treat; physical cause/origin and treatment expected
3	Difficult to diagnose or treat; other issues than physical causes interfering with diagnostic and therapeutic process

TABLE 9.5	Diagnostic/Therapeutic Challenge (Pediatric CB2)
Score	**Anchor points**
0	Uncomplicated diagnosis; treatment with few unpleasant side effects or risks
1	Clear differential diagnoses and/or diagnosis expected; noninvasive treatment with multiple components and/or minor but tolerable side effects
2	Difficult to diagnose but physical cause/origin expected; invasive treatment and/or multiple components with some risks and unpleasant side effects
3	Difficult to diagnose with interfering factors other than physical cause/origin; daily, complex, invasive, and/or cross-disciplinary treatment; potentially serious risks and toxic side effects

illnesses, their use of medical services and the number of treatments they undergo far exceeds the level of need based on illness present (Margalit & El-Ad, 2008).

In these patients, symptoms can be exaggerated (CB1), relationships with providers are typically poor (HHS2), coordination of care is difficult because of patient resistance even if desired by the patient's clinicians (CHS2), and vulnerability to iatrogenic medical complications (VB) can be considerable. While this is clearly a difficult group of patients with whom to work, their providers order and these patients use large numbers of unnecessary health services at great cost and are exposed to potential complications from tests, procedures, and medications (Margalit & El-Ad, 2008). Thus they are an important population served by case managers. In fact, case managers should always consider this condition when patients have many unexplained symptoms (HB2), jump frequently from physician to physician (CHS2), or are inconsistently taking many medications for obscure or ill-defined conditions (CP1).

For children/youth, an additional factor that can create a challenge to case managers is if the treatment is complicated, painful, or dangerous. Children/youth are less willing to put up with treatments that are inconvenient and/or uncomfortable. For instance, inhaled nebulizer treatments and chest percussion and postural drainage reduce complications of cystic fibrosis when consistently applied. However, unless treatments can be adapted to the youths' lifestyles (e.g., accommodating them to their active social and school lives), missed treatments will lead to complications, disability, and possible early demise. While this is also true for adults, adherence to treatment in adolescents may be compounded by their feelings of invincibility, especially if apparent symptoms are limited.

A final word about this item is that severity level 3 is used to identify patients in whom nonphysical conditions or reasons may be contributing to the diagnostic or therapeutic challenge. It could be that the patient is faking or exaggerating illness to get disability benefits (malingering), a common situation when litigation is found to accompany persistent or poorly delineated general medical symptoms (HB1). Perhaps more frequently, however, anchor point 3 is used to suggest that concurrent and contributing psychiatric illness has either been undiagnosed or is being ineffectively treated (CP2). In this case, physical treatment nonresponse is associated to a greater extent with persistence of psychiatric symptoms (e.g., depression) than with inappropriate treatment recommendations for the medical condition. Thus, the care manager will need to ensure that attention to psychiatric intervention is a part of the general medical therapeutic process.

VULNERABILITY

Complications and Life Threat (Table 9.6)

Taking the risks for biological complexity described in "Historical" and "Current State" items into account, vulnerability in the biological domain assesses the risk of recurrence, worsening health, or further impairment during the 3 to 6 months after returning the patient to standard care. This item measures the degree to which historical and current state barriers in the biological domain achieve maximum benefit and stabilization before the patient is returned to standard treatment. To a greater extent than with any other items in the adult or pediatric CAG, this is a clinical judgment made by the case manager. The intent is to protect the patient from future problems but not to the degree that he or she can no longer maintain health without case management supervision.

This is one of the reasons that from the first day, when the patient-case manager relationship is established, the case manager is training the patient to become self-sufficient. Clearly, there are some patients, such as those with dementia, no personal resources, or a nonexistent support system, in whom self-sufficiency cannot be expected. In a limited number of these patients, it may be necessary for the case manager to maintain a long-term relationship. Preferably, however, such patients are the ones in which significant attention is given to items within the social domain. Often, embellishing living arrangements, shoring up social support systems, and teaching interpersonal skills (e.g., HS2, CS1 and CS2) can provide the needed boost to allow return to standard care. In the case of children/youth, the need for case management activities may be greater for the caregiver/parent than for the child/youth (pediatric CS1). Focusing on addressing

TABLE 9.6	Complications and Life Threat (VB)

Score	Anchor points
0	Little or no risk of premature physical complications or limitations in activities of daily living
1	Mild risk of premature physical complications or limitations in activities of daily living
2	Moderate risk of premature physical complications or permanent and/or substantial limitations of activities in daily living
3	Severe risk of physical complications associated with serious permanent functional deficits and/or dying

parental needs and vulnerabilities may be critical in stabilizing the child's/youth's health.

PSYCHOLOGICAL DOMAIN

HISTORICAL

Barriers to Coping (Tables 9.7 and 9.8)

Patients' coping skills influence the way they experience mental and physical disorders, describe symptoms to their doctors, and adhere to treatment recommendations. These skills also affect the way that patients interact and work with health professionals and others who may come into contact with them during their journey to stabilized health. Knowing a patient's approach to dealing with problems through assessment of coping skills helps case managers understand the ability of the patient to deal with limitations in life circumstances due to illness, put up with the slow process of healing, and cooperate in their own care. For children/youth it is also helpful to understand coping mechanisms, not only as a reflection of how they might respond to and work with the case manager but also as a means of predicting long-term difficulties unless coping style can be altered.

An important prerequisite for effective coping is adequate cognitive processing. Patients with cognitive impairment and/or developmental delays may be limited in their decision-making capacity, resulting in impaired coping ability. When faced with stress, time constraints, or complicated tasks that require action, patients with restricted cognitive function do not have the ability to problem solve effectively. This leads to increased vulnerability and associated behavioral manifestations (e.g., increased anxiety, anger, and paranoia) when

faced with challenging circumstances, such as serious acute medical illness or chronic disease. These patients find it difficult to grasp the impact and consequences of their problems. Further, they may not recognize or as easily be able to follow advice or suggestions about how they can participate in improving their health.

Patients with certain personality traits or disorders can also find it difficult to respond appropriately to health problems or to the clinicians who evaluate them and administer treatment. Examples of personality traits that can get in the way of productive health behaviors are such things as procrastination, irritability, pessimism, resistance, paranoia, and contempt. If a person demonstrates a pattern of such traits or has a fixed pattern of ineffective and nonconstructive coping techniques as is seen in individuals with personality disorders, these should be factored into the approach that the case manager takes with the patient. For instance, patients with paranoid personalities typically place themselves at the center of the world, lack empathy, react with drama or quarrels, ignore problems, postpone solutions, and brood or blame others. In more extreme cases, personality disorders can manifest with gross neglect of health, self-mutilation, threats, and suicide attempts.

Another situation in which coping abilities can be impaired is when substances, such as alcohol, recreational drugs, or pharmaceuticals are used to alleviate the stresses related to illness or prevent personal action that would improve health. Substance abuse can be subtle, as when mind-altering prescribed medications (pain pills) are used in excess of that needed for the underlying illness. Alternatively, drug abuse can be blatant and demonstrable in the form of intoxication, tolerance,

TABLE 9.7   Barriers to Coping (Adult HPI)

Score	Anchor points
0	Ability to manage stresses/life and health circumstances, such as through seeking support or hobbies
1	Restricted coping skills, such as a need for control, illness denial, or irritability
2	Impaired coping skills, such as nonproductive complaining or substance abuse but without serious impact on medical condition, mental health, or social situation
3	Minimal coping skills, manifest by destructive behaviors, such as substance dependence, psychiatric illness, self-mutilation, or attempted suicide

TABLE 9.8   Barriers to Coping (Pediatric HPI)

Score	Anchor points
0	Ability to adapt to stresses/life and health circumstances, such as through talking with parents/peers, sports, clubs, or hobbies
1	Restricted coping skills, such as acting out with authority figures, dependency, or irritability; no anticipated long-term difficulties
2	Impaired coping skills, such as frequent conflicts with parents/teachers or substance abuse, but without serious impact on medical condition, mental health, or family/social situation; potential long-term difficulties
3	Minimal coping skills, manifested by destructive behaviors, withdrawal, and social isolation, such as substance dependence, mental illness, self-inflicted harm, or illegal behavior

social disruption, and continued use despite worsening health. This is also known as drug dependence.

The identification of poor coping skills leads to specific action, as discussed in Chapter 7. However, it can also influence the need to act on other items in all domains of the adult and pediatric CAG. For instance, patients with poor coping capacity may create crises at work or school (adult and pediatric HS1) or generate havoc in their relationships with others (adult and pediatric HS2). Impulsive behavior may lead to adversarial relationships with providers (HHS2). Manipulative behavior may limit communication among providers (CHS2). When these are traits of caregivers/parents (HS3), they can also have a detrimental effect on a child's/youth's involvement in their health.

While there is no quick solution for difficulties in coping, by recognizing restrictions in this area and taking steps to help the patient, including caregivers/parents, improve by connecting them with stress reduction and coping skills, therapists can potentially have immediate returns and prevent long-term problems. In the meantime, the case manager can work with the patient in addressing other problems and help move him or her toward health improvement.

Mental Health History (Table 9.9)

Patients with a history of mental health difficulties at any time in the past have an increased vulnerability for repeat episodes. This is why a positive mental health history is the only item that carries a lifetime risk. For instance, a woman in her 50s with a history of depression during pregnancy when 25, who is referred for signs and symptoms consistent with a diagnosis of breast cancer, is at an increased risk for a recurrence of depression. Therefore, observation for symptoms of depression and early intervention, if necessary, should be a part of her oncologic assessment. Screening for psychiatric comorbidity is often an afterthought during general medical evaluations, yet not doing so can

have negative consequences for both physical and mental condition outcomes.

In some patients with chronic psychiatric illnesses, such as bipolar depression, substance dependence, or dementia, symptoms may be currently present ("Mental Health Symptoms" [CP2]) yet have been present for an extended period of time. These patients will receive historical (HP2) and current state (CP2) scores reflecting the chronic nature of their mental health conditions. Such patients, however, also commonly exhibit risks in other items in multiple domains. For instance, impaired coping skills (HP1) commonly accompany psychiatric illness. Patients with chronic psychiatric conditions are also less likely to be able to maintain gainful employment (HS1). They have more difficulty in accessing general medical services (HHS1). If patients with mental health histories are able to find a reliable medical doctor to treat them but continue to have a need for specialized mental health services, they may discover that their physical and mental health clinicians do not communicate or coordinate care (CHS2). Thus the presence of a psychiatric history is often predictive of potential barriers to improvement that may need attention.

Finally, since past psychiatric difficulties are associated with future episodes, it is important to include a current assessment for mental health contributions to physical symptoms, particularly if the general medical conditions are poorly controlled or treatment resistant. This is an indication that psychiatric comorbidity may be playing a part in the somatic presentation, which requires documentation under other CAG items (CP1, CB2). Further, the presence of psychiatric symptoms is commonly off-putting to primary care providers, thus their interaction with the patient may suffer as a result (HHS2).

Cognitive Development (Table 9.10)

To a much greater extent than in adults, the presence of child/youth delay or arrest in cognitive development has special importance. Its presence signals a potential

TABLE 9.9	Mental Health History (HP2)

Score	Anchor points
0	No history of mental health problems or conditions
1	Mental health problems or conditions, but resolved or without clear effects on daily function
2	Mental health conditions with clear effects on daily function, needing therapy, medication, day treatment, partial program, and so forth
3	Psychiatric admissions and/or persistent effects on daily function

TABLE 9.10	Cognitive Development (Pediatric HP3)

Score	Anchor points
0	No cognitive impairment
1	Possible developmental delay or immaturity; low IQ
2	Delayed development; mild or moderate cognitive impairment
3	Severe and pervasive developmental delays or profound cognitive impairment

lifelong and costly need for assistance to the child/youth and his or her family. In addition to direct effects on the child's/youth's ability to effectively function, cognitive impairment at an early age can interfere with numerous other areas, creating complexity in multiple domains. For instance, there may be special home needs (CS1) in order for the family to be able to cope with the assistance and supervision required. School performance can lag (HS1 and CS4) and relationships with others, particularly peers, can be impaired (HS2) even if special education arrangements can be made. The ability to cope with change or stress may be limited (HP1), and mental health symptoms may spring up as a result (CP2).

Cognitive delays or impairment in children/youth can also be the result of adverse developmental events (HP4). The presence of any concerns about a child's development or learning should trigger rigorous assessment of early life incidents and exposures that might be treatable, and potentially attenuate or reverse some of the deficit, such as lead exposure. Insurance to cover the costs associated with special arrangements can also be a challenge (HHS1). This issue may be magnified when a child reaches the age of majority and transitions from pediatric to adult general medical and mental health care (CHS2). Often at this time, insurance coverage for the youth turned adult is lost because a preexisting condition is present as the youth's insurance product is also changed.

Adverse Developmental Events (Table 9.11)

Both biological and psychological adverse developmental events are often overlooked or poorly assessed as potential contributors to complexity in children/youth. These may include in utero exposure to toxins, such as is seen in fetal alcohol syndrome, maternal ingestion of prescribed and/or recreational toxic drugs, or exposure through the mother to various viruses (e.g., HIV). Other potential adverse events affecting development may include birth complications; acquired brain injuries; illnesses, such as encephalitis or meningitis; and even psychological and sexual traumas occurring during childhood and adolescence. All of these adverse events can result in long-term biological and mental health consequences that affect family and social adjustment.

Adverse developmental events have been included in the psychological domain, not because the etiology is psychological (though it can be), but because the consequences of the event often manifest in the form of mental health or cognitive symptoms. Importantly, when identified, adverse events are often associated with mental health symptoms that respond poorly to usual interventions (CP2). They can contribute to diagnostic dilemmas (HB2) and therapeutic challenges (CB2) when they have been poorly delineated and/or understood. They are associated with cognitive impairment (HP3) and can be associated with school (HS1 and CS4) problems, trouble forming relationships (HS2), and poor coping strategies (HP1).

CURRENT STATE

Resistance to Treatment (Tables 9.12 and 9.13)

Resistance to treatment evaluates the patient's interest in complying with treatment recommendations and his or her capacity to do so. If the patient adheres to treatment, outcomes improve. If not, he or she typically deteriorates. Active or passive volitional resistance to treatment, as implied by this item, is only one of many reasons for nonadherence (Exhibit 7.1). Nonetheless, it is an important issue that needs to be discussed directly with the patient and/or the child/youth and caregiver/parent. For instance, the patient or patient's family may not believe in Western (physiology-based) medicine but rather may prefer herbal approaches or homeopathic prevention and cure. In such patients, it may appear that they are collaborating with treatment whereas in reality suggested so-called healing prayer or alternative medicine techniques override allopathic interventions.

The patient's collaboration in his or her own care, however, is determined by multiple factors, such as:

- The patient's capacity to appreciate and respond effectively to problems ("Barriers to Coping" [adult and pediatric HP1, pediatric HS3], "Mental Health Symptoms" [adult and pediatric CP2], "Cognitive Development" [pediatric HP3])
- Earlier negative experiences with health care personnel ("Treatment Experiences" [HHS2])

Score	Anchor points
TABLE 9.11	**Adverse Developmental Events (Pediatric HP4)**
0	No Identified developmental traumas or injuries (e.g., physical or sexual abuse, meningitis, lead exposure, etc.)
1	Traumatic prior experiences or injuries with no apparent or stated impact on child/youth
2	Traumatic prior experiences or injuries with potential relationship to impairment in child/youth
3	Traumatic prior experiences with apparent and significant direct relationship to impairment in child/youth

TABLE 9.12	Resistance to Treatment (Adult CP1)
Score	**Anchor points**
0	Interested in receiving treatment and willing to cooperate actively
1	Some ambivalence though willing to cooperate with treatment
2	Considerable resistance with nonadherence; hostility or indifference toward health care professionals and/or treatments
3	Active resistance to important medical care

TABLE 9.13	Resistance to Treatment (Pediatric CP1)
Score	**Anchor points**
0	Parent/caregiver and/or child/youth are interested in receiving treatment and willing to cooperate actively
1	Some parent/caregiver and/or child/youth ambivalence though willing to cooperate with treatment
2	Considerable parent/caregiver and/or child/youth resistance with nonadherence; hostility or indifference toward health care professionals and/or treatments
3	Active parent/caregiver and/or child/youth resistance to important medical care

- The complexity of obtaining the treatments themselves ("Getting Needed Services" [CHS1])
- The coordination used among health care providers ("Coordination of Care" [adult and pediatric CHS2])

Any of these may play a role in the level of frustration felt by patients and their willingness to cooperate. The resistance, however, can be much more personal and direct. For instance, the patient may not like to take medication or may prefer alternative to traditional medicine but not share this with his or her allopathic providers. It could be that a caregiver/parent is irresponsible in the care of minor children or does not have the resources to follow through on treatment recommendations.

Mental Health Symptoms (Tables 9.14 and 9.15)

Related to this item, it is first important to differentiate patients with active manifestations of serious psychiatric conditions, such as schizophrenia, autism, substance dependence, bipolar disorder, eating disorders, etc., from those with mild mental health symptoms such as feeling tense or blue, having difficulty with concentration or memory, occasionally drinking too much, or finding it difficult to manage anger or impulses. In the former, there should uniformly be involvement by a psychiatrist or child psychiatrist, often working as a team leader with other mental health specialists, such as PhD-level psychologists, nurse clinicians, social workers, and so forth. For those with less severe mental health symptoms, focused mental health care can be provided by other behavioral specialists, such as masters-level psychologists, family therapists, counselors, and so forth, usually under the

TABLE 9.14	Mental Health Symptoms (Adult CP2)
Score	**Anchor points**
0	No mental health symptoms
1	Mild mental health symptoms, such as problems with concentration or feeling tense, which do not interfere with current functioning
2	Moderate mental health symptoms, such as an anxiety, depression, or mild cognitive impairment, which interfere with current functioning
3	Severe psychiatric symptoms and/or behavioral disturbances, such as violence, self-inflicted harm, delirium, criminal behavior, psychosis, or mania

TABLE 9.15	Mental Health Symptoms (Pediatric CP2)
Score	**Anchor points**
0	No mental health symptoms
1	Mild mental health symptoms, such as problems with risky behaviors or acting out, sadness, oppositionality, which do not interfere with current functioning
2	Moderate mental health symptoms, such as isolating, death preoccupation, defiance, or cognitive impairment, which interfere with current functioning
3	Severe psychiatric symptoms and/or behavioral disturbances, such as violence, self-inflicted harm, criminal behavior, severe autistic behaviors, psychosis, or mania

supervision of the more highly trained mental health personnel previously mentioned. This allows the case manager to be more confident that outcome-changing, specialist-based mental condition treatment is included. As mentioned in Chapter 5 (see section "Practitioners for Mental Health Disorders"), merely meeting with a mental health professional may not lead to effective management or resolution of mental health problems. Rather, the mental health professional's skill set must be matched to the patient's needs.

Mild and severe mental health symptoms are both of considerable importance, however, since they predict the degree to which patients can listen to and follow the advice of their general medical clinician and act on their own behalf to regain mental and physical health. More often than not, mild psychiatric symptoms, which influence daily functioning, are key factors in medical treatment nonresponse. For some, this shows up as poor follow-through on treatment or unhealthy behaviors. Even health system activities, such as filling out forms to obtain medical assistance ("Access to Care" [HHS1]), can become difficult. For others, mild to moderate symptoms interfere with social factors important in stabilizing health. Personal relationships, ("Family and Social Relationships" [adult and pediatric HS2]), can be affected and interfere with the availability of support ("Social Support"), whether for the patient or his or her caregiver/parent (adult CS2 and pediatric CS2 and CS3).

VULNERABILITY

Mental Health Threat (Tables 9.16 and 9.17)

As in the biological domain, taking the risks for psychological complexity described in "History" and "Current State" into account, mental health vulnerability, including special attention to cognitive delays or impairment in children/youth, assesses the risk of recurrence or worsening of barriers to improvement for mental function during the 3 to 6 months after returning the patient to standard care. Vulnerability assessment will influence the degree to which overcoming historical and current state barriers in the psychological domain has been accomplished before the patient is returned to standard treatment. Clinical judgment by the case manager is necessary for this to be done effectively. The intent is to protect the patient from future mental health problems but not to the extent that the patient or the patient's family or significant other does not ultimately reassume responsibility for continued health stability and return to standard care.

This item is one that requires special attention because mental health and substance use disorder services are typically difficult to access (adult and pediatric HHS1), are inconsistently provided and coordinated with other health services (adult and pediatric CHS1 and CHS2), and are geographically disparate from other health care (adult and pediatric CHS1). In patients who would benefit from mental condition care, the case manager will often have to personally find a provider, even when coping skills training is all that is desired (adult and pediatric HP1; pediatric HS3), and ensure that follow-through occurs so that the patient derives benefit from the services sought (CP2).

TABLE 9.16   Mental Health Threat (Adult VP)

Score	Anchor points
0	No mental health concerns
1	Mild risk of worsening of mental health *symptoms*, such as stress, anxiety, feeling blue, substance abuse, or cognitive disturbance with limited impact on function; mild risk of treatment resistance (ambivalence)
2	Moderate risk of mental health *disorder* requiring additional mental health care; moderate risk of treatment resistance
3	Severe risk of psychiatric disorder requiring frequent emergency room visits and/or hospital admissions; risk of treatment refusal for serious disorder

TABLE 9.17   Learning and/or Mental Health Threat (Pediatric VP)

Score	Anchor points
0	No mental health or intellectual deterioration concerns
1	Risk of mild worsening mental health or cognitive *symptoms*, such as home or school conflict, anxiety, feeling blue, substance abuse, or cognitive disturbance with limited impact on function; mild risk of treatment resistance (ambivalence)
2	Moderate risk of mental health *disorder* or impaired cognitive functioning requiring additional mental health care; moderate risk of treatment resistance
3	Severe risk of psychiatric disorder or cognitive impairment requiring frequent emergency room visits, hospital admissions, and/or specialized schooling; risk of treatment refusal for serious disorder

In patients with mental health or cognitive vulnerability, it is not sufficient for the case manager simply to ensure that the provisions of care are consistent. Often patients with psychiatric contributions to their complexity will also experience social barriers to improvement, such as housing problems or inadequate parental/caregiver supervision and support (adult and pediatric CS1), financial challenges due to job instability (adult HS1), school problems (pediatric HS1 and CS4), and relationship (adult and pediatric HS2) and social support (adult and pediatric CS2; pediatric CS3) problems. These issues will also require assessment and assistance when present.

SOCIAL DOMAIN

HISTORY

Job and Leisure; School Functioning (Tables 9.18 and 9.19)

This item addresses personal and social success in terms of employment, interactions with others, and the ability to participate in personally enjoyable activities. In children/youth, it reflects evidence of positive adjustment in school, academically, socially, and behaviorally. When problems are absent in these areas, improved outcomes related to health care can be expected. Patients who have historically been able to maintain active social lives, keep a job, or interact and perform well in school are more likely to have access to future support and financial resources (adult) or to complete educational pursuits and become contributors in society (children/youth). They are better equipped to respond to crises than those who do not possess these skills. Patients who read books or pursue hobbies with some regularity may also be more likely to actively participate in their personal treatment and maintain preventive health behaviors. On the other hand, those who spend the majority of their free time watching television or playing video games (passive activities) would not be included among those with leisure activities (adult) or productive behaviors (children/youth) since they require few social skills.

For clarification, a person has a job when an employer lists him or her as an employee. For instance, a patient who is on short-term disability, family leave, or is off duty because of a workers' compensation injury would be considered employed. Such patients have a job waiting for them when their health or family circumstances improve. When a person enters long-term disability, however (i.e., is away from work normally 6 months or longer), the patient is usually no longer on the employment roles since at that point the disability has persisted long enough that the employee is unlikely to improve to the point that he or she can return to his or her previous job. The employee on short-term disability or family leave would be similar to a student on summer break.

In the case of children/youth, they are considered students when they are expected to participate in a structured learning environment, either at an institution or in a home school, for the purposes of educational advancement. Both at home school and in the educational system, attendance is expected at educational activities and students are expected to prepare for those activities by reviewing assigned materials.

"School Functioning" (pediatric HS1) does not directly parallel "Job and Leisure" (adult HS1) since it includes historical disruptive behaviors at school as a manifestation of poor performance when complexity increases with this item, rather than just leisure activity. In the school setting, these historical behaviors are

TABLE 9.18   **Job and Leisure (Adult HS1)**

Score	Anchor points
0	A job (including housekeeping, retirement, studying) and having leisure activities
1	A job (including housekeeping, retirement, studying) without leisure activities
2	Unemployed now and for at least 6 months with leisure activities
3	Unemployed now and for at least 6 months without leisure activities

TABLE 9.19   **School Functioning (Pediatric HS1)**

Score	Anchor points
0	Performing well in school with good achievement, attendance, and behavior
1	Performing adequately in school but with some achievement, attendance, and behavior problems (e.g., missed classes, pranks)
2	Experiencing moderate problems with school achievement, attendance, and/or behavior (e.g., school disciplinary action, few social or school-related peer relations, academic probation)
3	Experiencing severe problems with school achievement, attendance, and/or behavior (e.g., home-bound education, school suspension, violence, illegal activities at school, academic failure, school dropout, disruptive peer group activity)

TABLE 9.20   Relationships (Adult HS2)

Score	Anchor points
0	No social disruption
1	Mild social dysfunction; interpersonal problems
2	Moderate social dysfunction, such as inability to initiate or maintain social relations
3	Severe social dysfunction, such as involvement in disruptive social relations or social isolation

a predictor for future difficulties and frequently parallel attendance and achievement problems. The attendance and "leisure" component in the adult HS1 has rather been captured in the current state "School and Community Participation" (CS4) item. It assesses the ability of the child/youth to effectively engage in educational and extracurricular efforts in the school and community.

Complexity on this item correlates with other items in the CAG. For instance, an adult or child/youth may also have increased risk for problems with "Barriers to Coping" (adult and pediatric HP1), "Mental Health History" (adult and pediatric HP2), "Cognitive Development" (pediatric HP3), and limited social support (adult and pediatric CS2). Those who are unemployed may have housing problems ("Residential Stability" [adult CS1]), no insurance ("Access to Care" [HHS1]), and difficulty in finding transportation to appointments ("Getting Needed Services" [CHS1]). Children/youth with school performance problems may have home situations ("Family and Social Relationships" [HS2] and "Residential Stability" [CS1]) that make it difficult to apply personal resources to educational pursuits.

Family and Social Relationships (Tables 9.20 and 9.21)

Conflict is a part of the human experience; however, repeated conflicts in several relationships—such as with a partner, with family members, at work, with classmates, or with friends—can be associated with increased risk of complexity. Such conflict could be associated with the stressors of having a child with high developmental needs (HP3), cognitive decline in the elderly ("Mental Health Symptoms" [HP2]), poor impulse control in a patient with ineffective personality traits ("Barriers to Coping" [adult and pediatric HP1]), or psychotic symptoms in a person with a psychiatric illness ("Mental Health Symptoms" [adult and pediatric CP2]). Regardless of the etiology, repeated involvement in disruptive social relationships or situations typified by repetitive physical aggression, threats, yelling, or psychological abuse should be taken into

TABLE 9.21   Family and Social Relationships (Pediatric HS2)

Score	Anchor points
0	Stable, nurturing home; good social and peer relationships
1	Mild family problems, minor problems with social and peer relationships (e.g., parent-child conflict, frequent fights, marital discord, lacking close friends)
2	Moderate level of family problems, inability to initiate and maintain social and peer relationships (e.g., parental neglect, difficult separation/divorce; alcohol abuse, hostile caregiver, difficulties in maintaining same-age peer relationships)
3	Severe family problems with disruptive social and peer relationships (e.g., significant abuse, hostile child custody battles, addiction issues, parental criminality, complete social isolation, little or no association with peers)

account as a care plan is developed since problems in forming relationships lead to isolation, abandonment, and/or increased restrictions of care. It can be reflected in aberrant "Treatment Experience" (HHS2) and lead to "Resistance to Treatment" (CP1).

Caregiver/Parent Health and Function (Table 9.22)

Caregivers/parents are important links to health for children/youth. This item is designed to document

TABLE 9.22   Caregiver/Parent Health and Function (Pediatric HS3)

Score	Anchor points
0	All caregivers healthy
1	Physical and/or mental health issues, including poor coping skills, and/or permanent disability, present in one or more caregiver, which do not affect parenting
2	Physical and/or mental health conditions, including disrupted coping resources, and/or permanent disability, present in one or more caregiver, which interfere with parenting
3	Physical and/or mental health conditions, including disrupted coping styles, and/or permanent disability, present in one or more caregiver, which prevent effective parenting and/or create a dangerous situation for the child/youth

their level of health and their ability to contribute to the support and well-being of those in their custody. Essentially, anything that impairs one or more of the child's/youth's caregivers from meeting their parenting responsibilities should be documented through this item. For instance, the physical or mental health of a caregiver/parent may limit his or her ability to assist with transportation to needed health appointments (CHS1). It may impair his or her ability to cope (HP1) with challenging child/youth physical (CB2) or mental conditions (CP2) or with disruptive behavior at school (HS1). In fact, either physical or mental conditions in a caregiver/parent may themselves contribute to health problems in the child/youth (CB1, HP2, HP3, or CP2) or to the inability of the child/youth, potentially limiting the child's and youth's own personal support network (CS1 and CS3).

In some caregivers/parents, it is not physical or mental conditions that affect their parenting capabilities. Rather, it is their personality or lifestyle. These factors may manifest as impaired ability to cope (e.g., excessive use of alcohol [adult HP1] or disruption in family relationship/activities [HS2]). They may also manifest as an unsafe home environment for the child/youth to live in (CS1; e.g., drug sales, prostitution, or illegal on-premises activities). In some instances, caregiver/parent challenges may herald the need for involvement of child protective services if the level of parenting is sufficiently limited or living circumstances are sufficiently dangerous. Even in homes with more than one responsible adult, pathology could be present in both or the dominance of one challenged parent may negate the beneficial effect of the other.

Parental ability to cope is also often stressed when the level of difficulties experienced or manifest by their child/youth is severe. In normal circumstances, they may employ good coping mechanisms, but they may become overwhelmed when significant child/youth challenges are faced. Thus, value judgments should be reserved regarding a parent's coping ability since he or she may be taxed beyond his or her limits by the behaviors and/or the situation of the child/youth.

In virtually all case management for children/youth, some assistance to caregivers/parents will be required in order for child/youth health and function to stabilize. While this is true, pediatric case management dictates that the target of management activities is for improvement in the child/youth, not the caregiver/parent, condition. Thus, if the level of personal challenge for the caregiver/parent equals or exceeds the needs of the child/youth, then part of the support for the child/youth may be connecting the caregiver/parent with social or mental health services, community resources, or his or her own case manager (when health issues are involved). In most situations, it is not intended that a pediatric case manager be responsible for the needs of an entire family; however, needs of family members affecting the health and function of the child/youth cannot be ignored.

CURRENT STATE

Residential Stability (Tables 9.23 and 9.24)

At the most basic level, adult "Residential Stability" assesses whether the patient has a stable place to live. It also focuses on whether a patient's living situation is appropriate for his or her care needs and is conducive to: (a) cooperation among the patient's clinicians, (b) the delivery of evidence-based treatment, and (c) attendance at health care appointments. For instance, in the case of an elderly patient with dementia or a physical handicap, independent living may only be possible when there is support available from a healthy partner or alternative

TABLE 9.23   **Residential Stability (Adult CS1)**

Score	Anchor points
0	Stable housing; fully capable of independent living
1	Stable housing with support of others (e.g., family, home care, or an institutional setting)
2	Unstable housing (e.g., no support at home or living in a shelter); change of current living situation is required
3	No current satisfactory housing (e.g., transient housing or dangerous environment); immediate change is necessary

TABLE 9.24   **Residential Stability (Pediatric CS1)**

Score	Anchor points
0	Stable housing and financial support for personal growth needs
1	Mild stress with multiple moves, school changes, financial issues
2	Moderate stress with unstable housing and/or living situation support (e.g., living in shelter, poor nutrition); change of current living situation is required
3	Severe stress with no current satisfactory housing (e.g., homelessness, transient housing, child/youth malnourished, or dangerous environment); immediate change is necessary

caregiver. As health needs increase, environments with higher supervision capabilities become necessary, such as through assisted living or nursing home facilities.

When a living situation is dangerous or very likely to lead to worsening health, such as living on the street, immediate action related to patients' living situations might become necessary. In the elderly, for instance, this could be related to filthiness or not being able to take care of themselves. Serious self-neglect can also be seen in patients with psychosis or addiction ("Barriers to Coping" [HP1] and "Mental Health History" [HP2]) or in children/youth in whom this is a problem for their caregiver/parent. It is evident that a poor and unstable housing situation does not contribute to a beneficial outcome of illness, specifically if close attention to self-care, such as in diabetes, is required (HB1 and CB1).

Housing is only one component of the needs of children/youth under "Residential Stability" (CS1). They also need housing that supplies safety and sustenance since, unless nearing the age of majority, they are unable to fend for themselves. When caregivers/parents move frequently, are unable to ensure adequate nutrition, or provide an unsafe environment, action on the part of the case manager becomes necessary. In exceptional circumstances, it may require involvement of child protective services.

An unstable, unsafe, and/or poorly organized home situation may also affect other areas of potential complexity, including the development of child/youth and caregiver/family support (CS2 and CS3), the ability to form and maintain lasting relationships (HS2), availability of health coverage (HHS1) or the ability to obtain and coordinate health services (CHS1 and CHS2), among others. If "Residential Stability" is a problem, other areas of complexity often need attention.

Social Support (Tables 9.25, 9.26, and 9.27)

While dysfunctional relationships (adult and pediatric HS2), ineffective coping mechanisms (adult and pediatric HP1; pediatric HS3), a transient living situation (adult and pediatric CS1), and chronic mental illness (CH2) can all be associated with poor social networking, some patients, whether adults or children/youth, just do not have the social skills or personality to maintain a safety net of individuals that can help them when they are having difficulties. Perhaps their family has moved to a different town, they have few activities outside of the home, or they do not speak the local language. All of these factors can play a role in creating a personal situation in which no one would be available to assist with personal support needs in a crisis. When situations such as these are present, indirect and direct

---

TABLE 9.25   Social Support (Adult CS2)

Score	Anchor points
0	Assistance readily available from family, friends, and/or acquaintances, such as work colleagues, at all times
1	Assistance generally available from family, friends, and/or acquaintances, such as work colleagues, but possible delays
2	Limited assistance available from family, friends, and/or acquaintances, such as work colleagues
3	No assistance readily available from family, friends, and/or acquaintances, such as work colleagues, at any time

---

TABLE 9.26   Child/Youth Support (Pediatric CS2)

Score	Anchor points
0	Supervision and/or assistance readily available from family/caregiver, friends/peers, teachers, and/or community social networks (e.g., spiritual/religious groups) at all times
1	Supervision and/or assistance generally available from family/caregiver, friends/peers, teachers, and/or community social networks, but possible delays
2	Limited supervision and/or assistance available from family/caregiver, friends/peers, teachers, and/or community social networks
3	No effective supervision and/or assistance available from family/caregiver, friends/peers, teachers, and/or community social networks at any time

---

TABLE 9.27   Caregiver/Family Support (Pediatric CS3)

Score	Anchor points
0	Assistance readily available from family, friends, and/or acquaintances, such as work colleagues/employer, at all times
1	Assistance generally available from family, friends, and/or acquaintances, such as work colleagues/employer, but possible delays
2	Limited assistance available from family, friends, and/or acquaintances, such as work colleagues/employer
3	No assistance available from family, friends, and/or acquaintances, such as work colleagues/employer at any time

case manager action may facilitate the identification of some support should a crisis arise or may prevent a crisis from happening in the first place.

In children/youth, a support system for both the caregiver/parent and the child/youth is important. For the caregiver/parent, characteristics of the support system would be similar to that of a patient in adult case management. Provisions for coverage of basic professional and personal responsibilities would be needed in the event that there was a school crisis or childhood illness. Such support could come from friends, relatives, significant others, coworkers, or social services agencies.

Support for children/youth comes from a variety of sources. While the primary starting place of support may be parents or other family members, it could also come from peers, clergy, coaches, or teachers. Youth,

all of whom are developing their own identities, not only require support during changes in life circumstances but also psychological support as they develop friendships (HS2), deal with personal conflicts (HP1), expand their social lives (CS4), and adjust to successes and failures (HS1). These factors are also important for adults but have special significance during the growth and maturation of childhood and adolescence.

School and Community Participation (Table 9.28)

Historical performance in the school setting is addressed in "School Functioning" (HS1), whereas current participation in school and the community are the focus of item CS4. Children/youth may have historically done well in school through the majority of their lives yet may have recently developed problems with attendance and/or demonstrated a significant reduction in their school and extracurricular activities. New changes in participation often suggest that acute, not long-term, factors are affecting the child's/youth's life. In such situations, it may not only be necessary to address recent school attendance issues, such as school phobias, or a child's/youth's personal isolation but also to assist with other components that could be influencing the change, such as frequent moves (CS1), disruptive family interactions (HS2), physical illness and/or symptoms (CB1), or unresolved stresses with limited coping capabilities (HP1).

VULNERABILITY

Family/School/Social Vulnerability (Tables 9.29 and 9.30)

In order to protect the patient from future worsening of health problems after discharge from case

TABLE 9.28	School and Community Participation (Pediatric CS4)
Score	Anchor points
0	Attending school regularly, achieving and participating well, and actively engaged in extracurricular school or community activities (e.g., sports, clubs, hobbies, religious groups)
1	Average of 1 day of school missed/week and/or minor disruptions in achievement and behavior with few extracurricular activities
2	Average of 2 days or more of school missed/week and/or moderate disruption in achievement or behavior with resistance to extracurricular activities
3	Truant or school nonattendance with no extracurricular activities and no community connections

TABLE 9.29	Social Vulnerability (Adult VS)
Score	Anchor points
0	No risk of need for changes in the living situation, social relationships and support, or employment
1	Mild risk of need for changes in the living situation (e.g., home health care); social relationships and support, or employment
2	Risk of need for social augmentation/support, financial/employment assistance, or living situation change in the foreseeable future
3	Risk of need for social augmentation/support, financial/employment assistance, or living situation change now

TABLE 9.30	Family/School/Social System Vulnerability (Pediatric VS)
Score	Anchor points
0	No risk from living situation; adequate social, personal, and developmental support, caregiver health, and function
1	Risk of need for additional living situation stability, social or school support, and/or family/caregiver intervention
2	Risk of need for temporary or permanent alteration in home, school, and/or family/caregiver/social environment in the foreseeable future
3	Risk of need for immediate temporary or permanent alteration in home, school, and/or family/caregiver/social environment (e.g., assist with foster home placement, referral to child protective services)

management, it is important to ensure that social item stability has been attained. Historical and current state family/social domain items primarily influence social vulnerability, but other items in the CAG can also play a role. For instance, poorly controlled medical and psychiatric illness (CB1 and CP2) can put the patient at great risk for job loss or poor school performance (adult and pediatric HS1) and the need for greater assistance with personal care (adult CS1). On the other hand, inadequate social support (CS2) and an unstable living situation (CS1) can foster worsening illness due to nonadherence to treatment recommendations (CP1). Lack of a job (adult HS1) and frequent moves (pediatric CS1) are harbingers for poor or no insurance (HHS1), difficulty in paying for health services and medications (adult and pediatric CHS1), and trouble finding doctors to care for them (adult and pediatric HHS1), let alone ones who will do so consistently and in a coordinated way (CHS2). As case managers work with patients, it is important to explore interaction of items when social vulnerability is assessed.

HEALTH SYSTEM DOMAIN

HISTORY

Access to Care (Table 9.31)

System-level difficulties in medical service access may vary as a function of differences in the health systems in which care is sought. Geography, language, payment for certain types of practitioners, and wait lists are more prominent system-level barriers to access in Canada and most European countries than is lack of insurance. For instance, specialty services may not be available in rural areas or there may not be practitioners who speak the language of the patient or understand his or her culture. These access issues require a good referral system and translation capability to maintain the level

TABLE 9.31   Access to Care (HHS1)

Score	Anchor points
0	Adequate access to care
1	Some limitations in access to care due to financial/insurance problems, geographic reasons, family issues, language, or cultural barriers
2	Difficulties in accessing care due to financial/insurance problems, geographic reasons, family issues, language, or cultural barriers
3	No adequate access to care due to financial/insurance problems, geographic reasons, family issues, language, or cultural barriers

of care needed for individual patients, and particularly those with health complexity. In some countries, long wait lists prevent timely service access and delivery.

In the United States, the most common and serious barrier to access is lack of insurance or having insurance benefits that are insufficient to support the type of care that is needed. For patients in this situation, their only option is to seek care through the emergency medical system, where care cannot be refused during a medical crisis. However, seeking services in the emergency setting does not allow follow-up treatment, whether by a general practitioner or specialist; support for elective tests; payment for medication; or screening and prevention. Even those who have full insurance under the law may, in fact, have no access because the type of insurance that they have remunerates for services at such a low rate that few practitioners are willing to accept patients covered by it.

Traditionally, case managers do not provide assistance to patients for whom the barrier to care is related to the type of insurance that they carry, the length of the wait list, or the availability of interpreters or specialists. In integrated case management, instead, these components are identified as major barriers to improvement and thus are considered a focus of basic case manager activities.

When system-level access problems prevent the delivery of effective health services, they can lead to interference in other complexity items. For instance, delayed improvement or nontreatment can affect work/school attendance or performance (adult and pediatric HS1). It can create difficulties in determining accurate diagnoses (HB2) since postacute evaluation consultations and testing cannot be completed because of limited follow-up and cost issues. When this happens, severity can progress so that impairment results (CB1) and the logistics of getting needed services (CHS1) becomes impossible. Often, emergency medical procedures exhaust financial resources and personal bankruptcy occurs. While patients then become eligible for public program insurance packages, this is often at the expense of residential stability (CS1) and the problems that emanate from that.

Treatment Experience (Table 9.32 and 9.33)

Simply put, this complexity item is a good predictor for the quality of future relationships with health care personnel. Adverse experiences with health care personnel or with the health system, such as with insurance companies or national health services, might negatively influence a patient's attitude toward health care personnel and the system, with a secondary impact on the outcome of care. Such a noncooperative attitude could be the result of the patient's own experiences but could also be related to experiences of their next of kin or good friends. In the case of children/youth, there is

TABLE 9.32	Treatment Experience (Adult HHS2)
Score	**Anchor points**
0	No problems with health care professionals
1	Negative experience with health care professionals (self or relatives)
2	Dissatisfaction or distrust of doctors; multiple providers for the same health problem; trouble keeping consistent and/or preferred provider(s)
3	Repeated major conflicts with or distrust of doctors, frequent emergency room visits or involuntary admissions; forced to stay with undesirable provider due to cost, provider network options, or other reasons

TABLE 9.33	Treatment Experience (Pediatric HHS2)
Score	**Anchor points**
0	No child/youth or parent/caregiver problems with health care professionals
1	Negative child/youth or parent/caregiver experience with health care professionals
2	Child/youth or parent/caregiver dissatisfaction with or distrust of doctors; multiple providers for the same health problem; trouble keeping consistent and/or preferred provider(s)
3	Repeated major child/youth or parent/caregiver conflicts with or distrust of doctors, frequent emergency room visits or involuntary admissions; forced to stay with undesirable provider due to cost, provider network options, or other reasons

double jeopardy. A bad experience could occur with the child/youth or with their caregiver/parent. It might stem from a misdiagnosis, lack of respect or understanding by a clinician, or the way terminal care was provided to a loved one. In fact, it could also be that the patient just did not get his or her way (e.g., support for disability or the refill of a controlled substance prescription).

A negative attitude about health practitioners need not be the result of a specific experience. It may also be that the patient harbors beliefs or attitudes about Western doctors (e.g., they are greedy, they are receiving favors or other incentives from drug companies, or they care only about the disease rather than the patient) that color their experiences. Regardless, the end result of a poor quality relationship between patient and provider can interact with or aggravate many other areas that influence outcomes of health care, such as adherence to treatment (CP1), progression of symptom severity (CB2 and CP2), or facilitation of communication among allopathic and naturopathic providers (CHS2). Because negative attitudes have this potential, they are considered an important contributor to complexity, potentially in multiple domains.

CURRENT STATE

Getting Needed Services (Table 9.34)

"Getting Needed Services" is complementary to "Access to Care" (HHS1) since it addresses the practical logistics of getting the care that leads to improvement if appropriate providers are available and the patient has coverage for services. For instance, in a patient who lives in a shelter with limited resources and a health problem that makes travel to a clinic difficult (e.g., diabetic foot ulcers or cognitive impairment) then

clinic visits will likely go unattended, even if there is a free community health clinic within blocks of where the patient lives. Costs of transportation, hassle factors, and the distance from the patient's residence may lead the patient to use ambulances and emergency rooms preferentially after medical crises arise, since they are free and logistically less complicated.

Similar problems are created for patients with numerous illnesses and needs from various clinicians. Since multiple clinical assessments performed on the same day are often excluded from payment by many insurance products, this problem is overcome by having patients show up for clinic visits on different days even if the service is provided in the same geographic location. This requires that patients and/or the caregivers/parents of children/youth miss work, find transportation, get childcare, and disrupt an already

TABLE 9.34	Getting Needed Services (CHS1)
Score	**Anchor points**
0	Easily available treating practitioners and health care settings (general medical or mental health care); money for medications and medical equipment
1	Some difficulties in getting to appointments or needed services
2	Routine difficulties in coordinating and/or getting to appointments or needed services
3	Inability to coordinate and/or get to appointments or needed services

busy schedule to maintain their own or their child's health. Again, this can become so onerous that patients stop going to appointments.

Inability to pay for services, medications, and medical equipment can also become a reason for non-adherence. Patients may have appointments and pre-scriptions but are not able to follow through on these components of treatment because out-of-pocket ex-penses are so great. For instance, patients may take half the dose of a medication in an attempt to save money by extending the time between refills. While it saves money in the short-term, predictably, symptom control falters, leading to emergency room visits and hospitalizations.

All of these factors are captured in this CAG item and can affect other complexity items, such as "Treatment Experience" (HHS2), "Barriers to Cop-ing" (HP1), and "Diagnostic/Therapeutic Challenge" (CB2).

It is not just geographic and financial factors that are implicated in this complexity item. The item con-tent also includes failure to access/obtain needed services because appropriate referrals for specialty service have not been made. Linked to coordination of care (CHS2), patients with untreated illness, such as depression or anxiety, can be prevented from receiv-ing needed services because an uninformed primary care physician fails to include a mental health assess-ment or treatment that would be expected to change the patient's outcome. In such situations, patients can remain untreated for extended periods and thus expe-rience worse medical (CB1) and mental health symp-tom control (CP2), treatment resistance (CB2), and the development of chronic health problems (HB1) with attendant social domain consequences.

Coordination of Care (Tables 9.35 and 9.36)

Good health care not only requires attention to the logistics of how services are provided (CHS1); it also requires coordination of services among health care providers. "Coordination of Care" has to do with the degree to which a patient's practitioners communicate with each other about the patient's health problems and their treatment. Within a given hospital and clinic system, there may be good access to information about the range of services provided to a patient, especially if there is a coordinated electronic medical record. When the patient, however, receives services from more than one practitioner working in different health systems or locations, communication becomes more difficult. This can show up as duplicate services (e.g., X-rays, prescrip-tions, etc.), conflicting recommendations by practitio-ners, health system abuse by patients with addictions, or other health service overuse syndromes, such as so-matization disorder.

Obtaining well-coordinated care is a particular challenge for patients who have both medical and psychiatric illnesses. Mental health and general medi-cal records are often stored separately and, in essence, hide important health information from other clini-cians involved in the patient's care. While there are rules that govern communication among clinicians and confidentiality of personal health information, in general, free communication about all health issues among the clinicians involved in a specific individual patient's care is the only way that the best treatment can be provided.

Protecting the privacy of personal health infor-mation is critical for all patients. At the same time, all practitioners working with a patient need to have

TABLE 9.35	Coordination of Care (Adult CHS2)
Score	Anchor points
0	Complete practitioner communication with good coordination of care
1	Limited practitioner communication and coordination of care; primary care physician coordinates medical and mental health services
2	Poor communication and coordination of care among practitioners; no routine primary care physician
3	No communication and coordination of care among practitioners; primary emergency room use to meet nonemergent health needs

TABLE 9.36	Coordination of Care (Pediatric CHS2)
Score	Anchor points
0	Complete practitioner communication with good coordination and transition of care
1	Limited practitioner communication and coordination of care; pediatrician coordinates medical and mental health services
2	Poor communication and coordination of care among practitioners; no routine pediatrician; difficulty in transitioning to age-appropriate care
3	No communication and coordination of care among practitioners; primary emergency room use to meet nonemergent health needs; systemic barriers to age-appropriate care transition

easy access to his or her health care information. When there is sensitivity related to the content of the condition being treated—whether it is erectile dysfunction, trauma related to spousal abuse, or psychiatric illness—appropriate discretion should be used in how information is documented, yet that information should remain accessible to the patient's clinicians, including case managers and others involved in trying to help the patient return to health.

Also included as a component of complexity under CHS2 are teens nearing the age of majority, and especially those with health complexity who are required to transfer their care from the pediatric medical community to the adult. Finding a family practitioner or a mental health practitioner willing to take on a patient with a suite of health needs and often a limited means to pay for them can be a significant challenge for the patient and for the practitioners working in the pediatric sector. Pediatric case managers can play an important role in transitioning youth to the adult health care system.

Lack of coordination of care affects many other items in multiple domains. For instance, lack of communication between a lung specialist and a psychologist, both treating an individual patient for shortness of breath and the anxiety associated with it, can lead to unnecessary tests and ineffective treatment (CB1 and CP2), worsening symptoms (CB1), and more difficulty in coping (HP1).

VULNERABILITY

Health System Impediments (Tables 9.37 and 9.38)

As with other vulnerability items, health system vulnerability assesses the risk of persistent and unresolved doctor-patient relational and health delivery navigational barriers to improvement that might lead to worse health outcomes during the next 3 to 6 months if the patient is returned to standard care. It will not be possible to discontinue individualized care through integrated case management until the risk of worsened outcomes due to access and coordination issues related to health system factors have been addressed or maximum case management benefit has been reached.

CHANGE MEASUREMENT AND CASE MANAGER CASELOAD ESTIMATION

CONSOLIDATED CASE MANAGER PATIENT PANEL SCORES

As mentioned in Chapter 3 (see section "Case Manager Caseload Limits"), the consolidated scores of managed patient panels can be used to estimate the number of patients that a case manager would be able carry while retaining effectiveness in providing case management services. Even with the introduction of the PIM-CAG, which has an item total scoring range of 0 to 75 compared to the range of 0 to 60 for the IM-CAG, it should be possible to use composite scores for patient panels to estimate case manager panel size. This should be true whether case managers work only with adults, only with children/youth, or with both.

While the authors recommend that this be subjected to confirmation through investigation (i.e., whether total IM-CAG and PIM-CAG scores are comparable in estimating panel size or whether combined total IM-CAG and PIM-CAG scores can be summed to determine panel size), the principle that individual levels of complexity

TABLE 9.37	Health System Impediment (Adult VHS)
Score	Anchor points
0	No risk of impediments to coordinated physical and mental health care
1	Mild risk of impediments to care (e.g., insurance restrictions, distant service access, limited provider communication and/or care coordination)
2	Moderate risk of impediments to care (e.g., potential insurance loss, inconsistent practitioners, communication barriers, poor care coordination)
3	Severe risk of impediments to care (e.g., little or no insurance, resistance to communication and/ or disruptive work processes that lead to poor coordination)

TABLE 9.38	Health System Impediment (Pediatric VHS)
Score	Anchor points
0	No risk of impediments to coordinated physical and mental health care
1	Mild risk of impediments to care (e.g., insurance restrictions, distant service access, limited provider communication and/or care coordination/ transition)
2	Moderate risk of impediments to care (e.g., potential insurance loss, inconsistent practitioners, communication barriers, poor care coordination/ transition)
3	Severe risk of impediments to care (e.g., little or no insurance, resistance to communication and/ or disruptive work processes that lead to poor coordination/transition among providers)

would correlate with the need for activity by the case manager should still hold true. Of course, absolute total scores cannot be suggested regardless of whether adults, children/youth, or both are to receive case management since the total score cutoff point would depend on targeted outcomes for the case manager, the objectives of the organization at which he or she works, and the directives of the purchasers of services.

From a practical standpoint, the total adult CAG score and pediatric score provides an opportunity to establish a number score for the overall complexity of a patient yet retain scores for individual items that will determine actionable clinical priorities. As a case manager works with the patient on action items in the cells of importance, he or she can use improvements in ongoing CAG subscores (Appendixes 4 and 5) to document change in the individual patient's status or when concerns related to the CAG items have been addressed (covered in the Chapter 11 section "Use of the CAG as a Global Assessment of Complexity Amelioration"). Changes in total CAG scores along with other measured clinical outcomes, such as HbA1c or PHQ-9 scores for patients with diabetes and depression, functional outcomes, total health care service use (from claims databases), quality of life, and patient satisfaction assessments, can be documented in the record of outcome measurements (**Table 9.39**; Appendix 11), which can help determine when movement toward graduation from case management should be initiated. Further, this composite forms a powerful way to document the value that case management, and even individual care by case managers, brings to patients.

CASELOAD ESTIMATION

One of the advantages of CAG methodology is that the sum of the total scores (all items added together; see right upper corner of IM-CAG and PIM-CAG) can be used to estimate the total case complexity of a case manager's patient panel. Thus, it has the potential to

---

TABLE 9.39   **Example of ROM (Record of Outcome Measures) With Sample Measures and Times**

OUTCOME MEASURES	BASELINE	FOLLOW-UP ASSESSMENTS		
Time period recorded	Initial *e.g., week 1*	2nd *e.g., week 4*	3rd *e.g., week 9*	4th *e.g., week 11*
Clinical measure **related to personal goal** *e.g., fewer headaches/week*				
Functional measure **related to personal goal** *e.g., soccer games attended*				
Health-related quality of life *e.g., # days healthy/month*				
Patient satisfaction *e.g. visual analogue scale score of 0–10*				
CAG score (total for period)				
Health care clinical measure *e.g., HbA1c*				
Health care clinical measure *e.g., PHQ-9*				
Health care functional measure *e.g., visual analogue scale score*				
Health care functional measure *e.g., # work days lost/month*				
Health care economic measure *e.g., # ER visits or hospital days*				

The record of outcome measures is a format that allows comparison of changes over time in clinical and functional measures. This is determined by the patient and case manager as they discuss what they consider important for a successful outcomes. This table shows sample measures and times that could be used with this tool.

approximate a case manager's active case panel size. For instance, one case manager may have 66 patients with average CAG scores of 28 in management for a total complexity composite of 1,848 (66 times 28). Another case manager may carry 84 patients with average CAG scores of 22 (composite also equals 1848). The two could have roughly comparable workloads depending on the populations that they serve. Thus, based on total complexity scores, a fixed caseload guideline could be determined to ensure that the time needed to perform case management activities is consistent with the number of patients carried. The absolute composite CAG score for the population served, the range, and the average score for individual patients will depend on the target population and the intended services for that population, as determined by the case management program in which the manager works.

REFERENCES

Boyd, C. M., Darer, J., Boult, C., Fried, L. P., Boult, L., & Wu, A. W. (2005). Clinical practice guidelines and quality of care for older patients with multiple comorbid diseases: Implications for pay for performance. *Journal of the American Medical Association, 294*(6), 716–724.

Denniston, P. L. (2009). *Official disability guidelines 2009* (7th ed.). San Diego, CA: Work Loss Data Institute.

Kathol, R., Saravay, S., Lobo, A., & Ormel, J. (2006). Epidemiologic trends and costs of fragmentation., *Medical Clinics of North America* (90(4), 549–572).

Katon, W. J., & Seelig, M. (2008). Population-based care of depression: Team care approaches to improving outcomes. *Journal Occupational Environmental Medicine, 50*(4), 459–467.

Kroenke, K., Jackson, J. L., & Chamberlin, J. (1997). Depressive and anxiety disorders in patients presenting with physical complaints: Clinical predictors and outcome. *American Journal Medicine, 103*(5), 339–347.

Kroenke, K., & Mangelsdorff, A. D. (1989). Common symptoms in ambulatory care: Incidence, evaluation, therapy, and outcome. *American Journal Medicine, 86*(3), 262–266.

Kroenke, K., & Rosmalen, J. G. (2006). Symptoms, syndromes, and the value of psychiatric diagnostics in patients who have functional somatic disorders. *Medical Clinics North America, 90*(4), 603–626.

Margalit, A. P., & El-Ad, A. (2008). Costly patients with unexplained medical symptoms: A high-risk population. *Patient Education & Counseling, 70*(2), 173–178.

Melek, S., & Norris, D. (2008). *Chronic conditions and comorbid psychological disorders.* Seattle, WA: Milliman.

Seelig, M. D., & Katon, W. (2008). Gaps in depression care: Why primary care physicians should hone their depression screening, diagnosis, and management skills. *Journal Occupational Environmental Medicine, 50*(4), 451–458.

Sheehan, D. V. (2002). Establishing the real cost of depression. *Managed Care, 11*(8 Suppl.), 7–10; discussion 21–15.

Smith, G. C. (2009). From consultation-liaison psychiatry to integrated care for multiple and complex needs. *Australia New Zealand Journal Psychiatry, 43*(1), 1–12.

Wagner, E. H. (1998). Chronic disease management: What will it take to improve care for chronic illness? *Effective Clinical Practice, 1*(1), 2–4.

Wagner, E. H., Bennett, S. M., Austin, B. T., Greene, S. M., Schaefer, J. K., & Vonkorff, M. (2005). Finding common ground: Patient-centeredness and evidence-based chronic illness care. *Journal Alternative Complementary Medicine, 11*(Suppl. 1), S7–S15.

CHAPTER 10

Using a Case Manager–Patient Dialogue for Complexity Assessment and Care Plan Development

OBJECTIVES

- To describe the use of open-ended questions and a patient-case manager dialogue in the performance of a relationship-based complexity assessment
- To list example open-ended questions that can be used to complete adult and pediatric integrated case management Complexity Assessment Grids (CAGs) so that all CAG content areas are covered
- To discuss special question-asking procedures for children/youth and caregivers/parents for use in pediatric complexity assessments
- To connect the integrated case management assessment with the development of a care plan
- To explain the importance of documentation methodology for outcome measurement, case closure, and communication with clinicians and other stakeholders in the patient's care

INTRODUCTION

This chapter is designed to detail two sets of open-ended questions, one used to complete the adult Complexity Assessment Grid (CAG) and one the pediatric CAG. The semiscripted interviews should allow the development of a relationship with the patient, facilitate anchoring (scoring) of all cells in the patient's adult INTERMED-Complexity Assessment Grid (IM-CAG) or Pediatric INTERMED-Complexity Assessment Grid (PIM-CAG) during the course of the interview, and support the creation of a comprehensive care plan. Through the use of these open-ended questions, rather than a series of grid item-specific, fixed-answer questions, a dialogue between the case manager and the patient or the case manager and the child/youth and/or caregiver/parent will systematically uncover complexity-based barriers to improvement while a relationship is being established.

The questions enumerated in this chapter provide a roadmap for completion of all items in the adult and pediatric CAGs. However, they are not intended to be used verbatim or even necessarily in the order in which they are listed. Rather, they provide guidance to otherwise experienced case management clinicians as they systematically assess the needs of patients with health complexity. The goal in listing the questions is to ensure coverage of all important areas in the complexity assessment process so that comprehensive care plans can be developed and patients

can be assisted through the hard work of regaining health.

Some clinicians consider the use of open-ended questions a luxury in this age of time efficiency and focused action because it is felt to be too time consuming to enter extended dialogues with patients. Traditional case management typically defines success by the number of calls made or the number of patient encounters completed, thus quick data gathering is highly valued. This is one of the important conceptual and practical differences between integrated case management and traditional case management.

Integrated case managers target high-cost and complicated patients with whom they will likely be working for weeks or months, initially with relatively frequent contact. Thus, time invested during early conversations in becoming personally acquainted with the patient can influence integrated case management success, which is measured in terms of improved health and the efficient use of health resources by managed cases, rather than the number of calls or patient encounters. In fact, investing time initially to build a relationship with the patient, the child/youth, or the caregiver/parent can speed outcome change by strengthening the case manager-patient alliance and collaborative resolve. In the integrated case management paradigm, more time spent in dialogue with the patient clarifying and correctly anchoring complexity item scores in real time is an investment in future progress. Further, at the completion of this dialogue-based assessment, the complexity grid will be fully scored and can be used as a tool to facilitate communication and prioritization of goals with the patient as a care plan is then developed.

Using open-ended questions, which by their nature take longer than completing a fixed number of check boxes in performing standardized interviews, does have some disadvantages. Many of the patients who enter integrated case management will have such significant health problems that they have lowered physical and emotional reserves. As a result, these patients may not have the energy or desire to complete an assessment that may last up to an hour even though it is personalized. Their health state and complexity is just too burdensome. For this reason, in such patients, it may be necessary to complete the initial assessment in installments. For many, if not most, only one interview will be necessary to complete the initial assessment. In some, however, such as in the mentally challenged or in frail elderly patients, without alternative information sources, the initial assessment may require three or more short contacts with the patient, taking no more than 15 minutes each.

Finally, the organization of questioning has been designed to find out about the *patient* before focusing on his or her diseases. The message is that the person is more important than his or her illnesses. Having said that, some patients will feel threatened if a stranger, the case manager, immediately launches into a number of personal questions unrelated to health and their health-related life situation. For this reason, case managers should open the dialogue (i.e., break the ice) by talking about the reason for referral, their general understanding of the patient's condition, the role of case management, and what the case management-patient interaction will entail. This should allow case managers to assess the patient's comfort level in talking with them and should determine the speed at which more personal questions can be asked. Ultimately, however, all content areas in the CAGs must be covered, using sensitivity and diplomacy when needed, so that a comprehensive care plan can be developed.

CATHY: AN EXAMPLE OF A PATIENT WITH HEALTH COMPLEXITY

The adult and pediatric CAG systematically address biological, psychological, social, and health system factors that create barriers to improvement in the lives of patients with health complexity. For instance, Cathy, a 53-year-old woman with heart failure, triggered positive (e.g. met triage criteria) for consideration of involvement in a newly developed clinic-based case management program because her doctors just could not get her water off (e.g. control her fluid balance)

and control her breathing despite aggressive medication adjustments and frequent appointments. In addition to being treatment resistant, she also triggered as a potential case management participant (see Figure 3.2) because she had been to the emergency room 12 times in the past 6 months and was admitted to the hospital 3 times in the past year. Her community health doctors, various supervised physicians-in-training providing service at Cathy's public clinic, did not know if she was taking her medications and were frustrated that she was often a no show for appointments. They knew she had congestive heart failure and some mental health problem for which she saw a psychiatrist. They liked Cathy as a person but were having no success in treating her.

Cathy's persistent and progressive heart condition was precipitated by a heart attack several years before. She had been receiving evidence-based treatment, or so her doctors thought. What their 15-minute follow-up appointments did not allow was gathering information in other than the biological domain.

Through integrated case management and use of a CAG assessment, it was possible to establish that Cathy had been living in a shelter for the past 9 months (CS1, "Residential Stability") and had no relatives and few friends to help with obtaining her medications or getting her to her frequent doctors' appointments (CS2, "Social Support"). When she traveled to the community health clinic, which was several miles away, she had to take a bus (CHS1, "Getting Needed Services"). Further, with a seventh-grade education, she had difficulty keeping track on her own of her many complicated and ever-changing medications (VS, "Social Vulnerability"). Even if Cathy understood the intervention directions given by her doctors, she was on public assistance with limited benefits and not enough money to purchase her medications or oxygen (HHS1, "Access to Care"; HS1, "Job and Leisure").

This became even more complicated by the fact that Cathy was also being treated for schizophrenia at the local mental health clinic, which had no connection to the community health clinic (CHS2, "Coordination of Care"). Her hallucinations had been in control for several years with some of the newer medications (HP2, "Mental Health History"), but she still had trouble coping with life's needs and personal stress (HP1, "Barriers to Coping") and had some heart-related side effects from her psychiatric medications (CB2, "Diagnostic/Therapeutic Challenge"). Her doctors never talked to her psychiatrists. The assertive community treatment (ACT) social worker assigned to her, who had a caseload of 250 county residents, focused only on keeping her out of the psychiatric hospital (CHS2, "Coordination of Care"). Without change, it could be predicted that inadequately controlled heart failure (CB2, "Diagnostic/Therapeutic Challenge") would persist and put her at risk for additional hospitalizations (VB, "Complications and Life Threat").

Since the ambulance picked her up when she took a turn for the worse (at no charge to Cathy), it was easier to get care in the emergency setting (CHS1, "Getting Needed Services"). By that time, she often required hospitalization. The severity of Cathy's heart failure clearly warranted attention (CB1, "Symptom Severity/Impairment") but it was the only piece of a complex puzzle that her clinic doctors were addressing. More was needed than oxygen, digitalis, and diuretics to transform Cathy from treatment resistant to a treatment success. Most of what Cathy needed, however, her clinic doctors could not give her. This chapter describes where to start and how to obtain the information summarized in Cathy's IM-CAG (**Table 10.1**, see page i4 for color version).

DEVELOPING A RELATIONSHIP USING OPEN-ENDED QUESTIONS

Obtaining information that will allow completion of the CAG is only half of the battle for a good case man-

ager. Equally important is the development of a relationship, an alliance, with the patient so that he or she is motivated to collaborate to achieve better health. The manager provides guidance, but the patient is the one who changes behaviors that lead to success in overcoming barriers (see Chapter 4). Unless a positive relationship is developed at the onset, particularly since the manager will be working with the patient for weeks to months, progress will be limited. That is why this manual uses open-ended questions and dialogue to gather information about the patient's needs. It is an attempt to help the patient and the manager connect, person to person, as the patient begins the journey to health.

OPENING THE CONVERSATION

The first encounter with the adult or the child/youth and caregiver/parent being referred for case management may occur through an introduction by the patient's primary or specialty care physician, from a telephone transfer by a case management enrollment specialist, during an acute hospital admission, or at the time of a scheduled call after an introductory case

TABLE 10.1	Cathy's IM-CAG						
Baseline	HEALTH RISKS AND HEALTH NEEDS						
Cathy	HISTORICAL		CURRENT STATE		VULNERABILITY		
Total Score = 44	Complexity Item	Score	Complexity Item	Score	Complexity Item		Score
Biological Domain	Chronicity **HB1**	3	Symptom Severity/Impairment **CB1**	2	Complications and Life Threat **VB**		3
	Diagnostic Dilemma **HB2**	1	Diagnostic/Therapeutic Challenge **CB2**	3			
Psychological Domain	Barriers to Coping **HP1**	2	Resistance to Treatment **CP1**	0	Mental Health Threat **VP**		2
	Mental Health History **HP2**	3	Mental Health Symptoms **CP2**	1			
Social Domain	Job and Leisure **HS1**	2	Residential Stability **CS1**	2	Social Vulnerability **VS**		2
	Relationships **HS2**	2	Social Support **CS2**	3			
Health System Domain	Access to Care **HHS1**	3	Getting Needed Services **CHS1**	3	Health System Impediments **VHS**		3
	Treatment Experience **HHS2**	1	Coordination of Care **CHS2**	3			
Comments							
Significant problems controlling congestive heart failure; controlled schizophrenia in a patient with little insurance, poor social support, and limited access to and coordination of care.							

management invitation letter. Before launching into the initial case management interview, it is important to provide a brief explanation of the case management program, why the patient is a candidate for participation, who referred the patient, which organization is sponsoring it, why it could be of value, and what it entails on the patient's part. If the management program is not linked to the patient's personal physician, the case manager should emphasize that the program focuses on helping patients who have complicated health issues that create barriers to receiving good care and achieving health.

The patient should be informed that at least one, but potentially several, interviews will help the manager to get to know the patient and to identify ways to be of assistance through the development and implementation of a care plan. The patient should also be told about confidentiality parameters and reporting requirements related to dangerousness. After the initial CAG assessment, the objective of the manager will be to assist the patient over weeks to months with specific health-improving activities that the patient and manager will begin together. Eventually, the expectation is that the patient will learn health navigation skills so that he or she can implement similar stabilizing strategies as those initiated with the help of the case manager, on his or her own. The manager and patient will collaborate in overcoming obstacles to successful treatment and optimal functioning prior to the patient's transfer back to standard care.

In patients with significant health problems that interfere with information gathering, it is helpful for the case manager to inquire whether a family member or significant other can help supply needed details. When this is not possible, then short iterative interviews over several days may be required before the initial assessment is complete. Sometimes it is necessary to obtain the majority of information from a relative, friend, or colleague or from clinician notes. Whenever possible, however, the patient should personally be a part of the fact-finding process.

When working with children/youth, even when they are nearing the age of majority or have been granted the status of an emancipated minor, the case manager should keep in mind that most assessments benefit by the input of one or more caregivers/parents. In part, this stems from the need in pediatric integrated case management for the case manager to obtain information about the child/youth and the caregiver/parent as well as the home, family, and school situation. Moreover, most children, even teens, do not have knowledge of many of the factors relevant to the complexity assessment, (e.g. adverse developmental events, caregiver's financial stability, etc.).

BREAKING THE ICE

Ideally, the case manager should have sufficient time between the identification of the patient for participation and the initial assessment to review clinical materials related to the patient's situation and to seek additional information from referring or treating practitioners. This allows the case manager to have an appreciation for the challenges and difficulties experienced by the patient and by the treating clinicians. Even when there is an imminent need to initiate case management assistance, it is important for the case manager to have a basic understanding of the reason for referral and the patient's health and personal situation. This allows them to respond to patient queries and sets the stage for launching into the complexity assessment and care plan development process.

The patient assessment itself starts with the case manager telling the patient what he or she understands about the clinical circumstances that led to the request for assistance. He or she shares the concerns of the clinicians working with the patient or other stakeholders (family, community agencies, employer, etc.) regarding the patient's health. The patient is allowed to react and correct the case manager and to dialogue about how case management involvement may improve the patient's situation in the future. From this initial discussion, it should be possible for the case manager to make a bridge with the patient and to begin the formal assessment process. Importantly, this preliminary dialogue can also be used to complete the portions of the complexity assessment (CAG) covered during the discussion. Often, but not always, the information covered relates to biological domain content and should not necessarily be aborted until a logical break creates an opportunity to move to obtaining information about the patient and his or her living situation (i.e., psychosocial issues).

ADULT AND PEDIATRIC COMPLEXITY ASSESSMENTS

ADULT ASSESSMENT INTERVIEW CONTENT

There is a tendency for busy traditional case managers to jump right into concentrated questions about illnesses, medications, and factors affecting adherence. This manual encourages a different approach. When possible, it incorporates psychosocial issues early in CAG assessment queries, first asking permission but then obtaining personal information about the patient's living situation and life circumstances. Through this process, the case manager tries to get to know the patient as a person. Further, they share the message that the person is more important than the illnesses that the patient is experiencing.

After initial social and general personal factors have been clarified, the case manager returns to CAG details about the patient's medical history, current illnesses and treatments, practitioners, challenges in obtaining health services, and experiences with and collaboration among providers. At the completion of this systematic questioning, most CAG items can be scored according to anchor point specifications and a care plan can be developed. The case manager better understands where barriers in specific areas of a patient's life need addressing to maximize improvement, minimize impairment, and make life happier, including:

- Personal issues (e.g., debilitated family member demands time and care)
- Social issues (e.g., few people to help)
- Physical issues (e.g., complexity of illnesses, treatments, complications)
- Financial issues (e.g., cannot pay rent, let alone for medication)
- Mental health issues (e.g., illnesses, symptoms, treatments or lack thereof)
- Health system issues (e.g., cannot find a specialist; long wait list for care; no insurance)

The only area that may remain to be elucidated is information about the patient's personality and coping mechanisms. Much can be gleaned from the responses that the patient gives about psychosocial, biomedical, and health system issues as the case manager appraises the patient's problem-solving approach and interactional capabilities. It is, however, helpful at this point to specifically ask how the patient sees him or herself and how he or she copes.

By this time, the patient should be familiar with the case manager and more comfortable with the assessment process. Thus, it is possible to finalize questions about the patient's personal habits (e.g., smoking and drinking) and about the way that the patient deals with stresses, acquaintances, and life situations. Further, it gives the case manager an opportunity to ask about the patient's greatest health concerns and to develop the patient's *personal* clinical symptom and functional activity improvement goals, on which the patient will work with the case manager.

None of the questions in the assessment dialogue are superfluous. The goal of the case manager is to listen to the patient, discuss and confirm problems, refine content information when needed, and identify health and life desires so that he or she can assist the patient with achieving a happier personal existence as efforts related to health are initiated. During the orientation and initial assessment, the case manager communicates a sense of optimism and assurance that he or she will be available to give support, suggestions,

and help. The patient, however, also learns that personal involvement is integral to the assistance process. The patient will be expected to understand his or her illnesses, to try new health behaviors, and to work closely with his or her personal doctors and the case manager as steps are taken to stabilize health.

Open-Ended Complexity Questions for Adults

Exhibit 10.1 contains 6 primary open-ended content model questions for adults with 7 to 10 potential follow-up questions under each content area. The 6 primary questions open discussion about: (a) general life circumstances; (b) physical health; (c) emotional health; (d) interactions with treating practitioners; (e) health system issues; and (f) potentially sensitive personal information. A 7th question allows the patient to add information at the end of the dialogue if they feel that something was missed.

Many, but not all, of the follow-up questions under the six main content questions are also open-ended—that is, they must be answered through dialogue rather than dichotomous (yes or no) answers. They complete the assessment information needed to fill in anchor points on the IM-CAG and jot notes about CAG items while the interview is in progress (Appendix E, see www.springerpub.com/kathol). The follow-up questions that can be answered with a "yes" or a "no" are intended to be followed with an explanatory query, which allows IM-CAG anchor point scoring. For instance, if follow-up question 2.3 in **Exhibit 10.1** is answered "yes" (medical assessments are underway), then the patient would be asked about the types of assessments he or she is getting since it is pertinent to a number of items in the IM-CAG, including HB2 ("Diagnostic Dilemma": repetitive evaluations), CB2 ("Diagnostic/Therapeutic Challenge": clear current diagnosis and/or needed treatments), HHS1 ("Access to Care": having insurance that pays for the services), and CHS2 ("Coordination of Care": pertinent clinicians aware of assessment).

While the questions are in quotes and have been specifically worded to help case managers actually verbalize questions that can be used to complete assessment interviews, they are not intended to be ordered as they are written or used verbatim. No two complexity assessments will be the same. Managers, in fact, should interject their own personalities and styles into the questions and the ordering of questions to allow the conversation to flow between them and their patients. It is truly a discussion between the case manager and the patient. What is important is that at the completion of the interview or sequences of interviews, all CAG item scores are correctly anchored, based on the conversation with the patient and that the foundation of a relationship between or among key participants has

EXHIBIT 10.1   Open-Ended Questions for Adults

QUESTION 1

Content Area: General Life Situation

"Is it okay to ask some questions to get to know you better before we focus on your current health situation?"

If okay, "Can you tell me a little about yourself, such as where you live, who you live with, how you spend your days, what your hobbies and interests are?"

Follow-up questions:

(The case manager can fill these in later if there is reticence to divulge personal information at this point.)

1.1 "What kind of job do you have?"
1.2 "Can you tell me about your financial situation/pressures?"
1.3 "Do you require assistance in getting out of the house?"
1.4 "Who helps you when a crisis arises?"
1.5 "Who are your friends?"
1.6 "How do you spend your free time?"
1.7 "Do you help take care of others—for example, a family member or a friend?"

QUESTION 2

Content Area: Physical Health

"How is your *(name main medical illness)* affecting you today?"

Follow-up questions:

2.1 "Have you had (other) physical problems or long-term conditions or illnesses?"
2.2 "Were these difficult to diagnose?"
2.3 "Are medical assessments underway?"
2.4 "What kind of treatments are you getting/have you received?"
2.5 "How have the treatments worked?"
2.6 "Have you had difficulty following through on recommended physical health treatments?"
2.7 "Do physical symptoms interfere with doing the things you like to do?"

QUESTION 3

Content Area: Emotional Health

"How do you feel emotionally, such as worried, tense, sad, or forgetful?"

Follow-up questions:

3.1 "Has your physical health situation affected your emotions (or your memory)?"
3.2 "Have you had mental health problems in the past?"
3.3 "Have mental health issues required treatment or hospitalization, such as for depression, anxiety, confusion, or memory problems?"
3.4 "What kinds of treatments are you getting/have you received and from whom?"
3.5 "Have you had difficulty in following through on past mental health treatments?"
3.6 "Are you receiving any treatment now?"
3.7 "Has treatment been helpful?"
3.8 "Do emotional factors interfere with doing the things you like to do?"

QUESTION 4

Content Area: Interaction With Treating Practitioners

"Can you tell me who you see for your health problems?"

Follow-up questions:

4.1 "Primary care physician/nurse practitioner?"
4.2 "Medical specialists?"
4.3 "Mental health providers, such as, psychiatrists, psychologists, social workers, nurses, etc.?"
4.4 "Other providers, such as, chiropractors, naturopath, church counselor, etc.?"
4.5 "Can you tell me how you get along with your doctors?"
4.5 "How do those giving you care talk with each other and coordinate your treatment?"
4.6 "Do you have difficulty communicating with them?"
4.7 "Are their offices near each other and easy to get to?"
4.8 "Have you had conflicts or disagreements with any of your doctors/providers, your hospital/clinic, or your insurance company that have led to bad feelings or mistrust?"

(Continued)

EXHIBIT 10.1   **Open-Ended Questions for Adults** (*Continued*)

QUESTION 5

Content Area: Health System Issues
"Can you tell me whether you have difficulty in getting the health care you need?"

Follow-up questions:
- 5.1   "What type of medical insurance do you have and does it cover the services you need?"
- 5.2   "Do you have trouble finding medical doctors who will accept you as a patient?"
- 5.3   "Do you need to go to separate clinics for mental health treatment?"
- 5.4   "Are there separate payment rules for mental health care?"
- 5.5   "Have you or your primary care physician had difficulty in finding a mental health provider for you?"
- 5.6   "How far do you live from the medical clinics and doctors you need to improve (control) your health?"
- 5.7   "Do you need a translator or someone from your culture to assist with health needs?"
- 5.8   "Can you afford your medical care, such as medications, needed tests, copays for appointments and hospital costs, needed medical equipment/devices, etc.?"
- 5.9   "Is transportation a problem in getting to your appointments?"
- 5.10   "Are there long waiting lists for the kind of care you need?"

QUESTION 6

Content Area: More Sensitive Personal Information
"What kind of person are you, such as outgoing, suspicious, tense, optimistic?"

Follow-up questions:
- 6.1   "Do you smoke?"
- 6.2   "On average, how many alcoholic beverages do you drink a day (week), such as glasses of wine, beer, etc.?"
- 6.3   "Do you use painkillers: how often, how long, more often than prescribed?"
- 6.4   "Do you use cocaine, marijuana, or other recreational drugs?"
- 6.5   "Have you ever been treated for substance abuse problems?"
- 6.6   "How do you handle difficult situations?"
   (Alcohol or drug use; become talkative or silent; or procrastinate?)
- 6.7   "What are your biggest health concerns at this time?"
- 6.8   "During the next 1 to 3 months, what about your health would you like to have under better control (*clinical*), such as have less foot pain, have no asthma attacks for a solid month, etc.?"
- 6.9   "What would you like to be able to do that you can't do now (*functional*), such as attend church regularly, participate in family events, return to work, etc.?"

QUESTION 7

Content Area: Additional Information From Patient
"What things did I not ask about that you think are important?"

---

been established (de Jonge, Bauer, Huyse, & Latour, 2003; de Jonge, Hoogervorst, Huyse, & Polman, 2004; de Jonge, Latour, & Huyse, 2003; Huyse, 1997; Slaets, Kauffmann, Duivenvoorden, Pelemans, & Schudel, 1997).

The Adult Assessment Interview

While there are 6 primary questions and nearly 50 follow-up questions listed in **Exhibit 10.1**, they do not all need to be asked. Case managers will find that complexity content in one area will often be covered while discussing related content from another question. For instance, the first question, "Can you tell me a little about yourself?" could provide information

about illnesses and treatments, difficulties with clinicians, insurance coverage, and so forth in addition to the social and personal issues that it is intended to review. When other complexity areas are discussed in the course of spontaneous conversation, IM-CAG anchor point scores can be established and notes related to them inserted without the need to reask questions related to them later.

Having said this, it is important for the case manager to sequentially step through the six content areas listed in **Exhibit 10.1**. These areas have been ordered from one to six deliberately. The first question clarifies details about the person and his or her life. While personal, most follow-up questions under Question 1 are not sensitive in nature (e.g., about job, friends, family, support system, living situation, etc.). Some can be sensitive, such as personal finances. In this content area, when the case manager finds that questions elicit discomfort, he or she should back off and return to the question later. In some interviews, it may even be necessary to spend more time on content area 2, physical health, to allow the rudiments of a relationship to develop before personal questions are asked.

Content areas 2 and 3, physical and emotional health, are core areas of traditional case management but are usually covered by managers working for different organizations or in separate sections of a single organization (e.g., medical and mental health). **Exhibit 10.1** should help those coming from either a medical background or a mental health background to pursue needed information in both areas. The questions, however, should be customized to the patient and the situation. For instance, when a patient's primary referral reason is related to a serious and persistent mental illness, such as schizophrenia, then the content of question 3 should likely precede question 2.

Often much information in the follow-up questions about physical and mental health can be filled in before the interview by reviewing clinician notes or claims databases. While this is helpful, it should not be relied on as the sole source of information. It is also important to obtain the patient's perception of his or her health situation. For instance, if a primary care physician's notes indicate that the managed patient's headaches are due to depression but the patient thinks that he or she may have a brain tumor, resolution of these conflicting viewpoints may influence whether intermittent emergency room visits persist related to this physical complaint.

Questions 4 and 5 clarify practitioner and health system details that influence whether the patient will be successful in receiving and adhering to treatments for conditions outlined by questions 2 and 3. Questions 4 and 5 are generally not a part of clinic personnel evaluations or a part of health-related databases. Information about these complexity areas can only be elicited through direct questions or dialogue with the patient.

Question 6 returns to personal and now more sensitive information about the patient. By this time, the case manager and patient will have covered most important content areas. Some personal, but not necessarily sensitive, questions will have been introduced during this process (e.g., how patients like their doctors, who helps them in crisis, whether they follow their doctors' recommendations, etc.). In question 6, personal and often sensitive questions explore the patient's personal habits, coping mechanisms, concerns, and desires.

There is no guarantee that the patient will be ready to openly and honestly answer the questions related to

this content area at the end of a 30- to 45-minute assessment. Nevertheless, he or she should be asked these questions, and answers should be recorded since they are pertinent to the long-term outcomes of the case management process. For those in whom questions in this and other areas remain uncertain or unanswered, they should be brought up at a later date, should be assessed based on the patient's behavior and/or further interactions with the case manager, or should be explored indirectly when talking with alternative sources of information, such as the patient's doctors or family members.

Finally, patients should always have an opportunity to provide feedback about the content of the interview, as is encouraged in question 7. It is not possible to address all areas of potential complexity even with an open-ended dialogue. This question allows additional areas of importance to be uncovered. It also tells the patient that his or her input is valued.

Near the completion of the interview, all open-ended content area questions should be reviewed to make sure that nothing has been missed (see listed questions in **Exhibit 10.1**). Further, notes taken during the interview about details in each of the six content areas and the seventh clarification question (Appendix E, see www.springerpub.com/kathol) can be used to consolidate the information in the IM-CAG and develop a care plan. The notes help to link items and to explain the rationale for anchor point scoring. Ultimately, they will also help communicate findings about barriers to improvement with the patient and the patient's clinicians through their inclusion in the IM-CAG scoring and documentation system.

Adult Assessment Duration

The time it takes to complete an initial complexity assessment varies based on a number of factors. First, assessments take longer as health complexity increases. For those with little or no complexity (i.e., IM-CAG scores of 15 or less), the initial assessment can take as little as 10 to 15 minutes. Few patients fall into this category since a complexity assessment is not needed in patients with no clinical suggestion of complexity. In those with mild to moderate complexity (i.e., IM-CAG scores of 16 to 30), assessments generally take 20 to 30 minutes. Patients with high complexity take the longest, ranging from 30 to 90 minutes because of the need for clarification about the number of conditions involved; the number of providers, medications and other treatments; the social support situation, financial circumstances; and many other factors that may require action on the part of the case manager and the patient. It is for this reason that sequential interviews are occasionally necessary to finalize an initial assessment.

Other factors also contribute to the duration of the assessment process. For some, there is distrust by the patient about the medical system and its practitioners, including case managers. In these instances, it takes time for pertinent information to come out as a trusting relationship between the case manager and patient grows. For others, the veracity of the patient can be in question, such as in those with substance abuse/dependency problems or those in the middle of disability litigation. Second source information gathering is often necessary to sort fact from fiction in these cases.

Some individuals/patients may welcome the opportunity to talk about themselves and their health situations. During their interviews, it is difficult to keep them on task related to the complexity questions. These patients take longer than those in whom responses track closely to the questions. Similarly, it may be challenging keeping an interview focused when working with elderly patients or those with cognitive impairment, but for a different reason. In these patients, the paucity of information shared or delayed responses prolong interviews. Since the case manager will be working with the patients for weeks or even months, it is important not to feel too rushed to obtain the final answer on every item in the IM-CAG assessment. The composite picture often provides excellent guidance in care plan development while waiting for additional evidence to trickle in.

Connecting Clinical Barriers With Measurable Outcomes

As information is gathered about the patient's physical and mental health conditions in questions 2 and 3, it is appropriate to ask the patient about and/or to check office or hospital notes so that pertinent baseline measures can be recorded (e.g., HbA1c levels in patients with diabetics, FEV1s in patients with emphysema or asthma, ejection fractions in patients with congestive heart failure, analogue pain scale scores). The same should be done related to baseline function (e.g., days of work missed, activity of daily living limitations, health care satisfaction, and quality of life). These measures can then be used as the patient is followed to document change in targeted clinical and functional factors, satisfaction, and quality of life over time. In some situations, it may be necessary to collaborate with the patient and the patient's clinicians in order to obtain the absolute measurements at the intervals desired.

The process of obtaining and recording baseline measures for mental health conditions, such as depression and anxiety, creates a special challenge since few primary care physicians, and even mental health professionals, consistently document symptom levels or record change over time. For this reason, if the patient describes discouragement, frustration, depression, or anxiety or is being treated for depression or anxiety, this is an opportunity for the case manager to fill out a Personal Health Questionnaire-9 (PHQ-9; Lowe, Unutzer, Callahan, Perkins, & Kroenke, 2004) if depression is a concern or a Generalized Anxiety Disorder-7 (GAD-7; Spitzer, Kroenke, Williams, & Lowe, 2006) if anxiety is a concern, presuming that the patient's clinician has not already done so. These standardized public domain instruments can then be used to assess symptom change over time for the most common mental health conditions seen in the primary care setting.

Documenting baseline measures is an important indirect message to the patient and the patient's practitioners (i.e., that the case manager takes outcomes seriously). It is also a vital activity for case managers since it will allow them to concretely assess the success that they are having in assisting patients through case management (see Appendices 11 and 12).

Identifying the Patient's Personal Clinical and Functional Goals

One of the important things from the patient's perspective is to accomplish goals that will have meaning and value to him or her. As a result, the case manager should help the patient define two specific goals (limit to two) that would be attainable with case management assistance that relate to health (see Table 9.39, "Clinical Measure Related to Personal Goal"), for example, getting up less often to go to the bathroom, having fewer headaches, and so forth and reducing impairment (see Table 9.39, "Functional Measure Related to Personal Goal"), for example, being able to walk to the store, playing with a granddaughter, attending football games, and so forth. By working with the patient on these tasks, it helps him or her learn how to set goals, to make changes, and to reach his or her own goals.

During this exercise, the case manager teaches the person how to make a goal manageable, so he or she can use the same technique or problem-solving logic in the future. For example, the case manager might say: "Stopping smoking cold turkey is a daunting task. How about trying to cut down to one or two cigarettes per hour first?" This helps the patient break up the longer-term goal into manageable pieces. It gives him or her ideas about how to structure and attain future goals.

In helping the patient identify a clinical goal, case managers should ask, "During the next 1 to 3 months, what about your health would you like to have under better control, e.g., have less foot pain, have no asthma attacks for a solid month, etc.?" and then give them a chance to respond. This should be followed by a similar query about a functional goal—for example, "What would you like to be able to do that you cannot do now, e.g., attend church weekly, go to the next family reunion, return to work, etc.?" These patient-directed goals should be realistic and within the time frame of work with the case manager, yet challenging enough that the patient will feel a sense of accomplishment if they are attained.

Personal goals will be monitored along with other patient-specific outcomes. They should be formulated in such a way that progress toward goal attainment can be easily tracked using quantitative indices (e.g., analogue pain scale scores, number of asthma attacks, number of times attended church in last month, attendance at piano recitals, days worked, etc.). The patient will need assistance in creating goals that are reasonable *and* measurable; however, *they should be consistent with what the patient values and wants to accomplish.* While the patient's goals may differ from the case manager's (e.g., to lower HbA1c levels, to have fewer visits to the emergency room, to take lower-cost medications, to go back to work, etc.), they will be the tunnel through which the patient and the case manager pass as they move toward health and function. Initially supporting patient-derived goals will help to elicit patient motivation and subsequent willingness to address goals that may be generated by the case manager (with the patient's input and collaboration).

While the patient's personal goals are one of the most important components of the patient-case manager relationship, they should also be flexible. Increased knowledge about the patient's clinical situation or changes, for better or worse, in his or her health status may require that goals be adjusted. Nonetheless, as refinements to goals are made, they should foremost remain the goals of the patient, not the case manager.

PEDIATRIC ASSESSMENT INTERVIEW CONTENT

The same systematic assessment process that is used for adults is used for children/youth. The pediatric assessment, however, requires alteration in how the information is gathered. The child/youth and the caregiver/parent are both important contributors to health or persistent illness and impairment. Once a child reaches the age where he or she is able to understand and communicate about the issues being discussed, his or her participation in the assessment, collaboration in the development of a care plan, and help in designing the action steps to recover health is important.

In young children (i.e., those between birth and around age seven), or in those with cognitive delays,

most complexity assessment information will be obtained from caregivers/parents. While young children can share how they feel physically and emotionally and general characteristics of their living situation, they are usually unaware of most other components that contribute to their personal health.

In most families, one caregiver/parent takes the lead in supporting and providing information about a child's/youth's health. Though it is acceptable to rely on a single caregiver's/parent's perspective, when possible, it is preferable to attempt to obtain information from each caregiver/parent. By doing so, it offers a more comprehensive picture of the child and his or her situation, as well as potential discrepancies in caregivers'/parents' views about how their child's/youth's health should be managed. It also allows the case manager to better understand the strengths and weaknesses that each caregiver/parent has, and how they affect the child/youth and his or her health status.

Involvement of children/youth after the age of seven in the assessment process increases in proportion to their ability to communicate and to understand the importance of their participation in improving their own health. The age of the child/youth also influences the degree to which concurrent and independent questioning of the caregiver/parent and the child/youth will take place. For instance, it is usually unnecessary to independently ask a child/youth about alcohol or drug use or about sexual activity before the age of 11 or 12 years. When he or she reaches or surpasses this age, however, it is also best to ask the questions during independent interviews with the child/youth and the caregiver/parent.

Sensitive questions, such as these, are difficult to answer for preteens and teens, let alone in the presence of their caregivers/parents. While there is no guarantee that such questions will be answered honestly, even in the absence of other family members, it does create an opportunity to compare youth and caregiver/parent responses. This, in itself, is sometimes informative.

Another factor that comes into play when conducting initial complexity assessments with children/youth is the relationship that they have with their caregiver/parents. The case manager should be cognizant of natural conflicts that arise as youth grow and transition from dependence to independence. In many families this transition creates tensions that can undermine efforts needed for the youth to engage in healthy behaviors (e.g., adherence with recommendations, reporting personal or social issues affecting health, etc.). The interpersonal dynamics of the caregiver/parent and child/youth relationship may also influence the way that the case manager asks questions (i.e., independently or with all present) and the approaches that are taken to overcome identified barriers. It is helpful for the case manager to share his or her perception about family interactions with the child's/youth's clinicians to see if they consider family dynamics an issue and agree with the case manager's conclusions.

The case manager should be sensitive during the interview to what information the child/youth has about his or her medical conditions (e.g., what has he or she been told by his or her caregivers/parents and the health care team?). Caregivers/parents often closely monitor the information the child/youth receives. It would not be helpful for a case manager to raise issues of which the child/youth is not aware. For this reason, it is often preferable for the case manager to interview the caregiver/parent before the child/youth to find out the level of information sharing within the family. If this is not possible, then general (e.g., "Do you have any health problems?") rather than specific questions (e.g., "Can you describe your cancer treatment?") about the child's/youth's illnesses are a better place to start.

Conflicting stories of the same event can be reported by caregiver/parent and child/youth. When disagreement occurs, then it is up to case managers to use judgment in deciding what to believe and how to proceed. Sometimes additional information from other sources is required. Sometimes reasking the question at another time brings clarity. In most situations, consensus emerges with time or interaction with the caregivers/parents or child/youth. The sorting process becomes important when different stories suggest the need for different case manager actions. When conflict cannot be resolved but action is necessary, it is best to err on the side of safety and potential value brought to the youth as PIM-CAG item scoring is performed.

Finally, as the case manager approaches the end of the assessment and attempts to delineate personal goals, the child/youth and caregiver/parent may voice differing desires. Since this patient-centered component of integrated case management enhances personal motivation, an attempt should be made to reconcile goals. If compromise, consensus, or prioritization of goals is not possible, then the case manager needs to decide whether to focus on achieving the caregiver's/parent's goals, the child's/youth's goals, or both. Fortunately, personal goals, whether the child's/youth's or the caregiver's/parent's, often correlate closely with the ultimate goals of case management (i.e., stabilized health and function). Thus, in most situations, goals should come into synchrony (e.g., the youth's functional goal is increased activities with friends, the parent's goal is better school attendance, and the case manager's goal is social situation stability). If any one goal is accomplished, all three should be possible based on the child's/youth's clinical condition.

Privacy and Reporting Laws

Before starting to work with children/youth and caregivers/parents, it is important to clarify for them that parts of the interviews will be performed with both parties present and parts with only the child/youth or caregiver/parent present. It is at this time that both should also be informed about how confidential information will be handled (see the Chapter 8 section "The Child/Youth and Caregivers/Parents Interview and Assessment"). If the child/youth is at the age of majority (18 or older in most locales), there is an obligation for the case manager to receive consent from both the parent and child to share information about their individual conversations with the case manager with others. Though there is no legal obligation to receive such consent in younger children/youth, it can be helpful to clarify confidentiality limits for them as well since the child/youth needs to know who will have access to the information they provide, particularly since the age of sexual consent is often several years younger than the age of majority.

Finally, both the caregivers/parents and children/youth should know that case managers, like other health professionals are under legal obligation to inform appropriate authorities about potentially dangerous situations (e.g., suicidal behavior, homicidal behavior, physical or sexual abuse, etc.) whether the object of concern is the child/youth or the caregiver/parent. Again, when the child/youth is at the age of majority and does not wish the caregiver/parent to know of even dangerous situations, the case manager may be required to inform authorities without telling the caregiver/parent. Clinical judgment is important in determining how this would be handled.

Open-Ended Complexity Questions for Children/Youth

Exhibit 10.2 contains similar primary open-ended model questions in the six content areas as used for adults. Each should be reworded to fit the age of the child/youth. For children/youth and caregiver/parents, the number of potential follow-up questions expands to nearly 80. As can be recalled from the section "PIM-CAG Items Peculiar to Children/Youth" in Chapter 8, the pediatric psychological and family/social domains now include additional items (HP3, "Cognitive Development"; HP4, "Adverse Developmental Events"; HS3, "Caregiver/Parent Health and Function"; CS3, "Caregiver/Family Support"; and CS4, "School and Community Participation"). As a result, the initial assessment dialogue necessarily swells to include questions on child/youth development and on family/social factors that affect both the caregiver/parent and the child/youth.

For children too young to answer for themselves, all information related to the initial assessment is obtained from the caregivers/parents. Children/youth able to provide information on their own should be involved in the assessment process to the extent possible. In general, this means that there will be a *combined interview* with the child/youth and the caregiver/ parent and *independent interviews* with each, the child/youth and the caregiver/parent.

In the *combined interview*, questions in unbolded print will be first addressed to the child/youth and second to the caregiver/parent except for questions in <u>underlined print</u>. For some families, <u>the content of the underlined questions may be sensitive</u> and can be skipped during the *combined interview* but then addressed in *independent interviews*. The decisions about when to ask the more sensitive, underlined questions are at the discretion of the case manager.

Questions in bold print are addressed to the caregivers/parents only and are used typically during their *independent interview*. When possible, it is helpful to confirm conflicting or uncertain findings with information from other sources, including health practitioners, teachers, peers, clergy, and so forth. Notes will be consolidated and anchor points scored in the PIM-CAG assessment instrument based on the best evidence from the information sources.

QUESTION 1

Content Area: General Life Situation

"Is it okay to ask some questions to get to know you better before we focus on your current health situation?"

If okay, "Can you tell me a little about yourself, such as, where you live, who your friends are, what you like to do (hobbies/interests, extracurricular activities), and with whom you like to do things?"

Follow-up questions:

(The case manager can fill these in later if there is reticence to divulge personal information at this point.)

1.1 "Can you tell me about the members of your family?"
1.2 "Who are your close friends or relatives?"
1.3 <u>"Whom do you[a] rely on when you need help?"</u>
1.4 "Can you tell me about how you like your school?"
1.5 <u>"How do you do in school?"</u>
1.6 "What things do you like to do outside of classes, such as, clubs, sports, music, etc.?"
1.7 "Have you had difficulty with attendance or getting along at school?"
1.8 <u>"Have you gotten in trouble in school, at home, or with the law?"</u>
1.9 "How do you spend your free time?"
1.10 **"Can you tell me about your spouse/partner?"**
1.11 **"Are there custody issues related to the child/youth?"**
1.12 **"Where does the child/youth live?"**
1.13 **"Have you moved often?"**
1.14 **"Who supervises and feeds your child/youth during nonschool hours?"**
1.15 **"What kind of job do you have?"**
1.16 **"Can you tell me about your financial situation/pressures?"**
1.17 **"Can you tell me about current stresses/changes in your family situation or things that are worrying you about the future?"**
1.18 **"Can you tell me about any physical or mental conditions or disability that you or your spouse/partner have?"**
1.19 **"Who helps you (the caregiver/parent) when a crisis arises?"**
1.20 **"How does your child's health situation affect your family?"**
1.21 **"Do you help take care of others, such as family or friends?"**
1.22 **"Can you tell me about behaviors, friendships, school, or legal concerns related to your child/youth?"**

QUESTION 2

Content Area: Physical Health

"How do you feel physically?"

Follow-up questions:

2.1 "Have you had (other) problems with your health for a long time?"
2.2 <u>"Are the doctors doing tests on you now?"</u>
2.3 "What kind of treatment are you getting?"
2.4 "Have you had difficulty doing what the doctors ask you to do?"
2.5 <u>"Have the doctor's treatments worked?"</u>
2.6 <u>"Do health problems keep you from doing the things you like to do?"</u>
2.7 **"How serious are your child's/youth's health problems?"**

(Continued)

2.8   **"Does your child/youth have any disabilities or limitations?"**
2.9   **"Were your child's/youth's health problems difficult to diagnose?"**

QUESTION 3

Content Area: Emotional Health
"How do you feel emotionally, such as worried, tense, sad, or forgetful?"

Follow-up questions:
3.1   "Do you get in trouble very often?"
3.2   "Have you ever seen a doctor or counselor because you got in trouble or because you felt so upset?"
3.3   "Have you gotten treatment for this or gone into the hospital?"
3.4   "Do you have trouble doing what your doctors ask you to do?"
3.5   "Has the treatment been helpful?"
3.6   "Do emotional factors or things that get you into trouble affect how you get along with others?"
3.7   "Do emotional factors or things that get you into trouble interfere with your ability to do the things you like to do?"
3.8   **"Can you describe if there were challenges in your child's/youth's development?"**
3.9   **"Can you describe if special services or school assistance was needed because of your child's/youth's cognitive development?"**
3.10   **"Has your child/youth had mental health problems, such as depression, eating disorder, severe anxiety?"**
3.11   **"Has your child/youth been treated for mental health or cognitive problems?"**
3.12   **"Can you describe if your child/youth experienced early life events that might have affected his/her health, such as head trauma, lead exposure, prenatal alcohol or drug exposure, abuse, or in utero infections?"**

QUESTION 4

Content Area: Interaction With Treating Practitioners
"Can you tell me who you see for health problems?"

Follow-up questions:
4.1   "Are your doctors (counselors) easy to talk to?"
4.2   "Do you trust your doctor (counselor)?"
4.3   "Have any of them done something that you do not like or disagree with?"
4.4   **"Pediatrician/nurse practitioner?"**
4.5   **"Medical specialists?"**
4.6   **"Mental health providers, such as psychiatrists, psychologists, social workers, nurses, etc.?"**
4.7   **"Other providers, such as, chiropractors, naturopaths, church counselors, etc.?"**
4.8   **"How do those giving your child/youth care talk with each other and coordinate his or her treatment?"**
4.9   **"Do you have difficulty communicating with them?"**
4.10   **"Are their offices near each other and easy to get to?"**
4.11   **"Have you (the caregiver/parent) had conflicts or disagreements with your child's/youth's doctors/providers, your hospital/clinic, or your insurance company that have led to bad feelings or mistrust?"**

QUESTION 5

Content Area: Health System Issues
"Can you tell me whether you have difficulty in getting the health care you need?"

Follow-up questions:
5.1   **"What type of medical insurance do you have for your child/youth and does it cover the services needed?"**
5.2   **"How do you find medical doctors who will accept your child/youth as a patient?"**
5.3   **"Do you need to go to separate clinics for mental health treatment?"**
5.4   **"Are there separate payment rules for mental health care?"**
5.5   **"Have you or your primary care physician had difficulty in finding a mental health provider for your child/youth?"**
5.6   **"How far do you live from the medical clinics and doctors you need to improve (control) your child's/youth's health?"**
5.7   **"Is transportation a problem in getting to your child/youth to appointments?"**

EXHIBIT 10.2   Open-Ended Questions for Pediatric Patients and Their Caregivers (*Continued*)

5.8 **"Do you need a translator or someone from your child's/youth's culture to assist with health needs?"**

5.9 **"Can you afford your child's/youth's medical care, for example, medications, needed tests, copays for appointments and hospital costs, needed medical equipment/devices, etc.?"**

5.10 **"Are there long waiting lists for the kind of care your child/youth needs?"**

5.11 **"Have you had difficulty in transitioning your child's/youth's care from his/her pediatric practitioners to adult doctors?"**

QUESTION 6

Content Area: More Sensitive Personal Information
"What kind of person are you,[b] such as outgoing, suspicious, tense, or optimistic?"

Follow-up questions:

6.1 "How do you handle difficult situations?" (talkative, silent, procrastinate?)

6.2 "What are your biggest health concerns at this time?"

6.3 "If I worked with you for the next several months, what would you most like me to help you make better about your health, such as no shots, stop being sick from meds, etc.?"

6.4 "What would you most like to be able to do that you cannot do now,[c] such as, play in the band, stay overnight with friends, lose weight?"

6.5 "Do you (think your youth) smoke(s)?"

6.6 "Do you (think your youth) use(s) alcohol?"

6.7 "Do other family members have alcohol or drug problems?"

6.8 "Do you (suspect that your youth) or your (his or her) friends use(s) drugs?"

6.9 "Have you (or your youth) ever been treated for substance abuse problems?"

6.10 **"What kind of person are you,[d] such as outgoing, suspicious, tense, or optimistic?"**

6.11 **"How do you[d] handle difficult situations?"**

QUESTION 7

Content Area: Additional Information From Patient or Caregivers/Parents
"What things did I not ask about that you think are important?

---

[a]*Note to case manager: The "you" in this question is the child/youth.*

[b]*Note to case manager: The "you" in this question is the child/youth. For the independent interview with the caregiver/parent, the question becomes "What kind of person is your child/youth, such as outgoing, suspicious, tense, or optimistic?"*

[c]*Note to case manager: Functional personal goals of the child/youth.*

[d]*Note to case managers: In the bold print questions such as 6.10 and 6.11, the "you" refers to the caregiver/parent.*

Not only is the initial pediatric assessment longer and more time consuming, it must also be performed in segments, as previously mentioned. For the three-part interview, it may take up to 2 to 2.5 hours to complete depending on the level of complexity and other factors mentioned in the adult section. First, it is recommended that the caregiver/parent and child/youth be interviewed together. If the child/youth is old enough and has the cognitive capacity to participate, he or she should be asked the common questions first (i.e., those with no underlining and not in **bold** from **Exhibit 10.2**). After the child/youth answers, the caregiver/parent can add to or clarify the information from the child/youth. Some follow-up questions listed in **Exhibit 10.2** may be unnecessary because of the child's/youth's age, the child's/youth's health issues, or the family circumstances.

During the second segment of the assessment, the caregiver/parent is interviewed alone. Many of the questions during this portion relate to information about which the child/youth will have little knowledge **(bolded questions)**, such as caregiver/parent health, early developmental traumas, and so forth. While the child/youth could sit in on this section of the assessment, it is not recommended. In addition to nonsensitive questions, there will also be sensitive questions asked of the caregiver/parent (underlined questions), such as whether he or she thinks the child/youth or his or her friends are using drugs or alcohol, whether there are school problems and why, and so forth. Thus, it is best for this conversation to be performed separately.

Segment three of the assessment is with the child/youth. During this discussion, the child/youth can speak more freely about his or her home and school situation, about his or her friends, about promiscuity or drug use, and so forth (underlined questions). When both segment two and three are completed, the caregiver/parent and the child/youth are given an opportunity to add to topics or information that may have been overlooked or poorly delineated.

SUMMARY STATEMENT

At the completion of the adult or pediatric interview, it is important to let the patient confirm what you heard. *Summarize* what you consider salient components of the interview, highlighting things that may make it more difficult to adjust or to cope with health issues, such as a poor social situation, major illnesses (biological and/or psychological), a limited patient understanding of the health situation, infrequent doctor visits (inadequate treatment and follow-up), and so forth. You can use the scored IM-CAG or PIM-CAG completed during the course of the patient assessment and the notes that you recorded in the "Adult or Pediatric Clinical Notes Documentation Sheets" (Appendix E and Appendix F, www.springerpub.com/kathol) to highlight and formulate your summary. Feedback from patients in response to discussion of the summary can be added to the note documentation sheet.

In pediatric assessments, there will be elements of the interview that are pertinent to both the caregiver/parent and the child/youth, only to the child/youth, and only to the caregiver/parent. The pediatric case manager, therefore, has an additional challenge in sorting information from the various sources, consolidating what can be told to each individual and to both, while formulating a care plan and finessing those items in which confidentiality needs to be respected.

Prior to closing the conversation, the patient should be told that between now and his or her next exchange, the case manager will synthesize the information and put it into a summary grid with some notes that will be sent to the patient and, in the case of children/youth, the appropriate parties based on the age of the child/youth and the consents given. It will be from this summary that the patient and the case manager can work in developing a plan of assistance. If there are things that can be done for the patient between the end of the assessment and the next contact, such as sending educational materials, attempting to find community resources, and so forth, they should be done. At this point, a face-to-face or telephonic follow-up appointment with the patient is made. Finally, the case manager should create a diary about the things promised to the patient between the completion of the assessment and the next meeting.

CARE PLAN DEVELOPMENT

As soon as the case manager finishes the assessment with the patient, his or her anchored CAG items should be reviewed and finalized (Appendix 4 [adult version] or Appendix 5 [pediatric version]). Additional comments should be added to the "Clinical Notes Documentation Sheet" if needed (Appendix E [adult version] or Appendix F [pediatric version]) to facilitate remembering the targeted considerations for which interventions will be developed. Comments should also be added to the CAG summary grid that will help the patient understand why each grid item received the score that it did. The comments should be worded so that they can be shared with the patient and, with informed consent, with the patient's clinicians. After this is completed, a draft care plan should be created using a paper and pencil (**Table 10.2**) or computer-generated template.

As the draft case management care plan is created, individual cells with item scores suggesting a need

TABLE 10.2   **Care Plan Development (CD)**

BARRIERS	GOALS		ACTIONS
CAG items	Personal followed by health care		Prioritized
	Short-term		
	Ultimate		
	Short-term		
	Ultimate		
	Short-term		
	Ultimate		
	Short-term		
	Ultimate		

for action (i.e., those scored 3 and 2) and action items that appear to be related should be inserted in the care plan template (**Table 10.2**). For instance, in the case described earlier in the chapter, Cathy's mental health history (**Table 10.1**; score of 3 for HP2) is lengthy but under control. Short goals for this area may be to make sure that she understands her illness, is taking her antipsychotic medication, and has good mental health follow-up.

Cathy's therapeutic challenge (score of 3 for CB2), however, is linked to a number of items. Perhaps the most important and immediate of these are the lack of funds to buy medications (score of 3 for CHS1), her unstable living situation (score of 2 for CS1), and insufficient personal support (score of 3 for CS2) to help her attend medical appointments regularly. To improve Cathy's ability to access and adhere to the treatments (short-term goal) that she needs for her heart disease, information relevant to CB2, CS1, CS2, and CHS1 may be inserted as linked items in the left hand "Barriers" column of **Table 10.2**. Actions related to the short-term goal of improved adherence to recommended treatment may include: (a) notifying her doctors about the confusion she has about her medications and the financial challenges leading to medication nonadherence and appointment nonattendance, (b) exploring inexpensive medication options with her doctors, (c) attempting to find alternative housing closer to the community health clinic and to obtain public transportation passes for appointments, and (d) checking with the ACT social worker to see if she is willing to monitor medical medication adherence along with her psychiatric medications when she visits Cathy. The ultimate goal will be consistent heart care and controlled symptoms.

It is not reasonable to think that tackling individual items or a couple of linked barriers alone will lead to control of Cathy's poor health and high service use. The care plan will involve connecting each of her high-scoring barriers, setting goals, and systematically working toward resolution or at least stabilization of each. Any one item can be the weak link in the chain. Over time, barrier resolution can be documented and transition back to standard care can be considered. The value of the IM-CAG is that it makes it possible to unravel the low and high intensity barriers, to communicate how they are connected to unstable health with the patient, to tie together the barriers, and to collaborate with the patient in setting and working toward goals.

While it is good for the case manager to develop his or her own draft care plan before going over the complexity assessment with the patient, it may be best not to share the draft care plan with the patient. Rather, after explaining the meaning of the patient's own CAG results to him or her, the case manager will work collaboratively with the patient to develop a mutually agreed-on care plan. Since the case manager has already thought through the primary barriers and how they are linked, he or she can help guide the patient, using motivational interviewing techniques, to facilitate the recognition of how his or her life situations can contribute to persistent health problems and the actions needed to correct them.

For young children/youth, the completed pediatric CAG can be shared with the caregiver/parent. If the youth is at or nearing the age of majority or even the age of consent, both should be given a copy of the grid, recognizing that confidentially shared material may need to be omitted. The child/youth can discuss it with his or her caregivers/parents prior to the return visit. It will help both better understand the situation, frame their questions, and initiate their work on creating a care plan that will help them return to health stability. If the youth is at the age of majority, then he or she will decide whether the caregiver/parent receives a copy. In most situations, sharing results with both is not an issue; however, when it is, the decision-making youth's rights must be respected.

INITIATING A CARE PLAN

The case manager should reconnect with the patient, preferably within a week of completing the initial assessment. This way the last conversation is fresh. He or she should thank the patient for the time and effort made in helping the case manager understand his or her health situation. If there is something in the free text notes recorded about the patient during the interview process that would allow a demonstration of interest in him or her (e.g., "How did your son's baseball game go?" or "Did your father get out of the hospital yet?") this is a good way to reinitiate the conversation.

If the patient has been sent a copy of their personal CAG results, the first order of business will be to explain what the grid does and how it helps the case manager work with patients who have complicated health needs. Before discussing the patient's personal report, the domains, the items within the domains, and the color-coded scoring should be explained. It is also helpful to share that the level of item complexity has been standardized and that each level is connected to concrete approaches to help. Importantly, the patient needs to know that it is not just the individual scores, but also the connections among scores, that will be used to work with the patient in identifying strategies to regain his or her health.

High CAG scores and notes related to the scores help identify and explain areas in which immediate assistance or education may be of benefit. Discuss these with the patient using motivational interviewing techniques. When interactions between high-scoring items and other items, even low-scoring ones, are identified, they should be connected and worked on together. For instance, in Cathy's situation, she is not at all resistant to treatment (CP1) yet does not take her medications as prescribed. Thus, therapeutic challenge (score of 3 for CB2) is also connected to mental health symptoms (score of 1 for CP2) since she cannot remember which medications to take and how to take them and has trouble getting needed services (score of 3 for CHS1) since she cannot pay for the medications. This would lead to educational and personal assistance goals that might include extra time in medication reconciliation and expanding existing home-based support to ensure that Cathy is taking her medications as her primary care physicians' desire. It could also mean enrolling her in an indigent patient drug benefit program.

Assistance should be prioritized to begin with the patient's most pressing needs, but it should always be connected to the patient's personal goals when possible. Sometimes it is helpful for the patient to understand that in order to reach his or her personal goals intermediate steps might be necessary. Do not overwhelm the patient. Listen when he or she directly and indirectly pushes back. This is where motivational interviewing techniques can be very helpful (e.g., "Would you like me to . . . ? Can I show you how to find . . . ? How do you think we should solve . . . ?").

Work through how breaking down barriers to improvement and prioritizing actions will be done and let the patient know that other less pressing needs may be tackled at another time. Remember, the intent is ultimately for the patient to be able to identify and address as many of these issues as possible for herself or himself. Always try to get the patient involved in the solution, so he or she can take ownership. The stepwise process through which this is done in integrated case management is further discussed in Chapter 11.

There are few changes in this general format for children/youth, though caregivers/parents will be an integral part of the intervention process. If possible, there should be agreement between caregiver/parent and child/youth as to initial goals for case management and the process for achieving these. When there is disagreement, attempt to come to a compromise. It may be necessary to create personal health and function goals for both the caregiver/parent and the child/youth to get uniform cooperation. Since interaction with the family will likely be for weeks to months, extra goals are a small sacrifice. Further, the child's/youth's and caregiver's/parent's goals can often be linked (e.g., if the child/youth can get out and play with his friends, he can also likely go to school).

GOAL-DIRECTED AND OUTCOME-ORIENTED INTEGRATED CASE MANAGEMENT

It is now time to systematically implement core case management procedures as the patient is educated and assisted in the illnesses of concern and helped to maximum benefit. A care plan should be completed with concrete goals (where the patient and case manager

TABLE 10.3	**Measurement of Progress (Care Plan MP3)**		
	GOAL	**ACTION**	**OUTCOME**
Barrier CAG Item(s) #____			
Barrier CAG Item(s) #____			
Barrier CAG Item(s) #____			
Barrier CAG Item(s) #____			
Barrier CAG Item(s) #____			

Three columns of information are entered for each problematic complexity item (or group of related items): goal, action, and outcome. This gives a tabulation of case management information for analyzing the patient's progress.

would like to be in one to three months) and associated actions (how to get there) coupled with individual and connected prioritized barriers to health uncovered during the complexity assessment. Importantly, they should lead to documentable outcomes (**Table 10.3**).

While this is a collaborative effort between the patient and the case manager, often the case manager has to guide the way by dividing the process into doable parcels (see Figure 3.3). Throughout the process, the case manager should be helping the patient to develop skills, based on his or her specific medical and mental conditions, so that he or she can fend for him or herself within weeks to months of entering the case management program. This may not be possible with all patients since chronic and persistent complexity may necessitate long-term case management involvement.

DOCUMENTATION

It is most convenient to insert the work processes into a customized case management software system, such as through CMSA's integrated case management documentation template, so that outcome documentation can naturally take place as a part of an internally consistent package. When this is not possible, documentation can also be done using the paper and pencil assessment and documentation templates available in Appendixes E, F, 4, 5, 10, 11, and 12 (see www.springerpub.com/kathol for online appendixes). It is important that case management documentation be done in such a way that other case management team members can see what is happening in the event that the primary case manager is not available when a patient calls with a question or is in crisis. Documentation must be customized to each case management system whether through computer software, on electronic file templates (e.g., Word or Excel documents), or in hard copy to facilitate analysis of clinical, functional, satisfaction, quality of life, financial, and patient-centered outcomes.

COMMUNICATION AMONG CARE MANAGEMENT PROGRAMS

Case management is a branch of care management that works with patients at the high end of the complexity and health care cost scale (see the Chapter 1 section "Case Management"). The goal of case management is to help patients with illnesses in which interventions are available, such that with assistance improved outcomes can be achieved. Based on the fact that complex patients are either high users of health-related services or at significant risk for becoming so, it is likely that they will have been participants in other care management programs (e.g., wellness, personal nurse, high-risk pregnancy, disease management, disability management, employee assistance, workers' compensation, etc.) before entry into case management. Additionally, many will require one or more of these resources after completion of case management. For this reason, communication capabilities between and among other management programs, access to data warehouses, and lists of health resources for patients is helpful for efficient progress to clinical improvement and effective transition from one program to another. The following are examples of coordinated management facilitators:

- Access to a list of health plan and management vendor benefits available to the patient through intranet or Internet Web-based applications
- Program summaries of all of the services available through each of the other management programs offered to the patient via intranet or Internet Web-based applications
- Contact numbers for each of the other management programs available to the patient that are readily accessible through intranet or Internet Web-based applications
- Ability to smoothly triage patients to other management programs either telephonically or through intranet or Internet Web-based applications
- System-wide informed consent procedures that do not impede communication among *clinicians* involved in the patient's assistance (e.g., Appendix 3)

For health plan patients with multiple management opportunities, there should not be a reason that personally signed informed consent is necessary for either physical or mental health clinical information sharing among clinicians helping the patient. On the other hand, procedures (including electronic security measures) should prevent personal health information from reaching nonclinical staff without an appropriate and legal reason to access or read it.

CASE GRADUATION

The entire case management process is one in which patients are assisted through complex, high-cost health care service need. The duration of case management may vary from weeks to months while disease management may be measured in days to weeks but occasionally months. All activities of highly trained and skilled case managers should be directed toward resolution of complex issues that are changeable; assistance with the development of the patient skills so that they can better deal with health complexity; and education about illness, outcomes, and resources. Motivational interviewing techniques should be used in all interactions with patients to facilitate maximum benefit.

Indicators (see Figure 3.4) that the patient is moving toward case closure include:

- Patient understands his or her illnesses and treatments
- Patient is adherent to treatments, diets, exercises, and so forth and is working with providers to achieve improved health and function
- The patient's personal, social, economic, and health system issues have been stabilized, though maybe not resolved (maximum benefit)
- The patient's clinicians and other health professionals are collaboratively working together on behalf of the patient
- The interaction of physical and mental conditions is being collaboratively addressed through the coordination of services
- The patient's physical and mental health symptoms and signs have stabilized or are resolving at expected rates
- All high-complexity CAG items have been addressed (though perhaps not resolved), and the patient's goals have largely been accomplished

Occasionally, patients will require long-term involvement (6 to 12 months or longer) from a health plan, county-based program, or clinic-based case manager. General clinical guidelines indicating a need for continued involvement include:

- Persistent complex combination of illnesses that require special integrated input to prevent poor clinical outcomes and continued high-cost service use

- Cognitive impairment with no family, significant other, or provider alternative, which prevents the patient from assuming responsibility for his or her health complexity (persistent vulnerability)
- Potentially very high-cost illness unless control is maintained (e.g., potential liver transplant in former alcoholic, etc.)

Contract requirements may also dictate a nonclinical reason for continuing the patient-manager relationship. With time, however, the intensity of involvement will decrease with long-term patients, which allows more time to be dedicated to those with greater need.

Since case management cases are by definition complex, they will often be candidates for participation in other management programs at the completion of their work with the case manager. The patient should be prepared in advance for transition from integrated case management to assistance by a personal nurse, disease manager, or other management staff. Further, as case management procedures close, it is important to assist the patient with reentry into the workplace or school. This can often be facilitated through involvement with the patient's company disability management firm or the employee assistance program that the employer uses to assist its employees with workplace reentry. For children/youth, school authorities and counselors should be involved so that transition stresses can be closely monitored.

At the completion of case management, the case manager should provide a summary of the initial adult or pediatric CAG, the final CAG, and the record of outcome measures (**Table 10.4**) to the patient, the child/youth and/or caregiver/parent, the patient's providers,

| TABLE 10.4 | Record of Outcome Measures (ROM) | | | | |

OUTCOME MEASURES		BASELINE	FOLLOW-UP ASSESSMENTS		
	Time period recorded	Initial	2nd	3rd	4th
Clinical measure (personal goal)					
Functional measure (personal goal)					
Health-related quality of life					
Patient satisfaction					
CAG score					
Health care clinical measure					
Health care clinical measure					
Health care functional measure (1)					
Health care functional measure (2)					
Health care economic measure					

and care managers who will be assuming a role in assisting the patient. These documents should be accompanied by a summary of the progress that has been made, ongoing interventions, and recommendations about continued needs for the patient. The patient should be informed whether or not the case manager is available to assist with future needs should they arise, and if so, how to make contact.

Sharing the results of the graduation CAG assessment in grid format with the patient's clinicians is helpful for them to understand areas of their patient's health that may impede the practitioners' future attempts to provide treatment about which they are unfamiliar. The grid may also add valuable content to the clinicians' records. As doctors and other health practitioners understand more about the value of case management and the assessments that are performed, the grids and care plans developed by them will ultimately become tools used to augment treatment plans since they address health issues often impossible to include in standard clinical practice.

REFERENCES

de Jonge, P., Bauer, I., Huyse, F. J., & Latour, C. H. (2003). Medical inpatients at risk of extended hospital stay and poor discharge health status: Detection with COMPRI and INTERMED. *Psychosomatic Medicine, 65*(4), 534–541.

de Jonge, P., Hoogervorst, E. L., Huyse, F. J., & Polman, C. H. (2004). INTERMED: A measure of biopsychosocial case complexity: One year stability in multiple sclerosis patients. *General Hospital Psychiatry, 26*(2), 147–152.

de Jonge, P., Latour, C. H., & Huyse, F. J. (2003). Implementing psychiatric interventions on a medical ward: Effects on patients' quality of life and length of hospital stay. *Psychosomatic Medicine, 65*(6), 997–1002.

Huyse, F. J. (1997). From consultation to complexity of care prediction and health service needs assessment. *Journal Psychosomatic Research, 43*(3), 233–240.

Lowe, B., Unutzer, J., Callahan, C. M., Perkins, A. J., & Kroenke, K. (2004). Monitoring depression treatment outcomes with the Patient Health Questionnaire-9. *Medical Care, 42*(12), 1194–1201.

Slaets, J. P., Kauffmann, R. H., Duivenvoorden, H. J., Pelemans, W., & Schudel, W. J. (1997). A randomized trial of geriatric liaison intervention in elderly medical inpatients. *Psychosomatic Medicine, 59*(6), 585–591.

Spitzer, R. L., Kroenke, K., Williams, J. B., & Lowe, B. (2006). A brief measure for assessing generalized anxiety disorder: The GAD-7. *Archives Intern Medicine, 166*(10), 1092–1097.

CHAPTER 11

Managing Adult and Pediatric Cases Using Integrated Case Management

OBJECTIVES

- To consolidate information shared in Chapters 1 through 10
- To synthesize the pieces of adult integrated case management and create the delivery package
- To describe how pediatric integrated case management differs from adult case management, including the value and the limitations
- To discuss the process of ongoing continuing education and supervision for integrated case managers
- To illustrate how outcome measurement can be performed for individual patients and for aggregate populations
- To portray integrated case management success for different stakeholders
- To review the process of patient graduation from case management services

INTRODUCTION

Integrated case management differs from traditional case management in several very important ways (**Table 11.1**). Chapters 1 through 10 present the building blocks that will now be put together in this synopsis, which describes how integrated case management is placed into action. Chapter 1 provides an overview of traditional case management and how it differs from integrated case management. Further, it introduces the concept of complexity as a means of identifying those most likely to benefit from integrated case management. Chapter 2 summarizes the importance of the interaction of illnesses, including general medical and mental health, as a predictor of poor outcome. It suggests that in the current health environment, it is difficult to service the needs of multimorbid patients effectively or efficiently.

Chapter 5 discusses the fact that case managers do not treat patients, but rather that they assist them in structuring their interactions with the health system and its providers in a way that allows them to overcome barriers to improvement. Thus, integrated case managers can and should effectively combine general medical, mental health, social, and health system domain assistance without transferring responsibilities to another (behavioral health) manager. To do this, it is necessary for professionals coming from general medical backgrounds to have a basic grounding in mental conditions and for those from mental health backgrounds to have basic grounding in physical

health conditions. Chapter 6 provides illness-related examples about how professionals from each disciplinary background can learn to provide interdisciplinary case management by accessing information about illnesses and their treatment through a variety of resources.

Chapter 3 opens the door to structural changes and work process adjustments that facilitate the use of integrated case management. It guides the reader through the reorganization of workflows, training needs, the enrollment process, patient stratification and prioritization, the implementation of integrated case management principles, and movement of the patient toward case closure. Chapter 4 reviews the importance of using motivational interviewing techniques while working with complex patients.

Chapters 7, 8, and 9 guide readers through the use of adult and pediatric INTERMED-Complexity Assessment Grid (IM-CAG and PIM-CAG) methodology (i.e., the systematic assessment of complexity) and its use in creating care plans for and with patients. These chapters describe the importance of domain item anchor points, the connection of anchor points to actions that would be taken to overcome identified health barriers, and the relation of anchor points to each other in the creation of a care plan. While the adult and pediatric CAG assessments are the documentation technique through which barriers to improvement will become disaggregated, Chapter 10 describes the use of open-ended questions as a means to elicit the information needed to score each item while developing a

TABLE 11.1   Traditional Versus Integrated Case Management

Traditional	Integrated
Illness-focused	Complexity-focused
Problem-based	Relationship-based
Diverse triggering methods	Complexity-based triggering
Case managers trained in general medical case management	Case managers trained in CAG multidomain methodology
Pediatric case management based on child/youth manager experience	Systematic pediatric case management capability based on complexity assessment
Mental health management support requires manager handoffs	Mental health management support without manager handoffs
Illness-targeted patient assessments and actions	Systematic actions linked to patient assessments in four complexity domains
Process orientation and measurement: cases touched, calls made	Outcome orientation and measurement: clinical, functional, fiscal, satisfaction
Manager caseload dictated by process targets	Manager caseload dictated by complexity levels and outcome expectations

relationship with the patient or the child/youth and caregiver/parent.

In Chapter 11, we put these pieces together, illustrating the stepwise process of adult and pediatric integrated case management. Integrated case management has several inherent advantages to other nonsystematic, nonintegrated case management techniques even before the case manager develops a care plan and starts working with and for the patient. Several of these advantages include:

- An initial assessment that allows the development of a relationship between the case manager and the patient
- Systematic identification of *actionable* barriers to improvement in four interactive health domains: biological, psychological, social (family/social in the pediatric), and health system
- A means of documenting total baseline patient complexity to guide interventions and to measure outcomes
- A method to estimate optimal case manager patient load
- The ability to assess, build a care plan, and work with patients who have only physical health prob-

lems, only mental health or substance use disorder problems, or both, using the same assessment and intervention procedures
- Differential individual item scoring that prioritizes action and indicates immediacy of need in both adult and pediatric populations

The advantage of integrated case management, however, becomes even more robust when the case manager starts working with the patient in developing a care plan, communicating issues that lead to difficulties in maintaining health between the patient and those working with the patient, collaborating to improve health, and documenting specific clinical, functional, economic, and satisfaction outcomes that result from case management activities.

ADULT INTEGRATED CASE MANAGEMENT

ENROLLMENT

Rubin's journey into case management began with a referral from his primary care clinical staff. They were seeing him for the first time for worsening back pain. Rubin, 57 years old, triggered an expanded case management alert system since he had no steady doctor and was on multiple medications, including narcotics; had been treated in the emergency room twice in the past month; and was asking that his long-term disability form be signed. He was afraid that he was going to lose his job and had left three doctors in 6 months because they would not prescribe his narcotic medications or fill out his forms.

Doctors and nurses in the clinic immediately recognized this as a challenge waiting to happen. Even though he had not yet been admitted to the hospital, his emergency room visits were escalating and he was at risk of losing his job (see Exhibit 3.3, Stratification Level II). Prior to this visit, his doctors had been focused on his back difficulties, examinations had been short, and physical and magnetic resonance findings had been inconclusive. Rubin was now desperate since he was at risk of losing his job, his insurance, and, as was found during the case management assessment, his family. He was willing to try to get things under control but did not know where to start. He was in the medium priority level for entry into the program (i.e., easy to contact with interest in change, improvement potential, and no history of case management participation; see Exhibit 3.4).

The clinic that took over Rubin's care was in phase two in the implementation of integrated case management. During the first phase, Rubin would not have been a candidate for individualized care through integrated case management. Prior to the addition of two more case managers due to the success of phase one of the program, case triggering was based on systematic review of the 12,500 patients in the four-doctor and two-nurse practitioner primary care clinic. In phase one, only patients who would have fallen in Stratification Level III or IV would have been candidates for entry. Enrollment was limited to established clinic patients with chronic multimorbid illness in whom many specialists were involved. The patients were on numerous medications, usually had had several recent hospitalizations, and often had contributing mental health symptoms according to the clinic doctors and nurses who referred them from their patient panels for case management.

During phase one, only the most difficult and challenging patients in the practice were entered since there were just not enough case managers to effectively assist everyone. In the two years of phase one, two case managers only worked with a total of 400 of the most complex 12,500 patients on the clinic's roles. Many of these patients, however, showed remarkable stabilization of their health and function with reduction of health care service use. Thus, expansion into phase two was begun. While most entering case management in phase two would also come from Stratification Level III and Level IV, some in Level II would also be entered in an effort to prevent them from advancing to Level III and IV. This was the situation for Rubin.

ASSESSMENT

Rubin was assigned to a case manager with an opening in her schedule. By now, the clinic had been able to establish that the optimal range for their case managers to deliver effective integrated services to their adult patients correlated with a total complexity score of their patient panel in the range of 600 to 1,000. Case managers were expected to document and record CAG change as they worked with their patients.

Rubin's IM-CAG (**Table 11.2**, see page i4 for color version) suggested that he needed work primarily in the health system and social domains though description of back symptoms were dramatic and interventions largely limited to pain medication (biological domain). A total score of 28 suggested low to moderate complexity. Rubin had a reasonable likelihood of improved clinical, functional, and economic outcome since he felt he was at the "end of his rope."

Even without knowing the details of Rubin's clinical situation, it is easy to see that physical issues are not the only or even the major reason that triggered Rubin into the case management system. Rubin's interaction with the health system and his social situation

TABLE 11.2	Rubin's IM-CAG						
Baseline	HEALTH RISKS AND HEALTH NEEDS						
Rubin	HISTORICAL		CURRENT STATE		VULNERABILITY		
Total Score = 28	Complexity Item	Score	Complexity Item	Score	Complexity Item		Score
Biological Domain	Chronicity **HB1**	0	Symptom Severity/Impairment **CB1**	2	Complications and Life Threat **VB**		1
	Diagnostic Dilemma **HB2**	1	Diagnostic/Therapeutic Challenge **CB2**	2			
Psychological Domain	Barriers to Coping **HP1**	0	Resistance to Treatment **CP1**	0	Mental Health Threat **VP**		0
	Mental Health History **HP2**	0	Mental Health Symptoms **CP2**	0			
Social Domain	Job and Leisure **HS1**	2	Residential Stability **CS1**	2	Social Vulnerability **VS**	2	
	Relationships **HS2**	1	Social Support **CS2**	3			
Health System Domain	Access to Care **HHS1**	2	Getting Needed Services **CHS1**	3	Health System Impediments **VHS**	3	
	Treatment Experience **HHS2**	3	Coordination of Care **CHS2**	3			
Comments							
Unrelieved back pain since lifting furniture at home; not working; kicked out of home by wife; living in hotel; three sets of family doctors for back pain treatment and disability support in four months; high deductible insurance.							

are contributing substantially to his problems. Rubin's IM-CAG scoring sheet suggests that he has had difficulty in finding and getting to the type of care that he needs (CHS1). This could be related to access difficulties from insurance or geographic factors (HHS1) but is more likely due to negative experiences with his doctors and the health system (HHS2). It is also apparent that those who care for him do not communicate with each other (CHS2). Of these IM-CAG items, all except access to care (HHS1) are red (see color plate for Table 11.2) and would be high in priority when working with Rubin. In fact, health system factors could be the main reason that Rubin creates a significant diagnostic challenge for his primary care clinicians (CB2) and has a high level of physical symptoms (CB1). Several of the cells in the social domain are also orange or red (HS1, CS1, and CS2). They raise concerns that Rubin's health system factors may be related to his economic and/or personal situation. The confluence of factors is affecting his current level of back pain complaints, disability, and rather restricted approach to treatment.

As the case manager works with Rubin, he or she will document the areas that have been addressed, outcomes from the assistance given, and goals that remain to be attained. With Rubin's initial CAG evaluation, it is possible to connect some of these dots and

form a combined strategy to improve Rubin's health using the grid as a visual communication device while following integrated case management procedures. The grid can be shared with Rubin as a means of helping to clarify the situation and move toward a solution. Further, the IM-CAG provides a convenient tool to use as the case manager and Rubin collaborate in developing a care plan (**Table 11.3**). It is also an easy way for the case manager to communicate about the actions to be initiated in the care plan with Rubin. When CAG capabilities are built into the case management documentation software, which is possible through agreement with the Case Management Society of America (CMSA), the process does not rely on paper and can work seamlessly with other documentation software used by the organization at which the case manager works. This also facilitates outcome and performance reporting.

One of the most important advantages of IM-CAG methodology is that it creates a total picture of the patient, uncovering most areas that may need actionable attention. In the preceding example, Rubin has no areas of concern in the psychological section, indicating that mental health issues and health behaviors are not a problem. On the other hand, the patient has no stable job or leisure activities, unstable housing, and no social

TABLE 11.3	Rubin's Care Plan Development (Baseline CD)		
BARRIERS	**GOALS**		**ACTIONS**
CAG items	**Personal followed by health care**		**Prioritized**
HHS2	**Short-term**	Collaboration between Rubin and providers in care	Assist Rubin in talking with clinic provider; attempt to develop an alliance
	Ultimate	Provider-patient relationship without conflict; adherence	Establish positive patient-provider relationship
CHS1 and CB2	**Short-term**	Medical home	Explore past treatments and treatment options; assist in reviewing acceptability of suggestions by doctor
	Ultimate	Single clinic, consistent doctor, outcome changing care	Confirm primary doctor; assist in obtaining county care management assistance
CB1 and CB2	**Short-term**	Understanding of back pain; logical treatment plan	Educate about back pain; confirm patient-physician-developed treatment plan
	Ultimate	Treatment that stabilizes and/or controls back symptoms	Ensure adherence to treatment plan; confirm symptom and functional change
CHS2	**Short-term and Ultimate**	Communication among providers	Obtain releases for records of earlier doctors and emergency room to medical home; establish consistent communication process
HS1, CS1, & CS2	**Short-term**	Money for living expenses; stabilized living situation	Seek public services support; investigate community resources; explore family counseling
	Ultimate	Safe living arrangements; financing for basic needs; reopen relationships with relatives/friends	Identify satisfactory and stable residence; check job situation; application for general assistance or job if appropriate; encourage old or new relationships

support system. While stabilizing Rubin's back pain is considered to be the first line of business, it is apparent from the IM-CAG that social needs will require attention soon, perhaps as a part of solving the health system issues. Importantly, unless social and health system issues are stabilized, the physical problems will likely not resolve. There is a significant chance that they will even escalate in the future.

MANAGING THE PATIENT

Figure 11.1 illustrates an iterative process that the case manager will go through as he or she works with Rubin. He or she and Rubin will together decide where to start and how to proceed. The case manager will utilize the grid information to help define the aggressiveness of his or her interaction with Rubin. In general, new patients will demand more manager time than cases in which the care plan has been delineated and activity is underway on several fronts. While the intent is for the patient to assume responsibility for his or her own care, typically, it is important for the case manager to initially demonstrate his or her value by demonstrating initiative (e.g., calling community resources, finding out about drug costs, checking about potential living situations, etc.). Thus, starting too many new cases at once is not advisable. If a case manager with the time to start a new patient is not available, it is better to facilitate support through standard care than to initiate the case management process. Overcommitted case managers lose effectiveness in improving health conditions when they cannot perform necessary functions.

Using complexity as the core of patient assessment helps case managers identify priority areas to target, develop an iterative strategy with patients and their families, address vulnerabilities, and overcome barriers to health. As case managers become more familiar with the use of the IM-CAG, they will recognize issues and themes in the grid that are interactive in terms of actions and outcomes. By addressing the cells contributing to these interactions jointly, rather than working on them as isolated health issues, it is possible to introduce efficiency as management services are provided (**Table 11.3**, e.g., CHS1 and CB2). The case manager can also work with the patient and the patient's family to help them understand how to fend for themselves in a complicated and sometimes hostile health care environment. One of the main goals in the case manager-patient interaction is for the patient and his or her family to understand the patient's illness (improving health literacy), to navigate the health system, and to get the type of treatment that leads to improved health. As the case manager works with Rubin, it is possible for him or her to assess the degree to which

barriers have been reversed and Rubin is increasingly taking ownership of his health issues (**Figure 11.2**). When he is nearing completion of his goals and has derived maximum benefit from case management assistance, it is time to consider return to standard care.

MOVING TOWARD CASE CLOSURE

Case managers cannot be expected to add to their caseload without graduating patients from their roles. They will lose effectiveness and will burn out in a job that can be very rewarding but is also grueling. Discharging patients, however, requires that case managers document improvement, gradually turn over responsibility for personal health to the patient or his or her family, and provide the patient's primary caregivers with an understanding of the big picture of their patient so they can assist the patient in maintaining and continuing to improve after the case management relationship has closed (**Figure 11.3**).

Use of the CAG as a Global Assessment of Complexity Amelioration

The IM-CAG has great potential to provide a longitudinal assessment of complexity amelioration as barriers to improvement are identified and actions are taken to reverse them. Many of the scores for both current and vulnerability items in the complexity grid can be expected to decrease if the patient has conditions or life circumstances that can be altered through case management assistance. For instance, if the case manager can facilitate communication among providers and coordination of care, CHS2 anchor point scores can change from 3 to 2 or even to 1. If poorly coordinated care led to health system vulnerability, then VHS scores would also drop.

With the exception of HHS1, absolute anchor point scores for historical items, by definition, do not change with case management complexity intervention. On the other hand, by addressing complex historical issues that predict poor outcomes (e.g., educating patients about their chronic illnesses and treatments), it is possible to decrease the impact that historical complexity will have on outcome. Therefore, a reasonable *rule for including historical complexity items* in outcome estimation would be to decrease absolute scores of 2 or 3 by one point if the case manager completed actions designed to lower their impact on outcome. Manual users should be aware that this has not yet been subjected to research scrutiny; however, it does provide case managers with a way to document their actions (Appendix 8) designed to alter outcomes related to identified historical barriers to improvement. Access to care (HHS1) is an exception to this rule because it is measured related to the preceding 6 months rather

FIGURE 11.1 Integrated case manager care plan: Initial and iterative intervention.

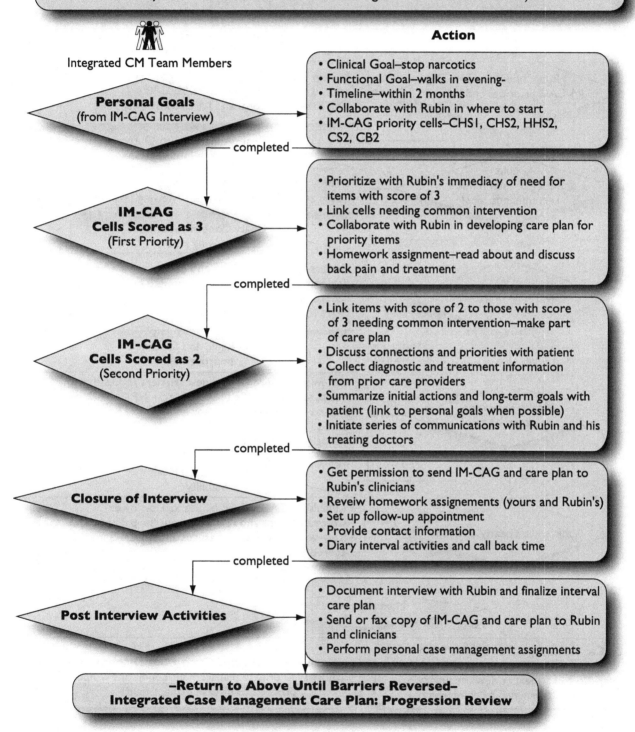

Initial & Iterative Case Management Intervention
(develop relationship and, with informed consent, share assessment results with Rubin, his family, his doctors; send illness and case management educational materials)

Integrated CM Team Members

Action

Personal Goals
(from IM-CAG Interview)

- Clinical Goal–stop narcotics
- Functional Goal–walks in evening-
- Timeline–within 2 months
- Collaborate with Rubin in where to start
- IM-CAG priority cells–CHS1, CHS2, HHS2, CS2, CB2

completed

IM-CAG Cells Scored as 3
(First Priority)

- Prioritize with Rubin's immediacy of need for items with score of 3
- Link cells needing common intervention
- Collaborate with Rubin in developing care plan for priority items
- Homework assignment–read about and discuss back pain and treatment

completed

IM-CAG Cells Scored as 2
(Second Priority)

- Link items with score of 2 to those with score of 3 needing common intervention–make part of care plan
- Discuss connections and priorities with patient
- Collect diagnostic and treatment information from prior care providers
- Summarize initial actions and long-term goals with patient (link to personal goals when possible)
- Initiate series of communications with Rubin and his treating doctors

completed

Closure of Interview

- Get permission to send IM-CAG and care plan to Rubin's clinicians
- Reveiw homework assignements (yours and Rubin's)
- Set up follow-up appointment
- Provide contact information
- Diary interval activities and call back time

completed

Post Interview Activities

- Document interview with Rubin and finalize interval care plan
- Send or fax copy of IM-CAG and care plan to Rubin and clinicians
- Perform personal case management assignments

–Return to Above Until Barriers Reversed–
Integrated Case Management Care Plan: Progression Review

FIGURE 11.2   Integrated case manager care plan: Progression review.

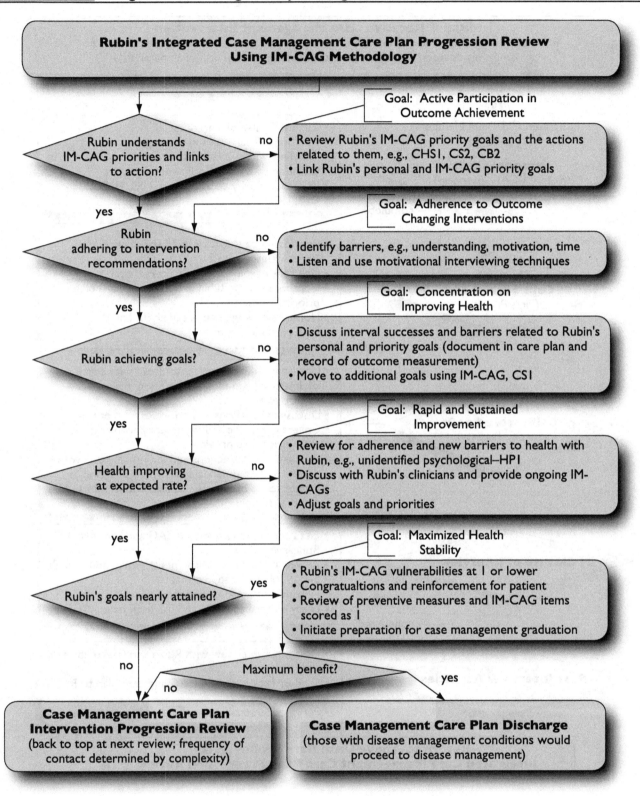

FIGURE 11.3 Integrated case manager care plan: Rubin's discharge.

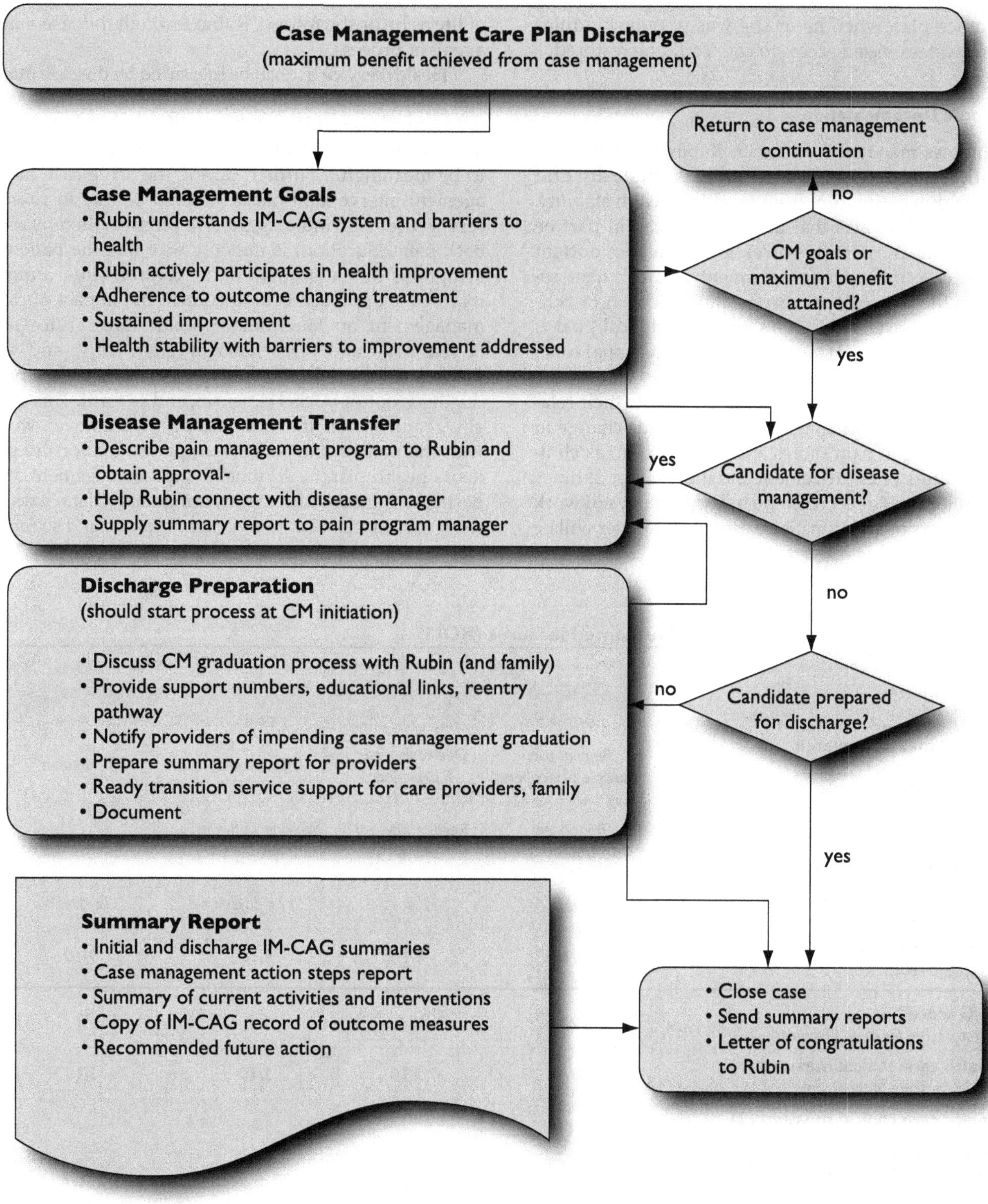

Case Management Care Plan Discharge
(maximum benefit achieved from case management)

Case Management Goals
- Rubin understands IM-CAG system and barriers to health
- Rubin actively participates in health improvement
- Adherence to outcome changing treatment
- Sustained improvement
- Health stability with barriers to improvement addressed

Return to case management continuation

CM goals or maximum benefit attained? — no / yes

Disease Management Transfer
- Describe pain management program to Rubin and obtain approval-
- Help Rubin connect with disease manager
- Supply summary report to pain program manager

Candidate for disease management? — yes / no

Discharge Preparation
(should start process at CM initiation)

- Discuss CM graduation process with Rubin (and family)
- Provide support numbers, educational links, reentry pathway
- Notify providers of impending case management graduation
- Prepare summary report for providers
- Ready transition service support for care providers, family
- Document

Candidate prepared for discharge? — no / yes

Summary Report
- Initial and discharge IM-CAG summaries
- Case management action steps report
- Summary of current activities and interventions
- Copy of IM-CAG record of outcome measures
- Recommended future action

- Close case
- Send summary reports
- Letter of congratulations to Rubin

than 5 years. Thus, it is possible to acutely change HHS1 scores based on case manager assistance. For instance, if a case manager can enroll a patient in an insurance plan when he or she was previously uninsured, system-based access to care could be restored.

Outcome Documentation

As the case manager works with Rubin, he or she systematically redresses the areas on the complexity grid that are preventing him from reaching health stability. **Table 11.4** illustrates that the IM-GAG can in part be used for this purpose; however, it is equally important for the case manager to document improvement related to the patient's primary health condition or conditions. For instance, Rubin's personal clinical goal is to stop his reliance on narcotics, and his personal functional goal is to be able to walk with his wife in the evening, presuming they are able to rekindle their relationship. The case manager also documents change in visual analogue pain scores and back flexion, as clinical indicators of improvement and the number of times per week Rubin gets out of the house and days of work as indicators of function. Since the case manager will be

working with Rubin and Rubin's doctors, it is possible to collect consistent outcome data. The case manager can also include a survey of satisfaction and/or quality of life as he or she follows Rubin through the case management process.

Health service use can be measured by the case manager and patient along with other measures; however, unless usage is significant, the timeframe for documenting improvement in this parameter is usually too short to be meaningful. Further, during the acute case management intervention phase, it could be that increased service use (e.g., more aggressive physical therapy and back pain education) is the only way that the patient's symptoms can be brought under control. Thus, a more reasonable approach is to document the impact of case management on longitudinal health care service use (1 year prior and 1 year after program entry) and, for that matter, other health-related costs, such as lost productivity, out-of-pocket expenses, and so forth. This usually requires that the case manager's employer work with the patient, the patient's employer, and/or the patient's health plan in documenting premanagement and postmanagement fiscal impact, using claims data, days of work missed, actual out-of-pocket expenses, and so forth.

TABLE 11.4   Rubin's Record of Outcome Measures (ROM)

OUTCOME MEASURES	BASELINE	FOLLOW-UP ASSESSMENTS		
Time period recorded	Baseline	Week 4	Week 8	Week 12
Clinical measure related to personal goal Off narcotics	Regular use; Multiple prescribers	Decreasing use; 1 prescriber	Off narcotics	Off narcotics
Functional measure related to personal goal Walk with wife in evening	Bedridden; traction	Regular physical therapy	Walking with wife 3 times a week	
Health-related quality of life # healthy days /month	3 days	12 days	21 days	23 days
Patient satisfaction (Scale 0–10)	2/10	6/10	9/10	9/10
CAG score (total score for period recorded)	28	24	20	18
Health care clinical measure (1) Average score on pain scale	9/10	7.5/10	5/10	3/10
Health care clinical measure (2) PHQ-9	8	—	—	—
Health care functional measure Back flexion	60 degrees	80 degrees	100 degrees	100 degrees
Health care functional measure Work days/week	0	4 hrs/3 dys; restricted activities	8 hrs/5 dys; restricted activities	8 hrs/5 dys; new job description
Health care service use Emergency room visits	4 per month	1 visit	0	0

Case Management Assistance Documentation

Practically speaking, at the beginning of case management, Rubin and the case manager work together to address red and orange (high complexity) issues. In the current state time frame, it should be possible to document improvement in the item scores. In the historical time frame, absolute scores would not change since they are reflections of historical health risks. For instance, Rubin's experience with prior clinicians would not change (HHS2). What would change is that there would be resolution of Rubin's expectations of his doctors and the doctors' focused attention on Rubin's back pain. Rubin and the case manager would work to improve Rubin's understanding of back pain and its treatment. The case manager would also encourage and support discussion between Rubin's clinicians and Rubin in hopes of improving the relationship between the two. Just as importantly, Rubin and the case manager would work with Rubin's employee assistance program to determine light duty potential or discuss alternative employment possibilities (HS1).

Part of Rubin's persistence of symptoms may relate to his desire to maintain disability income while not working. For historical items, therefore, ongoing IM-CAG scores would be adjusted based not on the absolute change in historical information but on the fact that issues related to the content area have been addressed. If a new or less vulnerable pattern of behavior results, then lower follow-up historical IM-CAG scores, rather than the absolute historical score, can be used to reflect the impact that case management intervention had on risk.

As historical and current state barriers to improvement are addressed and at least stabilized during the integrated case management process, it will be possible to revisit the vulnerabilities in each domain and think about the degree to which risk of poor outcome without individualized case management assistance has been reversed. In some situations, risk will remain high in selected vulnerability areas, yet return to standard care is appropriate since maximum benefit has been achieved. Thus, the case manager should be discussing return to standard care as soon as most vulnerability scores approach or reach 1 or 0. The process of graduation from case management, however, should begin well before the week of transfer back to standard care.

Finally, while integrated case management is an advancement in the way that patients can be approached and followed, it does not guarantee that every, or even most, patients will return to health. Patient motivation, the ability to change access to evidence-based services, the availability of health insurance, the natural course of illness, and many other factors play important roles. Further, even as patients improve there will always be new health needs that crop up. Not all issues in all cells on the IM-CAG can nor will be addressed in the time that a case manager-patient relationship can realistically be maintained, but a systematic process continues to be used in working with the patient toward barrier resolution (**Table 11.5**).

The case manager also needs to measure improvement, document stabilization, understand when maximum benefit has been attained, and know about the patient's health system and practitioner circumstances

TABLE 11.5   **Rubin's Measurement of Progress (MP3)**

	GOAL	ACTION	OUTCOME
Barrier CHS1, CB1, and CB2	*Medical home; educated about back pain; logical treatment*	*Rubin's education about back pain; establish stable physician relationship; ensure treatment and adherence; measure outcome*	*Community health center 3 miles from Rubin's home; Rubin working with respected doctor; following exercise and medication recommendations; less back pain and impairment*
Barrier HHS2	*Establish patient-doctor alliance*	*Talk with providers; identify and resolve conflicts*	*Establishing relationship with liked primary care provider who will coordinate health activity at community health center (reluctance because of workload, pay, and Rubin's complexity)*
Barrier CHS2	*Coordinate care*	*Establish communication link among providers and therapies*	*Coordinated appointments through primary care provider; shared notes with one specialist and physical therapy*
Barrier HS1, CS1, and CS2	*Improve living and financial situation*	*Involve employee assistance program; family counseling; look for alternative living arrangements*	*Move from hotel back home; return to light duty; family dispute improved*

once the patient is discharged from case management. For instance, Rubin has good commercial insurance but could lose it because of the duration of his time off work (long-term disability). After 3 months in case management, he now has ready access to and good communication among practitioners. His back pain is also under better control and he is back to work. His family difficulties are resolving with assistance from a family therapist. Improvement in Rubin's complexity score and improved clinical and functional parameters are important factors but only a part of the total puzzle. A truly successful case manager and his or her supervisors will understand the value of balance between supporting long-term existing cases and opening new ones.

SUMMARY COMMENTS

Rubin was lucky to have fallen into phase two of integrated case management dissemination at his new clinic. During the original rollout, only patients with Level III or Level IV stratification and moderate to high priority would have been considered for entry in the integrated case management protocol. Rubin, with an entry IM-CAG total score of 28, was less needy than other potential patients; however, within a relatively short period of receiving individualized care, it was possible to reverse a potentially costly progression of health complexity and the toll that it would have taken on Rubin's life. Those treated in phase one were not so lucky, as we will see in Chapters 12 through 14.

PEDIATRIC INTEGRATED CASE MANAGEMENT

The developers of the adult integrated case management program formulated the PIM-CAG in collaboration with pediatricians, child psychiatrists, child psychologists, and pediatric case managers to fill a void in the ability to assess and intervene for children/youth with health complexity. The instrument is new and is not yet validated in the child/youth population. Thus, less can be said about its construct and predictive validity and clinical utility. Nonetheless, it uses the same conceptual framework as the adult assessment process while recognizing that additional assessment and intervention needs are required to successfully lead a complex child/youth to stabilized health. That is why there are 25 rather than 20 items in the four complexity domains. Three-year-old Janet, who suffers from cerebral palsy after a bout of encephalitis at age 3 months, is an example (**Table 11.6**, see page i5 for color version). She has a

PIM-CAG score of 43 out of a possible 75 and has had a significant impact on the lives of her parents and siblings.

Basic adult integrated case management processes and procedures are equally applicable to children/youth. An initial assessment using open-ended, relationship-building questions that involve the parents/caregivers and the child/youth, when old enough, is completed (Chapter 10). The case manager works with the parents and the child/youth in the development of a care plan based on complexity scores. Goals and actions are outlined and outcomes are documented and measured. The process of case management may occur over weeks to months, depending on the level of complexity and needs of the child/youth. Ultimately, as in adult case management, the desire is for the family and/or child/youth to develop sufficient health-related knowledge and skills to be able to return to standard care.

Pediatric integrated case management targets the needs of the child/youth but recognizes that the needs of the caregiver/parent can sometimes be significant as well. For instance, Janet's parents were divorced 2 years after the traumatic medical event. Janet's mother is now on welfare since she has no source of income and her ex-husband is unemployed and thus is sending no alimony or child support payments. The mother is depressed and finding it hard to cope with the constant medical and psychological needs of her daughter and two other children. Janet and her family have moved three times in the past 2 years because of financial difficulties and have no other family or friends who provide support. Janet's mother has no health insurance and Janet receives support through the Children's Health Insurance Program (CHIP), but funding has recently been cut back.

With this type of complicated problem, there are certainly needs for Janet that require addressing; however, unless her mother's depression, financial situation, and social support improve, it is unlikely that Janet's mental and physical health issues will stabilize. Janet had been admitted to the county hospital two times in the past year because of behavioral difficulties and self-induced injuries.

It is hard to separate the needs of Janet from those of her mother. This creates a special challenge for pediatric case managers. In many situations, it is appropriate to assist both the child/youth and the caregiver/parent as a unit. In some situations, it is possible to activate additional assistance for the parent through community resources, such as social services. It is a judgment by the pediatric case manager what the most judicious approach would be.

TABLE 11.6   **Janet's PIM-CAG**

Baseline	HEALTH RISKS AND HEALTH NEEDS						
Janet	**HISTORICAL**		**CURRENT STATE**		**VULNERABILITY**	
Total Score = 43	Complexity Item	Score	Complexity Item	Score	Complexity Item	Score
Biological Domain	Chronicity **HB1**	0	Symptom Severity/Impairment **CB1**	2	Complications and Life Threat **VB**	2
	Diagnostic Dilemma **HB2**	1	Diagnostic/Therapeutic Challenge **CB2**	1		
Psychological Domain	Barriers to Coping **HP1**	0	Resistance to Treatment **CP1**	0	Learning and/or Mental Health Threat **VP**	2
	Mental Health History **HP2**	0	Mental Health Symptoms **CP2**	3		
	Cognitive Development **HP3**	2				
	Adverse Developmental Events **HP4**	3				
Social Domain	School Functioning **HS1**	0	Residential Stability **CS1**	3	Family/School/Social System Vulnerability **VS**	3
	Family and Social Relationships **HS2**	1	Child/Youth Support **CS2**	1		
	Caregiver/Parent Health and Function **HS3**	2	Caregiver/Family Support **CS3**	3		
			School and Community Participation **CS4**	0		
Health System Domain	Access to Care **HHS1**	3	Getting Needed Services **CHS1**	3	Health System Impediments **VHS**	3
	Treatment Experience **HHS2**	2	Coordination of Care **CHS2**	3		
Comments						
Cerebral palsy with cognitive impairment due to viral encephalitis at age 3 months.						

SHARPENING THE SAW

In Stephen Covey's (1989) *The 7 Habits of Highly Successful People,* habit seven is called "sharpen the saw." Rubin's and Janet's case managers recognize that the composite of problems of these two and the many other complex patients with whom they work, requires continuous learning, adaptation, and help. They must sharpen their saws to maintain a cutting edge that will maximize the benefit that they bring. As a result, managers should review the goals, actions, and outcomes weekly for their new and more complex patients with a general medical and psychiatric physician and with their case management supervisor. They should also discuss cases that are stabilizing and nearing graduation from case management. At the end of each month, they should receive feedback on the remainder of their patient panels.

In addition to review of personal patients, case managers working in clinics can hold case conferences fortnightly on one or more complicated patients or on a topic pertinent to the managers in their clinic and others in their health system. This allows discussion about approaches that can be taken with particularly thorny issues. It also allows case managers to continue to augment their knowledge about topics in their own discipline and others with which they are less familiar. While they will feel much more confident about the general approach they take with their patients each month, they will also readily recognize that there is always much more to learn.

MEASURING OUTCOMES

In our fragmented health system, each of the players has different goals and thus uses different parameters to measure success. For purchasers of health insurance, such as employers and public programs, success is measured in terms of dollars saved in health claims and administrative costs. Employers are also interested in fewer disability costs and a more productive workforce. Public programs, on the other hand, desire better health for their enrollees so that they use fewer county and state social services, stay out of the local jail system, and have less need for at-risk student school resources. For fund administrators, such as health plans, success is measured in terms of company profits and documentation of so-called value enhancements that will increase market share for future contracts. For public fund administrators, such as government programs or national health trusts, success is obtaining maximum health services within a fixed budget. For practitioners, it is giving good care and getting paid adequately for the health services provided. Finally, and most importantly, for patients, success is affordable health care that maximizes health.

With each stakeholder having different measures of success, which measures should the case manager rely on as management services are given? The interesting thing about integrated case management is that it brings success to all of the previously mentioned measures, but only if it starts by assisting complex patients with achieving better clinical outcomes. The first obligation of integrated case managers, therefore, is to help patients, selected because of their health complexity, regain health to the degree that the patient's illnesses and/or health situations allow. Since case managers work with complicated and high-cost patients, the potential for improving clinical health outcomes is great because of the background, skills, and knowledge base that they bring to the health equation.

Further, case managers, using the integrated case management approach, will address more than just disease-related parameters. They have the potential to help patients with the affordability of health care as well. For instance, helping a patient access a drug company- or government-sponsored medication payment program or working through his or her prescribing physician to help the patient obtain an affordable but equivalent generic product can be the difference in thousands of dollars a year (and health vs. illness). Plus, increased adherence to prescribed medications will lead to less cost in terms of health care service use and personal impairment downstream.

Patients entering case management are those who use the majority of health services. Thus, there is great potential for participants in case management programs to have and maintain lower total health care costs as their clinical problems improve. Studies to date document that when integrated programs are correctly organized, lower health care use and costs can be expected (see Exhibit 2.7 and Exhibit 2.8). In fact, return on investment can be substantial. Unlike other types of care management, savings for populations entering case management can be immediate through reduction in emergency room use, fewer readmissions to hospital, and fewer diagnostic tests and medications. This leads to immediate impact on general medical health plan profits if they have insourced mental condition support, integrated physical health and mental health business practices, and instituted integrated case management practices. As a result, such health plans should be able to offer added value with lower premiums to future potential purchasers. Further, studies suggest that claims costs continue to go down over time. It is thus important to include strategies to measure clinical, functional, satisfaction, and cost components as outcomes are altered.

There are also many secondary benefits for patients participating in integrated case management leading to improved health. Such patients will reenter the workforce more quickly and be more productive on the job. Since integrated case management does not restrict its assistance horizon to physical health, even patients in public programs will show benefits outside of total health care service use. States and counties should experience a reduction in educational, social services, and correctional institution costs for those who have been fortunate enough to enter case management. Health issues, and especially the behavioral and social components, play large roles in school success, reduction in reliance on county social support systems, and lower judicial recidivism.

It is not the case manager's responsibility to document all of the previously described parameters of success as he or she works with patients; however, it is the system's responsibility to document value that integrated case managers bring in as many areas as possible. The case manager can clearly follow changes in clinical and functional outcomes for the patients that he or she works with, both related to the IM-CAG scores and to mutually agreed-on clinical and functional parameters. He or she can also document improved quality of life and satisfaction.

If case managers work within a large clinical system or in a health plan, it is also possible to add aggregate health care service use and total cost of care subdivided into physical health, mental condition, and medication use before and after health management was initiated. Without too much sophistication, common clinical parameters, such as HbA1c, Personal Health Questionnaire-9 (PHQ-9) evaluations, daily weight measurements, FEV1 readings, and Generalized Anxiety Disorder-7 (GAD-7) evaluations; health care service use, such as emergency room visits, hospital admissions, and readmission rates; and total cost of care could also be compared between aggregates of those who enter and complete case management and a complexity-matched concurrent group that did not participate in case management though asked.

Employers and public programs can even become participants in the outcome measurement process. While personal health information needs to be protected with appropriate assurances, HIPAA allows aggregate assessment of employed populations on relevant measurements, such as disability costs, workers' compensation claims, absenteeism, and productivity. Public programs would be more interested in measuring aggregate participant use of other county, regional, or state programs, such as probation supervision, special education, and food stamps. Such measurement activities usually require a cooperative relationship among participants in the health of selected populations but will lead to future enhancements of intervention processes.

RETURNING PATIENTS TO STANDARD CARE

From the first day of case management, the case manager thinks about and prepares for the time when graduation from case management activities can take place. General parameters about the time that a patient may be working with a case manager can be derived from the integrated health management stratification level taken upon entry into case management services (Exhibit 3.3 and Appendix A, see www.springerpub.com/kathol). Other predictors however, are related to factors within the case management process that will influence progress, such as the cognitive abilities of the patient, insurance status, the social support system, and so forth. Regardless, it is imperative that the case manager: (a) have clear goals in mind for the patient at the completion of the initial integrated case management evaluation, (b) establish an alliance with the patient, the patient's family, and the patient's providers in moving toward these goals, (c) delineate expectations for the patient, and (d) document ongoing improvement and successes as well as failures.

As goals are met, the case manager should share these with the patient and his or her clinicians, discuss the graduation process, and prepare for transition back to standard care. For patients who enter case management with a high degree of complexity (IM-CAG scores greater than 30; PIM-CAG scores greater than 38),

transitioning the patient back to his or her primary care providers will be more of a challenge since it is likely that the personal relationship between case manager and patient will be stronger by the time he or she is ready to leave case management. Nonetheless, moving the patient to the next phase in his or her health maintenance program is as important for him or her as it is to free up time for the case manager to take on new patients. By the time the case management process is closed, interaction of the patient and case manager will have decreased so that they may not have contact with each other for weeks or even months.

While it is possible for the majority of patients to derive benefit and then leave case management assistance, there will be some very complex patients for whom assistance will become chronic or extended. While the frequency with which patient encounters occur may decrease, case closure is not possible since the patient will merely revert to prior poorly controlled health. It is in these cases that case manager, case management supervisor, and case management overseeing physician discussions can be helpful. The intent is for the patient to maintain health, sustain functionality, and control health care service use. When projected benefits of an extended relationship outweigh program costs, it is reasonable to continue long-term case management. This is also a good reason that measurement of outcomes is one of several important components of this manual (i.e., to document the value given).

Transition from case management back to standard care, with or without the assistance of other health management services, should be timely, systematic, and as nontraumatic as possible (**Figure 11.3**). It should include preparation of the patient and involvement of the care providers who will be continuing to work with the patient. Both should be given information about progress that has been made during the time the case manager has worked with the patient. They should also receive the current state of the patient with a summary of the original and follow-up IM-CAG assessments, an explanation of current action steps, and anticipated needs for the patient moving forward. Personal communication between the primary care provider and the case manager can be helpful in making the transition. Remember, while the patient may have made substantial progress, closing case management is a period of vulnerability, itself associated with risk of worsening health. A smooth transition will decrease this possibility.

CONCLUSION

Effective case management requires that barriers to health be systematically addressed. Integrated case management facilitates this process, helping to break barriers to health in patients with health complexity into component parts and to connect them with each other through the development of a prioritized care plan. Case management procedures are then used to assist the patient with altering areas of vulnerability and returning to better health. Once patients have achieved maximal benefit from case management services, they should transition back to standard care.

REFERENCE

Covey, S. R. (1989). *The 7 habits of highly effective people.* New York: Simon & Schuster.

CHAPTER 12

Assisting Lucinda: Depressed Diabetic Patient With Numerous Complications, Poor Control, and High Service Use

OBJECTIVES

- To illustrate implementation of the integrated case management complexity assessment using adult Complexity Assessment Grid (CAG) methodology for Lucinda
- To connect complexity assessment findings to the development of a care plan
- To demonstrate how to use the record of outcome measures for documenting patient and case manager-based performance
- To explain how to help Lucinda progress toward case graduation

LUCINDA'S STORY

The patient, Lucinda, is a 37-year-old overweight Mexican-American female referred for integrated case management by insurance reviewers specifically looking for patients who use many health services. She came to their attention because a request was being made for approval to remove a gangrenous toe. Lucinda has had numerous procedures, hospitalizations, and emergency room visits in the past 2 years. During the past 12 months, she has filled 32 prescriptions for eight different medications from six independent physicians, one of whom is a diabetic specialist, one a psychiatrist (for diazepam), and one a surgeon (for a pain medication). Three prescribers are primary care physicians. Lucinda has four other physicians who have submitted medical charges for her care in the past year. Her last admission was 2 weeks earlier for 2 days and she has been to the emergency room three times in the last month. During her hospitalization, At that time, she had blood sugar levels of 400+, a gangrenous toe, and a fever of 104 degrees Fahrenheit. Her last HbA1c was 9.2.

TRIAGE: ENROLLMENT SPECIALIST INTERACTION

The health plan utilization manager (insurance reviewer) identifies Lucinda as a potential high-impact, Level IV member since she triggers in the claims system because of recent hospitalization, being on numerous medications, and seeing many physicians in the past year (see Appendix 2). She has several complications of diabetes and is requesting approval for toe amputation by a local surgeon. She is taking psychotropic medications but not much is known about this. Last year, Lucinda's total claims costs were $20,726. This year's are already $47,725 and it is only April.

Lucinda is somewhat reluctant to talk with the enrollment specialist initially, but after the program is explained (see Appendix B, www.springerpub.com/

kathol), she opens up a bit. She agrees that her health is a problem and that she needs to change something (readiness for change VAS score = 9) but does not know what to do or how to do it (see Appendix B, www.springerpub.com/kathol). She has no confidence in making the changes herself (confidence in being able to change VAS score = 3) but is willing to try something new. Lucinda has tried many things in the past without success, thus she does not think anything will work.

Lucinda has a telephone and is home much of the time. She has a condition that, if in control, would be associated with better health, function, and lower cost. She has never been in a case management program before. This identifies her as a high-priority candidate for case management. The enrollment specialist directly transfers Lucinda to a case manager with an opening since Lucinda indicates that she has a little time to talk.

Before connecting Lucinda with the case manager, the enrollment specialist briefly tells the case manager, Ellen, about Lucinda's situation and explains that Lucinda understands only basics about case management.

INITIAL INTERVIEW

Ellen does not have time to review Lucinda's health records (claims) since Lucinda is immediately connected to her. Ellen introduces herself and describes what she does as a case manager. She tells her a little about her health-related background and how she works with people who find it difficult to control their illnesses in the complicated medical system. Ellen briefly describes what she has been told by the enrollment specialist about Lucinda's situation and asks if she is willing to allow her to help. Ellen answers several questions posed by Lucinda about the process, how Lucinda would work with her, and what kinds of things Lucinda would have to do if she agrees to participate. When these are answered, Lucinda gives approval but says that she will also be talking with her current doctors about whether she should participate.

Ellen notes that since she has not had time to look at Lucinda's insurance records she will do so after their conversation. She also tells Lucinda that she will try to talk with the Lucinda's primary physician or his staff to better understand Lucinda's health situation, to let Lucinda's doctors know what she does to help patients, and to find out if there are specific things that the doctors think would be helpful. Lucinda indicates that she only has 30 minutes to speak with Ellen.

Ellen indicates to Lucinda that she will be going into detail about Lucinda's health problems during her assessment but that she wants to get to know about Lucinda first. She outlines her legal reporting requirements related to what they discuss (e.g., about suicidal or homicidal comments that might come up) and then asks if it is okay to wait to ask more questions about Lucinda's illness until she knows a bit more about Lucinda and her living situation. Lucinda approves. As Ellen asks questions, she takes notes.

To help her organize her questions, Ellen has a printed copy of the standard questions on her desk in front of her (see Exhibit 10.1 and Appendix E, www. springerpub.com/kathol) and a blank INTERMED-Complexity Assessment Grid (IM-CAG) scoring sheet (see Appendix 4) with descriptions of the item anchor points (see Appendix 6). Ellen's health plan is putting templates of these into Ellen's case management documentation system but has not completed the process.

QUESTION 1: *"Can you tell me about yourself, e.g., where you live, who you live with, how you spend your days, what your hobbies and interests are?"*

Follow-up questions (Ellen can fill these in later if there is reticence by Lucinda to divulge personal information at this point.):

1.1 "What kind of job do you have?"
1.2 "Can you tell me about your financial situation/ pressures?"
1.3 "Do you require assistance in getting out of the house?"
1.4 "Who helps you when a crisis arises?"
1.5 "Who are your friends?"
1.6 "How do you spend your free time?"
1.7 "Do you help take care of others, i.e., family, a friend?"

Ellen's Notes

- Single mother of 14-year-old daughter and 9-year-old son
- Owns home
- Raised in U.S. with good English-speaking skills
- Divorced 7 years
- No boyfriend
- Works in a factory but missing much work (worried about keeping job, on short-term disability [STD])
- Extended family members live in town and help when they can (about once a week but supervise the two children when she is in hospital)
- Child support sporadic
- No current hobbies but likes to knit
- Kids doing well in school with usual problems
- Trouble making it to kids' school activities because of health problems
- Diabetes and its complications have always been a problem

The first question stimulates a conversation, which provides relevant information about Lucinda's living situation, job, family, and support network. To further clarify this general information, Ellen asks several follow-up questions that add the following information.

Ellen's Notes

- Sticks pretty much to family for support (few out-of-home friends)
- Mother diabetic (taken care of by father)
- Daughter (Anita, a 14-year-old); also overweight and has early diabetes managed by diet only but without complications so far; worried about her
- Financial pressures from high medication costs and medical copays
- Uncertainty about job and family household needs

- More trouble working when able, because of infections and eyesight problems (little sympathy at work)

Now that Ellen has a feel for Lucinda's personal and social situation, she tells Lucinda that she wants to better understand the difficulties that Lucinda has had controlling and living with her diabetes. She asks the following opening question.

QUESTION 2: *"Lucinda, you were referred to me because you have a serious complication of diabetes for which you need treatment. Can you tell me about your diabetes and how it is affecting your life?"*

FOLLOW-UP QUESTIONS
2.1 "Have you had (other) physical problems or long-term conditions or illnesses?"
2.2 "Were these difficult to diagnose?"
2.3 "Are medical assessments underway?"
2.4 "What kind of treatments have you received?"
2.5 "Have you had difficulty following through on recommended physical health treatments?"
2.6 "How have the treatments worked?"
2.7 "Do physical symptoms interfere with doing the things you like to do?"

Ellen's Notes
- Type 1 diabetes since high school
- Worse control in the past 3 years
- Seeing many different doctors, but they are not consistent since her primary doctor cannot always fit her in
- Appointments take time from work
- Last worked 3 months ago
- Now has hypertension, obesity, high cholesterol, early but progressive kidney disease, failing vision, back pain, leg pain (neuropathy), insomnia, and skin infections related to diabetes; acute problem is a gangrenous toe
- Takes 10 medications inconsistently (five regularly [*Ellen note: check insurance claims*]); different recommendations from different doctors; nondiabetic diet
- No exercise
- Checks sugars when she feels bad (often high) but records fictitious levels for her doctor (embarrassed about poor control)
- Medications too costly; occasionally misses insulin
- Had diabetic training years ago but does not remember much about it
- Things now out of control and she *feels defeated*
- Never treated for depression but takes an occasional diazepam to control nerves (doctors never ask about emotions during short visits; evaluations focused on medical complications)

The general discussion of Lucinda's experiences living with and trying to control her diabetes uncovers much useful information. There are several things, however, that did not come up. Ellen asks several additional questions about how the diabetes has affected her life and the things that she likes to do. Additional questions pertaining to Lucinda's financial situation, her marital status, and her work were also asked.

Ellen's Notes
- Cannot knit because of vision
- Does not date due to weight, health, and lack of interest
- Not working because of poor diabetes/health control
- Occasional visits to school functions and teacher meetings
- Ex-husband: no help since he lives in another city
- Alimony and child support sporadic

After hearing Lucinda's story about the progression of her illness, Ellen responds empathically by telling her, *"You sure have had your trials with your diabetes. It must be difficult for you not to be able to go to many of your kids' school activities and to be confined to the house."* Lucinda appreciates that Ellen recognizes that it is hard for her. This opens the door to finding out more about Lucinda's emotional health.

QUESTIONS 3: *"Has your diabetes affected your emotions, caused you to be discouraged or sad?"*

FOLLOW-UP QUESTIONS
3.1 "Has your physical health situation affected your emotions?"
3.2 "Have you had mental health problems in the past?"
3.3 "Have mental health issues required treatment or hospitalization, such as for depression, anxiety, confusion, or memory problems?"
3.4 "What kinds of treatments have you received and from whom?"
3.5 "Have you had difficulty in following through on mental health treatments?"
3.6 "Are you getting any treatment now?"
3.7 "Has treatment been helpful?"
3.8 "Do emotional factors interfere with doing the things you like to do?"

Ellen's Notes
- Sad all the time with little interest in doing things (Patient Health Questionnaire-2 [PHQ-2] positive)
- PHQ-9 (**Exhibit 12.1**) score was 19 without active suicidal ideation (moderately severe depressive symptoms)

EXHIBIT 12.1   **Lucinda's Depression Symptom Evaluation (Baseline)**

The following are Lucinda's responses to the depression symptom evaluation questionnaire:
Over the last 2 weeks, how often have you been bothered by any of the following problems?

Response Key: Not at all = 0 Several days = 1 More than half the days = 2 Nearly every day = 3

1.	Little interest or pleasure in doing things	**3**
2.	Feeling down, depressed or hopeless	**3**
3.	Trouble falling/staying asleep, or sleeping too much	**2**
4.	Feeling tired or having little energy	**3**
5.	Poor appetite or overeating	**2**
6.	Feeling bad about yourself, feeling that you are a failure or feeling that you have let yourself or your family down	**3**
7.	Trouble concentrating on things, such as reading the newspaper or watching television	**2**
8.	Moving or speaking so slowly that other people could have noticed. Or being so fidgety or restless that you have been moving around a lot more than usual	**1**
9.	Thinking that you would be better off dead or that you want to hurt yourself in some way	**0**
	Total Score for 1 to 9:	**19**

Scoring Key for PHQ-9: Minimal < 5; Mild 5–9; Moderate 10–14; Moderately severe 15–19; Severe >19

Impairment: If you checked off any problem on this questionnaire so far, how difficult have these problems made it for you to do your work, take care of things at home, or get along with other people?   **3**

Response Key for Impairment Question: Not Difficult at All = 0; Somewhat Difficult = 1; Very Difficult = 2; Extremely Difficult = 3

- Generalized Anxiety Disorder-7 (GAD-7; **Table 12.1**) score was 8 with no panic attacks (mild anxiety symptoms)
- Never treated for emotional problems and almost never asked about them by her doctors, though occasionally encouraged to see a counselor for acute mental health problems and given diazepam for "nerves" when she asked for something to calm her
- No other psychological problems
- Mother and sister have had depression; father is an alcoholic but currently is "on the wagon"

Most questions are answered related to symptoms that Lucinda has experienced or is currently experiencing, both related and not related to her medical diabetes and its complications. Since Lucinda's PHQ-9 score was high, Ellen asked Lucinda how she felt about treatment for depression if her doctors thought it would help.

Ellen's Notes
- Diazepam did not help
- Mother and sister got better with treatment
- Never tried counseling despite recommendations

Ellen is getting close to the 30-minute limit set by Lucinda at the beginning of the call. She indicates that she would like to ask Lucinda to tell her how limited she is in what she can do before their time is up. Ellen uses the company's 10-point functional impairment visual analogue scale, with 1 being the worst, to document Lucinda's score of 3. Ellen already knows that Lucinda has not been to work in past month. Thus the functional work scale was scored as "23 of 23 days missed" since Lucinda works 5-day weeks (with occasional overtime). Ellen fills in several items in the Record for Outcome Measures (**Table 12.2**) and anchors what she can on Lucinda's IM-CAG (**Table 12.3**, see page i6 for color version). After the call, Ellen will write notes at the bottom of the scoring sheet that can be shared with Lucinda when the IM-CAG is complete.

Ellen briefly summarizes what she has learned from Lucinda during the 30-minute discussion. As with many other patients with health complexity, clarifying Lucinda's barriers to improvement using defined item anchor points takes some time. Ellen is only halfway through the assessment. On the other hand, it is clear by the end of the first 30 minutes that Lucinda is feeling more comfortable with Ellen. Since it has been a dialogue, Ellen has been able to give examples of how others have attempted to change some of the problems that Lucinda describes. Ellen has also answered

TABLE 12.1 Lucinda's Anxiety Symptoms Evaluation (Baseline)

Over the last 2 weeks, how often have you been bothered by the following problems?	Not at all sure (Mark 0)	Several days (Mark 1)	Over half the days (Mark 2)	Nearly every day (Mark 3)
Feeling nervous, anxious, or on edge		1		
Not being able to stop or control worrying	0			
Worrying too much about different things			2	
Trouble relaxing		1		
Being so restless that it's hard to sit still	0			
Becoming easily annoyed or irritable			2	
Feeling afraid as if something awful might happen			2	
Add the score for each column	0	2	6	—
Total score (add column scores)[a]		8		

If you marked any problems, how difficult have these problems made it for you to do your work, take care of things at home, or get along with other people?

Not difficult at all	Somewhat difficult (Lucinda's response)	Very difficult	Extremely difficult

[a]For case management purposes, use total scores of 10 and above as significant levels of anxiety.

TABLE 12.2 Lucinda's Record of Outcome Measures (Interim ROM)

OUTCOME MEASURES		BASELINE	FOLLOW-UP ASSESSMENTS		
	Time period recorded	Interim			
Clinical measure (personal goal)					
Functional measure (personal goal)					
Health-related quality of life Number of days healthy/month					
Patient satisfaction (Scale: 0 low, 10 high)					
CAG score (Total for period)		25+			
Health care clinical measure HbA1c		9.2			
Health care clinical measure PHQ-9		19			
Health care functional measure Level of function (scale 0–10)		3			
Health care functional measure Number of work days lost/23 days		23			
Health care economic measure Number of emergency room visits in last 30 days		3			

TABLE 12.3   Lucinda's IM-CAG (Interim)

Interim	HEALTH RISKS AND HEALTH NEEDS					
Lucinda	HISTORICAL		CURRENT STATE		VULNERABILITY	
Total Score = 25+	Complexity Item	Score	Complexity Item	Score	Complexity Item	Score
Biological Domain	Chronicity **HB1**	3	Symptom Severity/Impairment **CB1**	2	Complications and Life Threat **VB**	3
	Diagnostic Dilemma **HB2**	0	Diagnostic/Therapeutic Challenge **CB2**	3		
Psychological Domain	Barriers to Coping **HP1**		Resistance to Treatment **CP1**	2	Mental Health Threat **VP**	2
	Mental Health History **HP2**	1	Mental Health Symptoms **CP2**	2		
Social Domain	Job and Leisure **HS1**	1	Residential Stability **CS1**	0	Social Vulnerability **VS**	1
	Relationships **HS2**	0	Social Support **CS2**	1		
Health System Domain	Access to Care **HHS1**		Getting Needed Services **CHS1**	2	Health System Impediments **VHS**	
	Treatment Experience **HHS2**		Coordination of Care **CHS2**	2		

Comments	
HB1	Long history of diabetes with multiple chronic complications
HB2	Easily recognized diabetes mellitus (DM) with complications
CB1	Eye, cardiovascular (CV), mental health (depression), renal, dermatologic, and neurological complications with HbA1c of 9.2; significant personal and functional limitations
CB2	Not following treatments, discouragement contributing to poorly controlled DM
VB	At risk for toe amputation and many other complications, possible early death
HP1	?
HP2	Family and probable personal history of untreated depression; history of alcoholism in father
CP1	Skeptical about potential change success but willing to try, not adhering to most diabetic interventions
CP2	Moderate to severe untreated depressive symptoms with mild anxiety symptoms
VP	Needs psychiatric assessment and treatment
HS1	Job waiting when healthy, on short-term disability for several months, risk of job loss, few social activities
HS2	Good family ties, few nonfamily friends; no significant home problems
CS1	Owns home
CS2	Family readily helps when Lucinda is having difficulties
VS	At risk for losing income and house if no improvement because of job loss, may need nursing care
HHS1 & HHS2	?
CHS1	Medications too costly to buy
CHS2	Many meds and docs, frequent hospital and emergency room use, poor access to consistent follow-up
VHS	?

a number of questions that Lucinda has about her diabetes. Lucinda has not been able to ask the same questions to her doctors because of limited time with them. For some questions, Ellen told Lucinda that she did not know the answer but that she would try to find out or help Lucinda frame questions for her doctor at her next visit.

INTERIM SUMMARY

"Lucinda, it sounds as though you have good family support and a chance to get back to work if you can get your health under better control. Your diabetes, however, has been getting the best of you. Your latest complication is the ulcer on your toe, but that is just one of many things that keeps you from doing things with your family and sends you to the doctor so often. Some of the things you told me raise concerns about your situation. It sounds like you are having difficulty following your blood sugars regularly. It also sounds like keeping up with your medication, diet, and the like is difficult. Part of the reason could be that you are so discouraged. You continue to try but have had limited success. The questionnaires I gave you (PHQ-9; GAD-7) about your emotions indicate that your discouragement itself could be helped with treatment. We know that frustration and discouragement are often seen in people with diabetes and may contribute to their inability to keep up with all the things that they have to do to control their diabetes. This could also be true for you. If I can get a hold of your doctor, do you mind if I ask if he feels that this is a problem?"

Lucinda agrees that discouragement may be contributing but says that the cost and side effects of medication, the time and cost of going to the doctor, and the cost of diabetic monitoring equipment are also involved. Lucinda is also concerned about not having a consistent doctor that knows and follows her.

When queried about important things not asked so far, she indicates that she is worried about her daughter Anita's relationship with a boy that Lucinda does not like. Because she is confined to home, she is not able to monitor what her daughter is doing as well. Her son (9-year-old, Manuel) is doing fine.

INTERIM SUPPORT

Since the assessment must be completed in two sections, Ellen checks if there is something that she can do to start helping Lucinda before their next meeting. *"From our discussion, it appears that there are several areas in which I may be able to assist you, for instance, giving you some information on diabetes or helping find sources for help in buying your medication and diabetic supplies. It is important, however, that you would like to get assistance with these things. Are there things related to your health*

that you would like me to start helping you with today? Can I send you some recent materials on diabetes care and a glucose level diary? Do you prefer English or Spanish?"

Lucinda is willing to have the information sent in English. The things that she would really like help with, however, are getting one doctor to really get to know her and assistance in getting to appointments. Any ideas about places to get medication and supplies paid for would also be helpful.

Ellen says, *"Is it okay for me to talk with the nurse in your doctor's office? Perhaps, I can see if there is a way that one of the doctors can follow you regularly and work with the specialists who are needed for your care, such as the surgeon, the eye doctor, etc. I will also share some of the things that we talked about today. It is important that they know that I will be working with you."*

LUCINDA GIVES PERMISSION

In preparation for the next contact, Ellen indicates, *"When we talk again, we will go into greater detail about the problems you may be having in obtaining the treatments you need for your diabetes and its complications. It has been a pleasure to get to know you during this initial discussion. Can we set up a time for another call?"* Lucinda sets a time later in the week for the second interview.

After the call is ended, Ellen reviews her notes, confirms that anchor point scoring is accurate based on the information shared by Lucinda, and formulates her thoughts about the development of a preliminary care plan (**Table 12.4**). Ellen will be talking with Lucinda within days, but she already knows that Lucinda, with a long history of illness (HB1), has not had a review of diabetes treatments and preventive measures (CB2) for some time. Lucinda also has poorly controlled diabetes with multiple complications and functional impairment (CB1) and symptoms consistent with depression (CP2) that are untreated and could be contributing to the poor diabetic control (VB). Finally, Lucinda is not getting needed services because of cost (CHS1) and poor communication among her doctors and with her (CHS2). For these issues Ellen creates an initial care plan, which will be further completed after the next interview with Lucinda.

FOLLOW-UP INTERVIEW

Ellen calls Lucinda at the agreed-on time. She asks if everything went all right at Anita's band recital and if Manuel scored any goals in his recent soccer game. She also indicates that some materials have been sent to her about new treatments and approaches for diabetes. When the materials arrive, Ellen will be happy to go over them and answer questions. Ellen also asks how Lucinda's toe is doing.

TABLE 12.4   Lucinda's Care Plan Development (Interim CD)

BARRIERS	GOALS		ACTIONS
CAG items	Personal followed by health care		Prioritized
HB1 and CB1	**Short-term**	*Improve illness understanding*	*Send educational materials on diabetes; review with Lucinda at second or third interview (teach and learn)*
	Ultimate	*Participate in self-care*	*Help incorporate materials sent into health activities*
CB2, CP2, and VB	**Short-term**	*Communicate Ellen's participation in Lucinda's care; understand provider's goals; get depression treated, if needed*	*Ask primary treating physician(s) to allow case management assistance; query about prescription goals; share baseline PHQ-9 score*
	Ultimate	*Case manager to collaborate with care providers; physical and mental health symptom control*	*Send letter and brochure about case management (see Appendix C and D, www.springerpub.com/kathol); establish relationship(s) with treating physician(s)*
CHS1 and CHS2	**Short-term**	*Financial support for needed services; communication among practitioners*	*Medication procurement support program identification; generic prescriptions; get names of all practitioners working with patient; flex benefits*
	Ultimate	*Consistent use of needed medications and treatments*	*Medical home with understanding of needs and coordination of care*

Ellen tells Lucinda about the conversation that she has had with Lucinda's clinic office nurse. Since the enrollment specialist had gotten a consent signed by Lucinda, it was possible to have office notes faxed to Ellen. Ellen has reviewed them. Ellen states that she now understands why Lucinda was so interested in getting a steady doctor. There have been nearly 15 doctors involved in her care in the last year, not counting emergency room and inpatient doctors.

Ellen asks Lucinda if anything has happened since their last conversation and answers several questions that Lucinda has. She then starts to complete the remainder of the assessment.

QUESTION 4: *"Can you tell me which doctor knows the most about you and whether you like working with him or her?"*

FOLLOW-UP QUESTIONS
4.1 "Primary care physician/nurse practitioner?"
4.2 "Medical specialists?"
4.3 "Mental health providers, e.g., psychiatrists, psychologists, social workers, nurses, etc.?"
4.4 "Other providers, e.g., chiropractors, naturopaths, church counselors, etc.?"
4.5 "Can you tell me how you get along with your doctors?"
4.6 "How do those giving you care talk with each other and coordinate your treatment?"
4.7 "Do you have difficulty communicating with them?"

4.8 "Are their offices near each other and easy to get to?"
4.9 "Have you had conflicts or disagreements with any of your doctors/providers, your hospital/clinic, or your insurance company that have led to bad feelings or mistrust?"

Ellen's Notes
- No consistent doctor that follows all problems or sees Lucinda regularly
- Doctor teams from her general clinic take care of acute problems (many different ones seen in past year); they often change her medications; 10- to 15-minute visits for focused problem; most lab tests and X-rays done at clinic; likes Dr. Sanchez, a Spanish-speaking doctor, but she is usually too busy to see Lucinda
- Diabetic specialist prescribes insulin, talks about diet and exercise; occasional lab tests; no diabetic diary
- One surgeon for toe ulcer; wants to operate
- Other doctors: eye doctor (4 years ago); kidney doctor (9 months ago); psychiatrist (seen in emergency room one time); neurologist (for leg pain but medications from general clinic); heart doctor (saw in the emergency room during chest pain episode and gave Lucinda psychiatric referral)
- Other providers: herbalist friend; occasional chiropractor for back pain
- Medical/surgical clinics in a big complex two miles away; virtually never sees two doctors on the same day

- Five to ten office visits per month with some additional emergency room visits
- No conflicts with doctors but none seem to care about Lucinda, just her illnesses and the poor control; does not trust some
- Has to keep job or Lucinda loses her insurance; not insurable with other coverage until bankrupt when she qualifies for general assistance plan with poor access to care; does not trust insurance company (Ellen excepted, so far)

Ellen's reading of the clinic notes and insurance claims are confirmed. Lucinda truly has no medical home. She has a clinic at which much of her care is given; however, her appointments are made with any doctor that is available since the doctors in the clinic work many places. There is no diabetic teaching, no encouragement to use a blood sugar diary, and only occasional laboratory tests performed during an acute problem. No one makes sure that preventive services are being given. Doctors always express concern about Lucinda's poor control and change her medications. Lucinda does not have the heart to tell them that she often misses her medications and occasionally her insulin. She frequently does not know which or how much medication she should be taking. Different doctors make conflicting recommendations (e.g., ACE inhibitors, water pills, statins, antibiotics, etc.).

QUESTION 5: *"Why has it been so difficult to find a doctor to take a special interest in your care?"*

FOLLOW-UP QUESTIONS
5.1 "What type of medical insurance do you have and does it cover the services you need?"
5.2 "Do you have trouble finding medical doctors who will accept you as a patient?"
5.3 "Do you need to go to separate clinics for mental health treatment?"
5.4 "Are there separate payment rules for mental health care?"
5.5 "Have you or your primary care physician had difficulty in finding a mental health provider for you?"
5.6 "How far do you live from the medical clinics and doctors you need to see to improve your health?"
5.7 "Do you need a translator or someone from your culture to assist with health needs?"
5.8 "Can you afford your medical care, i.e., medications, needed tests, copays for appointments and hospital costs, needed medical equipment/devices, etc.?"
5.9 "Is transportation a problem in getting to your appointments?"
5.10 "Are there long waiting lists for the kind of care you need?"

Several of the questions about health system issues that are creating a barrier to improvement at the practitioner level have already been answered. There is poor coordination of care and little communication among Lucinda's doctors. Few know about the difficulty that Lucinda has in getting to appointments and paying for her medications. She does have insurance but still has many copays that add up. Plus, now that she has been out of work for three months, she is at risk of losing her job. Loss of insurance through her large employer would be devastating.

Ellen's Notes
- Good medical insurance with limited copay for services, but medications still cost a lot; mental health copays are high and coverage is limited since her employer is not required to conform to parity laws
- Chose a community clinic close to home because of difficulty traveling, but there are too few doctors for the number of patients
- Trouble driving because of toe problem; family helps
- Doctors see Lucinda and "bill a lot" but none follow through on care and outcomes
- No medical record sharing among primary doctors/clinics and specialists as far as Ellen can tell

QUESTION 6: *"What kind of person are you, e.g., outgoing, suspicious, tense, or optimistic?"*

FOLLOW-UP QUESTIONS
6.1 "Do you smoke?"
6.2 "On average, how many alcoholic beverages do you drink a day (week), e.g., glasses of wine, beers, etc.?
6.3 "Do you use painkillers: how often, how long, more often than prescribed?
6.4 "Do you use cocaine, marijuana, or other recreational drugs?"
6.5 "Have you ever been treated for substance abuse problems?"
6.6 "How do you handle difficult situations?" (alcohol or drug use, talkative, silent, procrastinate?)
6.7 "What are your biggest health concerns at this time?"
6.8 "During the next 1 to 3 months, what about your health would you like to have under better control (clinical), e.g., have less foot pain, have no asthma attacks for a solid month, etc.?"
6.9 "What would you like to be able to do that you can't do now (functional), e.g., attend church regularly, participate in family events, return to work, etc.?"

Much has already been discussed. *Several reasons for not taking medications:* too complicated, inconsistent directions from different doctors, medications cost too much (does not always have them to take), side effects (not discussed with doctor or doctor's staff), meds not seen as working, chiropractor and family told her she takes too many medications. *Several reasons for not attending follow-up visits:* too many visits and not enough time or money to get to them, mixed messages from different doctors, does not trust some doctors, family conflicts, discouraged (depressed). *Reasons for not exercising, following diet, completing diary:* too much trouble; does not work anyhow; too hard; does not feel like doing it.

Ellen has developed a respect for Lucinda's challenges due to her health and family responsibilities, but she still needs to better understand why Lucinda has so much difficulty in keeping her medical situation under control. When Ellen talked with the office nurse at the clinic Lucinda usually attended, Ellen expressed concern about the possibility of depression since the depression symptom scale (PHQ-9) had been so high. The nurse stated that the last two doctors mentioned similar concerns but had done nothing since it was so difficult to obtain psychiatric and psychological help. In addition to other personal questions related to this content area, Ellen returned the focus of the conversation to Lucinda's overwhelming feelings of discouragement and discussed the possibility that depression could be contributing to Lucinda's uncontrolled medical condition.

Ellen's Notes

■ Easygoing and optimistic most of the time but recently just cannot keep up with demands
■ Depression could be contributing since it ran in Lucinda's family; Lucinda was willing to get assessed and treatment, if necessary
■ Does not smoke or use drugs; drank to excess and used marijuana while married (thinks it contributed to her divorce) but has not been drunk for over 5 years; drinks occasionally
■ Uses nonnarcotic pain killers for back and legs; prescribed diazepam but rarely uses it
■ Turns to relatives when stressed
■ Tends to procrastinate or just let nature take its course in difficult situations; Lucinda is not pushy

Ellen now reaches one of the most important parts of the evaluation—the point at which she finds out what Lucinda considers her personal goals in working with Ellen. Ellen now has a good idea about the challenges that Lucinda faces and has already formulated in her own mind the things that she thinks that Lucinda needs to do to bring her health under better control, but it is time to listen to and to hear what Lucinda thinks.

Ellen says, *"I now understand about the difficulties you are having controlling your diabetes and also how it affects you and your family. Before ending this discussion, I also want to make sure I am helping you accomplish the things that are important to you. To do this, I would like you to tell me what your personal goals would be during the next several months while I am working with you. What about your health would you like to have under better control, such as your foot pain, your blood sugars, your discouragement? Also, what would you like to be able to do that you can't do now, such as do more with your daughter, go to work, knit?"*

Ellen helps Lucinda through the decision-making process. Lucinda chooses the following two goals:

■ Clinical Goal: to resolve the middle toe ulcer without surgery (baseline measurements 1.3 cm in diameter and 0.2 cm deep; this goal needs to be confirmed with Lucinda's diabetes doctor and surgeon to ensure that it is safe and possible. If it is, it will require coordinated effort by Lucinda, Ellen, the diabetologist, her surgeon, and perhaps a podiatrist.
■ Functional Goal: to return to work.

Ellen also helps Lucinda rate her satisfaction with the health care she has received. It is 5 on a scale of 10 with 10 being the highest (see the following visual analogue scale). Lucinda also indicates that she has had no "healthy days" in the past month (health-related quality of life). *Rate your satisfaction with the health care you are currently receiving, all things considered, on a scale of 1 to 10, with 10 being the highest:*

$$0 - 1 - 2 - 3 - 4 - 5 - 6 - 7 - 8 - 9 - 10$$

ASSESSMENT SUMMARY

It took another 45 minutes to complete the second half of the health complexity assessment with Lucinda. Before closing the discussion, Ellen asks Lucinda if she can summarize what she heard during the two discussions they have had so that she can be sure that she does not miss any important items. Ellen says, *"There is no question that you have many problems related to your diabetes. You are being treated for heart and blood vessel, infectious, eye, and nerve complications. High blood fats are also being treated. Your kidneys are okay but are being monitored with blood tests. You have trouble following through on your treatments because you see so many different doctors and receive inconsistent advice. You do not trust some of your doctors, but you feel that the more important problem is that none of the doctors really know your entire health situation. The cost of the treatments is sometimes more than you can afford, and you have trouble getting to all your appointments. This sometimes necessitates emergency room visits. You are just flat discouraged, perhaps depressed, about all the problems you are having with your health. It saps your energy and makes it difficult to do things with your family. It is even hard to do what your doctors recommend. Your greatest interest is in having your toe heal without surgery and getting back to work.*

Lucinda agrees that this is accurate and confirms that she is at a loss about where to start to change things. Ellen asks, *"What things did I not ask about that you think are important?"* Lucinda does not have additional things to add.

Here Ellen and Lucinda discuss the fact that the diabetes has to come under better control and Lucinda's energy has to improve in order for her to accomplish her personal goals. Using motivational interviewing techniques, Ellen suggests that a plan for change may include:

1. Getting control of blood sugars back on track
2. Good foot care
3. Treating depression
4. Coordinating provider involvement
5. Seeing if light duty is available at work when Lucinda is stabilized enough to return

Ellen recommends that Lucinda and she make an appointment in about a week, after Ellen has had a chance to put her thoughts together, to discuss the barriers that Ellen has uncovered that are contributing to Lucinda's poor health. They can then work together on a strategy that will allow Lucinda to stabilize her health and achieve her personal goals. In the meantime, Lucinda will have had a chance to glance through the material the Ellen sent earlier in the week. Ellen also said that she would try to contact Lucinda's clinic to see if there was a way for Lucinda to work with a single primary doctor, perhaps Dr. Sanchez.

Ellen says that she would like to send a summary of the assessment to Lucinda and asked if there is a confidential way to get it to her without others seeing it. Lucinda said that the best way would be to mail it to her. Ellen and Lucinda set up an appointment to talk again in ten days. By that time, Lucinda's IM-CAG should arrive at her house.

COMPLEXITY DOCUMENTATION, BASELINE RECORD OF OUTCOME MEASURES, CARE PLAN DEVELOPMENT

Based on the information provided by Lucinda, Ellen scored the remaining items in the IM-CAG (**Table 12.5**). She also added and changed comments to the scored items from the preliminary grid to help clarify for Lucinda the reason that different cells were represented by the various colors (bottom of **Table 12.5**, see page i7 for color version). Four cell scores were changed from the preliminary IM-CAG to the final initial

assessment based on additional information from the second interview (CB1 from 2 to 3; HP2 from 1 to 2; CHS1 from 2 to 3; CHS2 from 2 to 3). Lucinda's total score was 38 (upper left hand **Table 12.5** and color version). Ellen put a copy of the scored IM-CAG in the mail as instructed by Lucinda so that she would have a chance to review it before Ellen and Lucinda's next telephone call.

Ellen was expected to document the value that she brought to her patients and the health plan. For this to occur, her supervisor and employer expected several items associated with the complexity assessment to be tracked through the course of case management in the record of outcome measures. These included the total IM-CAG score, personal and health clinical and functional goals, health satisfaction, quality of life, and cost outcomes. Ellen placed Lucinda's scores into the baseline record (**Table 12.6**).

The presence of multiple red zones (see color version) with a total score of 38 on the CAG suggests that there are significant problems for Lucinda in the biological and health system domains. She has multiple chronic illnesses (many related to diabetes) with significant symptoms and impairment but treatment that is not controlling her health. Lucinda is not adhering to treatment, in part because of poor coordination of her care and in part because of her financial problems. Lucinda also likely has untreated depression that is contributing to nonadherence.

Red indicates a need for *immediate* action, thus with the Lucinda's permission and collaboration, early intervention will be intense and focused on the red areas (HB1, CB1, CB2, VB, HHS2, CHS1, CHS2, VHS). To the extent possible, red zone interventions will be done in such a way that correction of orange (HP2, CP1, CP2, VP, HHS1) and yellow (HP1, HS1, CS2, VS) zones will occur at the same time or follow naturally in the case management process. It will also have the ultimate focus on maximizing the possibility for Lucinda to avoid surgery on her toe and to get back to work, her primary goals.

The initial time spent with Lucinda will focus on helping her understand her personal complexity assessment, how it was scored, and its implication for specific actions that may be of assistance to her. From this, Ellen and Lucinda will work on a final care plan together. Since Ellen has taken the time to document complexity-based barriers and to link them with each other already in a care plan draft (**Table 12.7**), she can help guide Lucinda through the process using motivational interviewing techniques.

Early activity will include confirming Lucinda's understanding of her illnesses and their treatment, establishing coordination of care by a more limited number of Lucinda's doctors, addressing treatment

TABLE 12.5   Lucinda's IM-CAG (Baseline)

Baseline	HEALTH RISKS AND HEALTH NEEDS					
Lucinda	**HISTORICAL**		**CURRENT STATE**		**VULNERABILITY**	
Total Score = 38	Complexity Item	Score	Complexity Item	Score	Complexity Item	Score
Biological Domain	Chronicity **HB1**	3	Symptom Severity/Impairment **CB1**	3	Complications and Life Threat **VB**	3
	Diagnostic Dilemma **HB2**	0	Diagnostic/Therapeutic Challenge **CB2**	3		
Psychological Domain	Barriers to Coping **HP1**	1	Resistance to Treatment **CP1**	2	Mental Health Threat **VP**	2
	Mental Health History **HP2**	2	Mental Health Symptoms **CP2**	2		
Social Domain	Job and Leisure **HS1**	1	Residential Stability **CS1**	0	Social Vulnerability **VS**	1
	Relationships **HS2**	0	Social Support **CS2**	1		
Health System Domain	Access to Care **HHS1**	2	Getting Needed Services **CHS1**	3	Health System Impediments **VHS**	3
	Treatment Experience **HHS2**	3	Coordination of Care **CHS2**	3		

Comments	
HB1	Long history of diabetes with multiple chronic complications
HB2	Easily recognized DM with complications
CB1	Eye, cardiovascular (CV), mental health (depression), renal, dermatologic, and neurological complications with HbA1c of 9.2; significant personal and functional limitations
CB2	Not following treatments, untreated depression contributing to poorly controlled DM
VB	At risk for toe amputation and many other complications, possible early death
HP1	Passive acceptance of health situation; history of substance abuse
HP2	Family and probable personal history of untreated depression; history of alcoholism in father, abuse in patient
CP1	Skeptical about potential change success but willing to try, not taking most diabetic interventions
CP2	Moderate to severe untreated depressive symptoms with mild anxiety symptoms
VP	Needs psychiatric assessment and treatment and assistance with pushing health system to stabilize
HS1	Job waiting when healthy, on short-term disability for several months, risk of job loss, few social activities
HS2	Good family ties, few nonfamily friends; no significant home problems
CS1	Owns home
CS2	Family readily helps when Lucinda is having difficulties
VS	At risk for losing income and house if no improvement because of job loss, may need nursing care
HHS1	Poor mental health benefits in plan
HHS2	Distrust of some doctors; no bad experiences other than apparent disinterest by doctors; frequent emergency room visits and admissions
CHS1	Medications and diabetic supplies too costly to buy; challenge to get to uncoordinated appointments; no mental health referral by primary physicians
CHS2	Many meds and docs, frequent hospital and ER use, poor access to consistent follow-up
VHS	Persistent problems anticipated without consistent and coordinated medical and mental health care

TABLE 12.6   Lucinda's Record of Outcome Measures (Baseline ROM)

OUTCOME MEASURES		BASELINE	FOLLOW-UP ASSESSMENTS		
	Time period recorded	*Baseline*			
Clinical measure (personal goal) *Heal toe ulcer without surgery*		*1.3 cm diameter; 0.2 cm depth*			
Functional measure (personal goal) *Return to work*		*Full short-term disability*			
Health-related quality of life *Number of healthy days/month*		*0*			
Patient satisfaction *(Scale: 0 low, 10 high)*		*5*			
CAG score *(Total for period)*		*38*			
Health care clinical measure *HbA1c*		*9.2*			
Health care clinical measure *PHQ-9*		*19*			
Health care functional measure *Level of function (scale 0–10)*		*3*			
Health care functional measure *Number of work days lost/23 days*		*23*			
Health care economic measure *Number of emergency room visits in the last 30 days*		*3*			

adherence and consistency, and making sure that the psychiatric symptoms experienced by Lucinda are not overlooked. These activities will be connected to Lucinda's personal goals since through them her goals can be achieved. Lucinda's social situation appears fairly stable; however, there may be some challenges in getting back to normal function (e.g., back to work) when health-related aspects improve.

CASE MANAGEMENT

CASE MANAGEMENT PROCESS

When Ellen and Lucinda complete the initial care plan (adapted from **Table 12.7**), identified needs and actions are fairly overwhelming. Ellen explains that everything will not be corrected in a day or even a week. Thus, Lucinda and Ellen prioritize goals and actions, first to maximize the potential for Lucinda to achieve her personal goals. Ellen explains that it is a step-by-step process, broken into bite-sized pieces. Together they will decide where to start and how to proceed. Since achieving these goals necessarily requires that Lucinda's health and general function have to improve,

many other goals can simultaneously be pursued in relation to the personal goals.

Ellen systematically works with Lucinda to reverse the high-priority red and orange item goals (see color templates). As the process gets underway, indirect or unexpected barriers are identified (e.g., resistance by Lucinda's daughter and mother in accepting the need to treat depression in Lucinda). It is critical that Lucinda fully understands and embraces the *why* and the *how* of the actions being taken. For instance, if she cannot explain the rationale for her own depression treatment to her family, they may talk her out of it. Thus, Ellen must work closely with Lucinda to make sure Lucinda understands why one illness (depression) affects another (diabetes and its complications). Lucinda, in a sense, must become a complex case manager herself because case management assistance won't be available forever. Lucinda needs to fully grasp the critical importance of thinking dually, mind and body, and having an outcome orientation. Such dialogues are an inherent part of the motivational interviewing skills discussed in Chapter 4.

Ellen works for a health plan. Thus, she has been given some latitude to flex benefits. Ellen uses the big

TABLE 12.7	Lucinda's Care Plan Development (Baseline CD)*

BARRIERS	GOALS		ACTIONS
CAG items	Personal followed by health care		Prioritized
HHS2 and CHS2	**Short-term**	Identify active practitioners	1. TALK WITH HEALTH PLAN MEDICAL DIRECTOR ABOUT CALLING DIABETOLOGIST, SURGEON, AND DR. SANCHEZ (PODIATRIST?) 2. COORDINATE PRACTITIONER INVOLVEMENT WITH LUCINDA'S HELP
	Ultimate	Prevent toe amputations	1. MAXIMIZE SKIN CARE
HS1	**Short-term**	Help Lucinda get back to work	1. HAVE LUCINDA MAKE AN APPOINTMENT WITH COMPANY EMPLOYEE ASSISSTANCE PROGRAM REPRESENTATIVE 2. CHECK ON LIGHT DUTY POSSIBILITIES AT WORKSITE
	Ultimate	Return to work	1. LOOK INTO WORK REENTRY OPTIONS
HB1, CB1, CB2, CP2 and VB	**Short-term**	Improved illness understanding; confirm consistency of treatment program	1. Send and go over educational materials on DM and depression 2. DISCUSS THE RELATIONSHIP OF POOR CONTROL TO LUCINDA'S PERSONAL GOALS (TOE HEALING AND BACK TO WORK) 3. Work through steps to control DM and depression 4. Medical director and primary provider discussion about Lucinda's experience with docs, adherence due to cost, depressive symptoms, RELUCTANCE TO AMPUTATE TOES, and maximizing health plan support for Lucinda's treatment and goals (with permission)
	Ultimate	Coordinated diabetes management and depression treatment	1. Assist with follow-through on agreed-on treatment plan
CB1, CB2, CP1, & VB	**Short-term**	Improve adherence to treatment	1. Review medications (duplications, difficulties, costs); review 3 months of provider contacts (include emergency room visits, admissions, physical therapy, etc.) 2. Review diary keeping for blood sugars 3. REVIEW WOUND CARE PROCEDURES
	Ultimate	Improve diabetic control and outcomes	1. Help Lucinda list meds and accurate blood sugars so she can talk with primary provider and diabetologist 2. Set time to talk with them about extra appointment time (soon)
HHS1, CHS1, & VHS	**Short-term**	Improve access to and payment for care	1. Three-way call with Lucinda and health plan to clarify medical and mental health benefits and options 2. Attempt to get benefit exceptions to formulary medications or copays 3. Help coordinate treating providers; medication reconciliation 4. Investigate medication payment assistance
	Ultimate	No access or financial disincentives to appropriate care	1. Outline medical and mental health benefits and medication payment options for Lucinda

*Actions directly linked to Lucinda's personal goals are in small caps.

health picture to improve Lucinda's situation, which, without assistance, will continue to lead to high health service use unless her clinical condition stabilizes. As a problem solver with Lucinda, Ellen obtains a formulary exception on copays and approval for an out-of-network but more readily available psychiatrist to work with Lucinda.

Some of Ellen's help is just practical advice. For instance, she encourages Lucinda to write a list of questions for her providers before each visit and take it with her to appointments. These can be used to stimulate more productive discussions with her doctors.

In the long run, the list is more efficient for Lucinda *and* for her providers since it prevents calls to office staff or, worse, nonadherence with treatment leading to emergency room visits. Ellen also suggests that Lucinda might consider bringing a trusted family member with her to her appointments, as a second set of ears. This could reduce confusion about the details of the treatment plan. These tips help Lucinda feel more in control of her health care and provide a faster track to health.

Ellen and Lucinda talk nearly daily for about 2 weeks after they have agreed on the care plan with established priorities. Thereafter, progressively less time is required as stabilization of Lucinda's doctors, treatments, finances, and ultimately condition occurs. The effects of better health reduce Lucinda's use of health services and help her to return to a maximum level of function. When Lucinda approaches the point where case management assistance is no longer needed, Ellen is only in contact with her every second or third week.

Ellen notes that some things required finesse. For instance, as Lucinda accepted the need for depression treatment, Ellen had to work with Lucinda, Lucinda's primary care physician, and her psychiatrist to make sure there was communication among them and coordination of Lucinda's mental health care with her medical care. Further, there was some disagreement between the psychiatrist and the family medicine doctor, Dr. Sanchez, about who should prescribe the medication for depression and how related symptoms should be monitored. Ultimately, Dr. Sanchez prescribed medications suggested by the psychiatrist, who consulted in the background. Ellen performed periodic PHQ-9 evaluations to document change. Over time, Dr. Sanchez became comfortable in doing her own PHQ-9 evaluations and often saw the link between PHQ-9 scores and HbA1c levels in her other diabetic and chronically ill patients.

Lucinda graduates 3 months after entering case management. Before returning her to standard care, Ellen ensures that Lucinda is up to date on preventive measures for her illnesses (e.g., eye examinations, renal function tests, etc.), that she is moving toward increased function, such as experiencing work success and doing more with her family, and that she has learned and is using the techniques that Ellen has been sharing as they worked together.

FOLLOW-UP AND MEASUREMENT

The IM-CAG helped guide Ellen as she and Lucinda identified areas in which action could be taken to address specific goals. At the end of 6 weeks, IM-CAG (**Table 12.8**, see page i8 for color version) items were rescored using follow-up scoring rules (see the Chapter 11 section "Use of the CAG as a Global Assessment of Complexity Amelioration"), and the notes related to items were updated at the bottom. To measure progress (**Table 12.9**), goals, actions, and outcomes were revised and discussed. Progress toward Lucinda's personal goals was reviewed and the steps taken to move toward them were adjusted based on the clinical situation. For instance, Lucinda reentered the workplace in a restricted capacity much earlier than anticipated as her diabetes stabilized and toe ulcer started to heal. Lucinda and Ellen celebrated Lucinda's success. They

added the functional goal of increasing the number of times Lucinda left her house for social activities (i.e., making it to her son's soccer games, volunteering at school). Lucinda's goals remained primary and were Ellen's catalyst to improve the bigger picture (i.e., better health and function with reduced service use).

In addition to documenting and updating the IM-CAG and care plan measurement of progress, Ellen also recorded the level of global function (visual analogue scale and number of days of usual activity missed), clinical improvement (ulcer size, PHQ-9 score, HbA1c level [done every 3 months]), satisfaction, and quality of life (**Table 12.10**).

COMPOSITE ASSESSMENT OF THE CASE MANAGERS AND CASE MANAGEMENT

Ellen will not know for months what health service use outcomes the assistance she provided to Lucinda yielded. In fact, for Lucinda personally and for Ellen, total health care service use is not an issue unless it creates personal financial hardship (out-of-pocket expenses or cost of insurance premiums) or possibly leads to uninsurability for Lucinda in the future. On the other hand, it is of considerable import to purchasers of care (employers and government programs) and to health plans, such as the one for which Ellen works.

As a result, Ellen knows that her health plan has already established Lucinda's: (a) total health care costs, subdivided into medical service use, mental condition service use, and pharmacy use; (b) number of emergency room visits; (c) number of hospitalizations; and (d) number of days of hospitalization for the year preceding the date of entry into case management. During the next 2 years, the health plan will track Lucinda's and other case management participants' quarterly service use and total health care cost. These individuals will be compared to a similar population that is not exposed to case management. The financial outcome assessment will be coupled with global complexity, clinical, functional, quality of life, and satisfaction scores for patients who participate in the case management program to assess for Ellen's performance compared to the aggregate of case managed cases, each of the case managers, and the teams of case managers. Composite outcomes will also be evaluated in relation to as many measured outcomes as possible in a complex, but non-case managed, control group. Most of these comparisons will relate to claims since in few of these comparison patients will clinical, functional, satisfaction, and quality of life parameters be retrievable.

STEPS TO CASE GRADUATION

Case management graduation begins with the development of a relationship between Ellen and Lucinda

TABLE 12.8   Lucinda's IM-CAG (Week 6) Using Follow-up Scoring Rules for Historical Items

Week 6	HEALTH RISKS AND HEALTH NEEDS					
Lucinda	**HISTORICAL**		**CURRENT STATE**		**VULNERABILITY**	
Total Score = 21	Complexity Item	Score	Complexity Item	Score	Complexity Item	Score
Biological Domain	Chronicity HB1	2	Symptom Severity/Impairment CB1	2	Complications and Life Threat VB	2
	Diagnostic Dilemma HB2	0	Diagnostic/Therapeutic Challenge CB2	2		
Psychological Domain	Barriers to Coping HP1	1	Resistance to Treatment CP1	0	Mental Health Threat VP	1
	Mental Health History HP2	1	Mental Health Symptoms CP2	1		
Social Domain	Job and Leisure HS1	1	Residential Stability CS1	0	Social Vulnerability VS	1
	Relationships HS2	0	Social Support CS2	1		
Health System Domain	Access to Care HHS1	1	Getting Needed Services CHS1	0	Health System Impediments VHS	2
	Treatment Experience HHS2	2	Coordination of Care CHS2	1		

Comments	
HB1	Long history of diabetes with multiple chronic complications (6 weeks: re-education about diabetes and complications complete)
HB2	Easily recognized DM with complications
CB1	Eye, cardiovascular (CV), mental health (depression), renal, dermatologic, and neurological complications with HbA1c of 9.2 (6 weeks: diet, exercise, blood sugar diary being used; toes healing, surgery less likely; sugars and lipids improving; blood pressure controlled) significant personal and functional limitations (6 weeks: restricted work)
CB2	Not following treatments (6 weeks: medications reconciled and Lucinda taking; better control), untreated depression contributing to poorly controlled DM (6 weeks: understands link of depression to poor DM control)
VB	At risk for toe amputation and many other complications (6 weeks: coordination of care, adherence and communication among providers decreases risk), possible early death
HP1	Passive acceptance of health situation (6 weeks: Lucinda more assertive about clarifying health and treatment needs); history of substance abuse
HP2	Family and probable personal history of untreated depression; history of alcoholism in father, abuse in patient (6 weeks: understands vulnerability to mental health symptoms)
CP1	Skeptical about potential change success but willing to try, not taking most diabetic interventions (6 weeks: active participation in personal care, adherent; happy about improvement)
CP2	Moderate to severe untreated depressive symptoms with mild anxiety symptoms (6 weeks: depression improving with medication)
VP	Needs psychiatric assessment and treatment and assistance with pushing health system to stabilize (6 weeks: active psychiatrist involvement with intermittent assessments to handle treatment resistance)
HS1	Job waiting when healthy, on short-term disability for several months, risk of job loss, few social activities (6 weeks: working part time at desk job with foot elevated)
HS2	Good family ties, few nonfamily friends; no significant home problems
CS1	Owns home
CS2	Family readily helps when Lucinda is having difficulties (6 weeks: more independent)
VS	At risk for losing income and house if no improvement because of job loss, may need nursing care
HHS1	Poor mental health benefits in plan (6 weeks: flexed provider [out-of-network increased pay for non-face-to-face time with Lucinda] and medication benefits, Lucinda learning about limitations of benefits and options)
HHS2	Distrust of some doctors; no bad experiences other than apparent disinterest by doctors; frequent emergency room visits and admissions (6 weeks: one general practitioner [Dr. Sanchez] coordinates treatment)
CHS1	Medications and diabetic supplies too costly to buy; challenge to get to uncoordinated appointments; no mental health referral by primary physicians (6 weeks: flexed benefits make out-of-pocket expenses affordable; many fewer doctor appointments)
CHS2	Many meds and docs, frequent hospital and emergency room use, poor access to consistent follow-up (6 weeks: no emergency room visits or hospitalizations, communication through Dr. Sanchez with all providers)
VHS	Persistent problems anticipated without consistent and coordinated medical and mental health care (6 weeks: insurance support and single coordinating physician improves potential outcome)

TABLE 12.9   Lucinda's Measurement of Progress (Week 6 MP3)*

	GOAL	ACTION	OUTCOME
Barrier HHS2 and CHS2	• Stable and coordinated care	1. Assist in getting unique desired doctor 2. Help Lucinda establish plan for toe healing 3. Improve communication among providers	1. Dr. Sanchez designated primary physician 2. DIABETOLOGIST AND PODIATRIST GIVE DR. SANCHEZ AND LUCINDA WOUND HEALING PLAN; LUCINDA FOLLOWING IT
Barrier HS1	• Return to work	1. Help connect Lucinda with employee assistance program 2. Help Lucinda find out about light duty	1. APPOINTMENT MADE 2. JOB DESCRIPTION RECEIVED 3. LIGHT DUTY AVAILABLE 4. BACK TO WORK PART TIME
Barrier HB1, CB1, CB2, CP2, and VB	• Illness understanding; participation in personal health • Coordinated diabetes and depression treatment	1. Send materials on diabetes and depression 2. Discuss educational materials 3. Review and flex Lucinda's insurance benefits 4. Help Lucinda make appointment with psychiatrist 5. Medical director to connect Dr. Sanchez and psychiatrist	1. Glucose diary, diet, care of toe ulcer; depression treatment started, PHQ-9 score 12 2. One general practitioner understands Lucinda's problems (paid for time of case review) 3. Lucinda refused cognitive behavioral therapy, started on citalopram, understands depression/DM connection
Barrier HHS1, CHS1, and VHS	• Insurance that meets health needs; • Able to pay for services	1. Review insurance contract 2. Discuss flexing benefits with employer 3. Get payment for out-of-network provider and adequately for Dr. Sanchez	1. Lucinda understands insurance benefit limits 2. Medications changed to generic or formulary expanded to cover needed meds 3. One prescriber (Dr. Sanchez) with risk-based payment bonus
Barrier CB1, CB2, CP1, and VB	• Control of symptoms • Getting needed services	1. Review medications in Lucinda's medicine cabinet 2. Have Lucinda review med list with Dr. Sanchez 3. Coordinate primary care, specialists, and psychiatrist visits 4. Connect office visit notes	1. Discarded 17 pill bottles after review with general practitioner, reduced monthly cost of meds by $235, currently one office visit/week, no emergency room visits 2. Sugar range: 75 to 315, usual 185 3. DIAMETER 1.0 CM, DEPTH 0.2 CM; CLEAN AND NON-INFLAMED

*Actions directly linked to Lucinda's personal goals are in small caps.

on day one. Through numerous initial calls with Lucinda, her family, and her providers, Lucinda and those important in her care should come to understand her illnesses, how they interact, *and* the things that can be done to reverse her downward spiral. Using the IM-CAG as a guide, it becomes easier to understand the components contributing barriers to improvement and to communicate the steps that can be taken to reverse them. Ellen's initial focus was on Lucinda's hot spots.

Ellen helped Lucinda coordinate the efforts of multiple physicians who rarely talked with each other and often did not even understand what treatment Lucinda was receiving (barriers related to CHS1, CHS2, and HHS2). Through collaboration with Lucinda and the one physician that Lucinda liked, Ellen essentially created a medical home for Lucinda with a central point of care. She also connected practitioners through

shared notes and summaries. In addition, she assisted Lucinda in coordinating visits and services.

Saving Lucinda's toe was identified as a major goal; however, it only represented the degree to which Lucinda's diabetes was out of control (barriers related to HB1, HB2, CB1, CB2, HP2, and CHS2). Through addressing her concerns about her toe, it was possible for Ellen to help Lucinda see and connect diabetic complications with diet, exercise, and taking medications. Adding a podiatrist helped ensure that Lucinda's primary clinical goal was met, but it was only a small part of the total effort on the way to graduation.

Before Ellen became involved, no one had asked Lucinda about depression, even though several considered that it might be contributing to the poor outcomes that she was experiencing. It was necessary for Ellen to talk with Lucinda, Lucinda's family, and

TABLE 12.10	Lucinda's Record of Outcome Measures (Week 6 ROM)				
OUTCOME MEASURES		**BASELINE**	**FOLLOW-UP ASSESSMENTS**		
	Time period recorded	*Interim*	*Week 6*		
Clinical measure (personal goal) *Heal toe ulcer without surgery*		*1.3 cm diameter; 0.2 cm deep*	*1.0 cm diameter; 0.2 cm deep*		
Functional measure (personal goal) *Return to work*		*Full short-term disability*	*Works part-time*		
Health-related quality of life *Number of days healthy/month*		*0*	*8*		
Patient satisfaction *(Scale: 0 low, 10 high)*		*5*	*8*		
CAG Score *(Total for period)*		*38*	*21*		
Health care clinical measure *HbA1c*		*9.2*			
Health care clinical measure *PHQ-9*		*19*	*12*		
Health care functional measure *Level of function (scale 0–10)*		*3*	*6*		
Health care functional measure *Number of work days lost/23 days*		*23*	*10; 4 hrs/day*		
Health care economic measure *Number of emergency room visits in the last 30 days*		*3*	*0*		

Dr. Sanchez (through the health plan medical director) to discuss and explain the rationale for including depression treatment in the overall plan.

With Ellen's help, Dr. Sanchez learned how to find and work with a psychiatrist in dosing antidepressant medication, how to decrease Lucinda's and her family's resistance to depression treatment, and how to follow her through to resolution of symptoms. At graduation, not only was Lucinda's diabetes better, she also felt better about herself and the future. Graduation, in fact, took a positive spin. She knew better what she needed to do and had the energy to do it when Ellen moved on to assist other patients.

Through the treatment provided to address her toe ulcer, Lucinda also learned the importance of adherence to treatment and diabetic control, including both testing her blood sugar with finger pricks and monitoring her HbA1c's; learned how to keep a medication, diet, and sugar diary; and came to understand the guidelines for complication prophylaxis. Family members were enlisted to help, including Lucinda's children, so that they would be a support to their mother, who could now do more with them. Lucinda also learned how to save money on medications by using less expensive brands. Plus, she was making more money since she was back to work.

At the core of Ellen's initial activities was education about diabetes and depression. Lucinda read nothing of the materials that were sent to her. The fact that she had the pamphlets that were sent, however, allowed Lucinda and Ellen to spend time on the phone building a relationship while learning about the things that would make her better. Never did Lucinda feel that Ellen was mad at her for not reading the materials. Long ago, Ellen learned that sent materials were rarely read.

In traditional case management programs, the primary and often the only goals are clinical improvement. Integrated case management, using IM-CAG methodology, recognizes that health is connected to function. Unless Lucinda was able to resume doing the things that she liked and the things that made her life more stable (e.g., work or participation in family activities) health was unidimensional. Right from the beginning, Lucinda worked with Ellen to achieve both clinical and functional goals. Of course, Lucinda picked a functional goal that was consistent with one her employer would want (i.e., returning to work). Even if she had not done so, encouraging a patient to return to social functioning usually contributes to the potential for that patient to regain her work productivity. The fact that Lucinda owned the goal made working toward it a lighter burden. In the process, she learned how employee assistance could be helpful and that a light duty transition back to work made it easier.

Finally, integrated case management allows measurement of outcomes (**Table 12.11**). Lucinda and Lucinda's providers could measure Lucinda's progress concretely with the help of Ellen. This provided a sense of accomplishment and recognition that Lucinda and her doctors were reaching a point where they could take it from here.

During the process, Lucinda learned about how to make sure that her doctors talked with each other, how to access community resources, and how to follow through on preventive diabetic care, including for her eyes, kidneys, nerves, and heart. The 3-month IM-CAG (**Table 12.12**, see page i9 for color version) and the record of outcome measures made it apparent that it was time for Lucinda and her doctors to take over her care.

Ellen consolidates and summarizes Lucinda's education and the approaches that has been taken to address her behaviors and illnesses. She congratulates Lucinda on the degree to which she has taken over her self-care (i.e., medication monitoring, diaries, appointment making and coordinating, formulating questions for doctor, and personal care of diabetic complications). Further, Lucinda's doctor and family, with Lucinda's permission, were filled in on the progress that Lucinda had made and what steps could be considered for the future.

At graduation, Lucinda and her active providers received a copy of the initial and final IM-CAG, the care plan measurement of progress, the record of outcome measures, and a summary of anticipated future needs, which had previously been agreed on with Lucinda. Ellen thanked Lucinda for being such a good sport and a hard worker. She noted that it was a pleasure to work with her. Finally, Ellen gave Lucinda her office phone number and e-mail address in case she wanted to touch base. She wished her God's speed.

TABLE 12.11   Lucinda's Record of Outcome Measures (Week 12 ROM)

OUTCOME MEASURES	BASELINE	FOLLOW-UP ASSESSMENTS		
Time period recorded	*Interim*	*Week 6*	*Week 8*	*Week 12*
Clinical measure (personal goal) *Heal toe ulcer without surgery*	*1.3 cm diameter; 0.2 cm deep*	*1.0 cm diameter; 0.2 cm deep*	*0.5 cm diameter; surface*	*Closed*
Functional measure (personal goal) *Return to work*	*Full short-term disability*	*Works part-time*	*Full days, restrictions*	*Full days, No restrictions*
Health-related quality of life *Number of healthy days/month*	*0*	*8*		*23*
Patient satisfaction *(Scale: 0 low, 10 high)*	*5*	*8*	*8*	*9*
CAG score *(Total for period)*	*38*	*21*		*15*
Health care clinical measure *HbA1c*	*9.2*			*7.8*
Health care clinical measure *PHQ-9*	*19*	*12*	*10*	*9*
Health care functional measure *Level of function (scale 0–10)*	*3*	*6*	*7*	*9*
Health care functional measure *Number of work days lost/23 days*	*23*	*10; 4 hrs/day*	*5; 8 hrs/day*	*0*
Health care economic measure *Number of emergency room visits in the last 30 days*	*3*	*0*	*0*	*0*
Health care economic measure *(annual cost of care)*	*$67,577*			

TABLE 12.12   Lucinda's Graduation IM-CAG (Week 12)

Week 12	HEALTH RISKS AND HEALTH NEEDS					
Lucinda	HISTORICAL		CURRENT STATE		VULNERABILITY	
Total Score = 15	Complexity Item	Score	Complexity Item	Score	Complexity Item	Score
Biological Domain	Chronicity **HB1**	2	Symptom Severity/Impairment **CB1**	1	Complications and Life Threat **VB**	1
	Diagnostic Dilemma **HB2**	0	Diagnostic/Therapeutic Challenge **CB2**	2		
Psychological Domain	Barriers to Coping **HP1**	1	Resistance to Treatment **CP1**	0	Mental Health Threat **VP**	0
	Mental Health History **HP2**	1	Mental Health Symptoms **CP2**	0		
Social Domain	Job and Leisure **HS1**	1	Residential Stability **CS1**	0	Social Vulnerability **VS**	1
	Relationships **HS2**	0	Social Support **CS2**	1		
Health System Domain	Access to Care **HHS1**	1	Getting Needed Services **CHS1**	0	Health System Impediments **VHS**	1
	Treatment Experience **HHS2**	2	Coordination of Care **CHS2**	0		

	Comments
HB1	Long history of diabetes with multiple chronic complications (6 weeks: re-education about diabetes and complications complete)
HB2	Easily recognized DM with complications
CB1	Eye, cardiovascular (CV), mental health (depression), renal, dermatologic, and neurological complications with HbA1c of 9.2 (6 weeks: diet, exercise, blood sugar diary being used; toes healing, surgery less likely; sugars and lipids improving; blood pressure controlled; 12 weeks: toe ulcer healed, sugars and lipids controlled); significant personal and functional limitations (6 weeks: restricted work; 12 weeks: doing things with family, full work)
CB2	Not following treatments (6 weeks: medications reconciled and Lucinda taking; better control), untreated depression contributing to poorly controlled DM (6 weeks: understands link of depression to poor DM control)
VB	At risk for toe amputation and many other complications (6 weeks: coordination of care, adherence and communication among providers decreases risk), possible early death (12 weeks: consistent treatment and adherence anticipated)
HP1	Passive acceptance of health situation (6 weeks: Lucinda more assertive about clarifying health and treatment needs); history of substance abuse
HP2	Family and probable personal history of untreated depression; history of alcoholism in father, abuse in patient (6 weeks: understands vulnerability to mental health symptoms)
CP1	Skeptical about potential change success but willing to try, not taking most diabetic interventions (6 weeks: active participation in personal care, adherent; happy about improvement)
CP2	Moderate to severe untreated depressive symptoms with mild anxiety symptoms (6 weeks: depression improving with medication; 12 weeks: depressive symptoms essentially gone, on medication)
VP	Needs psychiatric assessment and treatment and assistance with pushing health system to stabilize (6 weeks: active psychiatrist involvement with intermittent assessments to handle treatment resistance; 12 weeks: recognizes need to stay on medication, watching weight)
HS1	Job waiting when healthy, on short-term disability for several months, risk of job loss, few social activities (6 weeks: working part time at desk job with foot elevated; 12 weeks: back to work without restrictions, doing things with family)
HS2	Good family ties, few nonfamily friends; no significant home problems
CS1	Owns home
CS2	Family readily helps when Lucinda is having difficulties (6 weeks: more independent)
VS	At risk for losing income and house if no improvement because of job loss, may need nursing care
HHS1	Poor mental health benefits in plan (6 weeks: flexed provider [out of network increased pay for non-face-to-face time with Lucinda] and medication benefits, Lucinda learning about limitations of benefits and options; 12 weeks: considering different insurance benefits next year with better mental health coverage)
HHS2	Distrust of some doctors; no bad experiences other than apparent disinterest by doctors; frequent emergency room visits and admissions (6 weeks: one general practitioner [Dr. Sanchez] coordinates treatment)
CHS1	Medications and diabetic supplies too costly to buy; challenge to get to uncoordinated appointments; no mental health referral by primary physicians (6 weeks: flexed benefits makes out-of-pocket expenses affordable; many fewer doctor appointments)

(Continued)

TABLE 12.12	Lucinda's Graduation IM-CAG (Week 12) *(Continued)*
CHS2	*Many meds and docs, frequent hospital and emergency room use, poor access to consistent follow-up (6 weeks: no emergency room visits or hospitalizations, communication through Dr. Sanchez with all providers; 12 weeks: full communication among a limited number of doctors, no emergency room use or hospitalizations)*
VHS	*Persistent problems anticipated without consistent and coordinated medical and mental health care (6 weeks: insurance support and single coordinating physician improves potential outcome; 12 weeks: low risk for problems but still has a significant number of chronic illnesses)*

CHAPTER 13

Assisting Robert: Disabled Employee With Chronic Lung Disease, Panic Attacks, and Alcohol Abuse

OBJECTIVES

- To augment case management skills using complexity assessment and integrated care plan techniques for an employee of a large manufacturer
- To uncover health complexity and reverse its impact on workplace absence and productivity
- To coordinate health improvement with workplace reentry and improved social support

ROBERT'S STORY

Robert is a 49-year-old electrician for a large manufacturer who has been identified through the employer's disability management report. The disability management company at Robert's worksite notes that he has been on short-term disability for 4 months and would be a candidate for long-term disability soon. Robert's disability manager, Charlene, is concerned that if Robert is placed on long-term disability, which has more rigorous definitions of what constitutes disability, he will not remain qualified for disability support. Robert would then find it difficult to obtain alternative employment because of his health history. Charlene indicates to her supervisor that Robert has been seen in the emergency room five times in the last 2 months and has been in contact with his personal doctor twice monthly. He is on five medications, all prescribed by his general practitioner, Dr. Couch, who, as a retired surgeon, is supplementing his income doing general practice during a challenging economy.

In addition to chronic lung disease, Robert has a long history of anxiety with panic attacks. There is, however, no mental health professional involved in his care. Since the company's contracting health plan changed 3 years earlier, Robert has been forced to see Dr. Couch because his old primary care doctor was not in the new health plan network. Dr. Couch is. For three years, Robert's work performance record has deteriorated. Disability and family leave time tracking indicate that he has taken time off for breathing problems, chest pain, back pain, headaches, anxiety, and flu-like episodes. This is, however, the first extended leave that he has taken. Dr. Couch, who signs Robert's disability forms, projects that he will be permanently disabled according to a discussion he has had with the disability plan's medical director.

Since his early 20s, Robert has been treated for anxiety disorder with panic attacks, a condition that runs in his family, but has stopped going to a therapist or psychiatrist because he can save out-of-pocket expenses by getting all of his care from Dr. Couch. Robert's last admission of 2 days was 6 months earlier for chest pain. At that time, oxygen saturation was 91% and FEV1 was 58% of predicted. Despite a normal heart tracing and little other evidence of a cardiac origin for his chest pain, Robert refused to leave the emergency room because he thought he was going to die. He smokes two packs of cigarettes per day.

A TRIGGERED CASE

Robert has been identified as a candidate for case management since he triggered numerous items on the disability company's red flag system. He has concurrent physical and mental health difficulties for which he receives no mental health services. Robert is, however, consuming many medical services. He has been hospitalized in the last 6 months and has been seen in the emergency room at least two or more times each month for the past several months. Though his treatment is with a single physician, he is on numerous and changing medications. None are being taken regularly for anxiety despite notation of symptoms in emergency room discharge reports. Charlene, Robert's disability manager, asks if Robert would be willing to work with a health specialist associated with his insurance company who could, perhaps, help him get better control of his health and hopefully back to work. Robert agrees.

TRIAGE: ENROLLMENT SPECIALIST INTERACTION

Robert does not answer the phone to talk with the case management enrollment specialist two times before she finally connects. He states that he was afraid it was his boss wanting him to return to work. Robert likes his job and wants to work, but he says, "I just couldn't." When he went to work before, he was afraid he would have a "breathing spell," make a mistake, and possibly hurt himself or someone else. Since he is an electrician, this is a real possibility. He has been on short-term disability for the past 4 months. Robert will go on long-term disability in a couple of months. His income would drop in half when this occurs and his job with his current employer will no longer be guaranteed should he improve and wish to return. At age 49, he does not want to stop working. Robert was good at what he did. The workplace was also his social outlet and the area of his life that made him feel good about himself.

Robert notes that his breathing and anxiety symptoms had been in good control before he started care with Dr. Couch. According to Dr. Couch, Robert does not need mental health services. Dr. Couch considers chronic bronchitis the main reason for Robert's being unable to work.

Robert had a good work history up to 3 years ago and wants to change his current condition (Appendix B, "Readiness for Change Scale," 11 on a scale of 10, see www.springerpub.com/kathol) but has little confidence in being able to do so (Appendix B, "Readiness for Change Scale," 3 on a scale of 10). He

also does not know where to start. Robert has never been in case management before; has a telephone, which he indicates he would answer if someone can really help him; and has health conditions that are reversible and have been controlled in the past. This identified him as a high-priority candidate for case management.

During the past several years, Robert has noted a dramatic increase in his out-of-pocket expenses for health services, including emergency room visits, medications, tests, and short hospitalizations. Last year, he breezed through his $4,000 high deductibles by mid-March. Luckily, the company's insurance covered most expensive health events, such as emergency room visits, ambulance costs, and inpatient stays, after he reached his deduction limits. This year Robert reached his $4,500 deduction limits in February and has used over $55,000 in health benefits. Not only are his health problems high cost because of medical expenses, he has also been absent from work at least a third of the year. Lost productivity and disability costs are also adding up. His composite picture stratifies him into Level IV for consideration of case management. He is a highly complex patient.

The enrollment specialist obtains the necessary permissions and then transfers Robert to a case manager, Martin, who is free to add a case. She wants to make sure that the connection with Martin is made immediately because Robert has been difficult to get a hold of during the triage process.

INITIAL CONTACT WITH THE CASE MANAGER

The enrollment specialist fills in Martin briefly about the issues that Robert is having and his current health challenges. In addition to connecting Robert to Martin, the enrollment specialist forwards claims data, to which she has access, for Martin to review. She also sends the disability notes from Charlene. While Martin glances at the claims material and notes during the initial discussion, he does not spend much time on them because he wants to make sure that he connects with Robert.

Martin starts his interview by summarizing the case management program and answering Robert's questions. He gives a bit about his background and tells Robert how the program works. In short, Martin helps patients who have complicated problems, not just with their medical treatment but also with anything that makes it difficult for them to regain health, including insurance, finances, transportation, and doctor issues. Robert confirms that he understands and is willing to proceed. He says that he has a little time but has already been on the phone for 15 minutes.

Martin summarizes what he has heard from the enrollment specialist about Robert's difficulties with breathing problems, chest pain, and other health complaints. He also mentions Robert's prior treatment for anxiety. Robert confirms these problems and adds that his health has worsened during the last year. He is at the end of his rope but does not know what to do.

Martin assures Robert that he thinks that he can help but wants some time to go through records of Robert's care before he starts what Martin called a "complexity assessment." Further, Martin wants to set up a call when he and Robert will have enough time to go through all the details about Robert's health problems. Martin says that this usually takes about an hour to complete and can be done over the phone. Robert and Martin agree on a telephone appointment two days later.

INITIAL INTERVIEW

Martin calls Robert at the chosen time. Robert has some additional questions for Martin about how his working with Robert will affect Robert's disability, how long they will be working together, and why Robert has been chosen to be managed. Martin has already answered some of these same questions during the opening call but reinforces his prior answers. He encourages Robert to talk with Charlene regarding Robert's concerns related to his disability rights. Martin indicates that he does not have anything to do with Robert's employment or his employer. Martin's focus will be on helping Robert improve his health and, if possible, get back to work. Martin mainly works with disability managers, such as Charlene, when the people he helps got to the point that they were ready for work reentry. Sometimes it is helpful to work with the disability manager in finding out about whether the worksite can accommodate work restrictions.

When Robert's questions have been answered, Martin indicates to Robert that he will be going into detail about Robert's health problems during his assessment but that he wants to get to know about Robert first. He asks if it is okay to wait to ask more questions about Robert's illness until he knows a bit more about Robert and his living situation. Robert says okay. As Martin asks questions, he takes notes in the updated case management software.

Martin uses a copy of the standard assessment questions open in a separate window on his computer to help him progress through the interview with Robert (see Appendix E, see www.springerpub.com/kathol). A blank adult CAG scoring sheet (see Appendix 4) is open on the main screen, which has automatic pop-ups for the adult anchor points, the ability to score each CAG item as it is being discussed, and a note documentation section that can be edited and used to communicate the findings and rationale related to complexity items with Robert. While the following questions are organized so that all areas needed for a complexity assessment will be covered, Martin feels no need to follow them closely. He has learned long ago that pertinent information spontaneously comes out at various points in each interview. It is more important to let the conversation itself partially direct which questions need to be asked and which do not.

QUESTION 1: *"Can you tell me about yourself, e.g., where you live, who you live with, how you spend your days, what your hobbies and interests are?"*

FOLLOW-UP QUESTIONS

Martin can fill these in later if there is reticence for Robert to divulge personal information at this point.

1.1 "What kind of job do you have?"
1.2 "Can you tell me about your financial situation/pressures?"
1.3 "Do you require assistance in getting out of the house?"
1.4 "Who helps you when a crisis arises?"
1.5 "Who are your friends?"
1.6 "How do you spend your free time?"
1.7 "Do you help take care of others, i.e., family, a friend?"

Notes

- High school education with electrician technical school and nearly 25 years of experience as an electrician with the same company
- Is a good electrician with many years experience, but it is "unsafe" to do the job with his current symptoms, that is why he has been on short-term disability for the last 4 months
- Bad divorce 12 years ago, now little social support since parents are dead, siblings live in other states, and few friends
- About twice a year, sees his two children (a 15-year-old and an 18-year-old) who live in another city with his wife (who has remarried), misses seeing his children, up-to-date on alimony
- Fewer visits to kids, church, sports events in the past two years because it is too much trouble and there are few people to go with him, plus he gets "panicky" in crowds
- No hobbies or activities
- Used to go to church (Lutheran), but no longer attends

- Over 100 pack/year history, currently smoking 2 packs a day
- Living alone in an apartment; no relatives or friends rely on him for help; "sort of a loner"
- Worried about losing job but gets panicky every time he goes to work, which is unsafe with the kind of work he does
- No need for assistance with activities of daily living
- Does not have much help when health problems happen, so he goes to the emergency room
- Spends his free days in a sports bar with friends and is an avid football and basketball fan; has rarely done this in the past 2 months
- He and other family members have had trouble with anxiety and depression for years but treatment has only been marginally effective (according to him)
- Does not like Dr. Couch but does not feel he has much choice because of his company's insurance change and a new doctor network; costs for out-of-network doctor, and especially a psychiatrist, are exorbitant on his salary; at least he can get in to see Dr. Couch
- Used to like model airplanes but has not done this for years

QUESTION 2: *("Robert, you were referred to me because you have had a lot of problems going to work due to your breathing problems. Can you tell me about your breathing and how it is affecting your life?")*

FOLLOW-UP QUESTIONS
2.1 "Have you had (other) physical problems or long-term conditions or illnesses?"
2.2 "Were these difficult to diagnose?"
2.3 "Are medical assessments underway?"
2.4 "What kind of treatments have you received?"
2.5 "Have you had difficulty following through on recommended physical health treatments?"
2.6 "How have the treatments worked?"
2.7 "Do physical symptoms interfere with doing the things you like to do?"

Notes
- *Chronic bronchitis:* has been coming on for years and now causes shortness of breath and coughing, especially when he gets a cold; smoking seems to "help" but has been told he needs to stop smoking (Dr. Couch has not talked about smoking with him); treatment with bronchodilators (terbutaline, Atrovent, theophylline); intermittent antibiotics (tetracycline, others in medicine cabinet); never steroids; spirometry (FEV1s 50% to 65% of predicted) and oxygen saturation (91% to 93%) when in emergency room in past 6 months (luckily Robert had been keeping his emergency visit summaries and had this information); never used O_2 at home though came close after hospitalization a year and a half ago
- *Chest pain:* comes on over 15 to 20 minutes, is sharp, and goes away slowly; his dad died of a heart attack; doctors have given him nitroglycerin tablets "just in case" (rare; gets headache); more often treated with diazepam when in the emergency room with a small prescription for use after discharge; heart tracings (electrocardiograms) all normal
- *Hyperlipidemia:* diet, exercise (none), statin (last cholesterol high; high-density [good] lipids low)
- *Headache:* when he has too much to drink, which is about 2 to 3 times a week (to excess by his report); at least 2 to 3 drinks every day; more than 20 for a week; anti-inflammatory agents, such as ibuprofen
- *Other:*
  □ Back pain: occasional problem when he doesn't watch what he picks up; anti-inflammatory agents, such as ibuprophen; chiropractic manipulation and acupuncture; not much problem now that he is not working
- *Treatment adherence:*
  □ Occasional missed medications: does not think he needs them when symptoms not present; too expensive
  □ Occasional missed doctor's visits: limited value of visits to Dr. Couch (mainly to get disability forms signed and medication refills)
  □ Preventive measures: not asked to stop smoking (may not be able to anyhow); not counseled about at-risk drinking; not asked about diet and exercise
- *Effect on life:* high medical service use with occasional hospitalizations; essentially home bound though gets out to shop; buys pre-prepared foods; doesn't do yard work or other maintenance tasks; *forced* by company to go on short-term disability because they were afraid that he would hurt himself or others when working with "hot" wires; often on ladders and is worried about falling if he has one of his breathing or anxiety spells. Though many episodes at work are like his old anxiety attacks, when he is in the painting section of the company, he predictably develops wheezing and has to leave.
- Anxiety makes breathing worse since he gets a feeling that he will die; this causes him to go to the emergency room; most of the time Robert gets antibiotics and breathing treatments (inhalers) at the emergency room and then is sent home; this scares him a lot and he becomes panicky
- "Panicky" means attacks where he feels out of control, can't catch his breath, and feels like he could black out, lose his balance, or lose coordination (can't do electrical job with these symptoms)

- Scheduled appointments with Dr. Couch are 4 months apart but he has numerous unscheduled visits
- Says that Dr. Couch has little understanding of his anxiety symptoms when he has breathing problems or chest pain

Overall, Robert's main problem is ostensibly chronic lung disease with frequent episodes of chest pain, but this is made incapacitating by his anxiety. Other potential problems include substance abuse (at least at-risk drinking; see Chapter 6 section "Summary of Alcohol Abuse and Dependence") and back pathology. Depression needs to be excluded.

QUESTIONS 3: (*"Robert, you have mentioned several times that you have difficulty with anxiety. Can you tell me how this started and how it affects your life?"*)

FOLLOW-UP QUESTIONS

3.1 "Has your physical health situation affected your emotions?"

3.2 "Have you had mental health problems in the past?"

3.3 "Have mental health issues required treatment or hospitalization, such as for depression, anxiety, confusion, memory problems?"

3.4 "What kinds of treatments have you received and from whom?"

3.5 "Have you had difficulty in following through on mental health treatments?"

3.6 "Are you getting any treatment now?"

3.7 "Has treatment been helpful?"

3.8 "Do emotional factors interfere with doing the things you like to do?"

Notes

- Anxiety: "comes out of the blue"—for example, he can't go to sporting events because he gets anxious in crowds, becomes short of breath, dizzy, and weak. Once, a buddy had to take him home. Also happened at work.
  - Treatment: intermittent diazepam (uncommon since Dr. Couch does not like to use it; uses alcohol as a replacement)
  - Alcohol seems to help but it also makes Robert sleepy
- Anxiety was treated and controlled with scheduled doses of medication for 25 years but only sporadically for the last 3 years by Dr. Couch; no history of psychotherapy or psychiatric hospitalization
- Dr. Couch studiously avoids discussion about anxiety or other mental health or substance abuse issues

- At-risk alcohol use: never treated, never talked with Dr. Couch about it
- Treated for depression 5 years ago
- Patient Health Questionnaire-2 (PHQ-2) score was 1 of 2 (loss in interest in going to work but still interested in doing things with friends); PHQ-9 was completed (see **Exhibit 13.1**) and found to be 9 (mild depression)
- Generalized Anxiety Disorder-7 (GAD-7) score was 19 with panic attacks and severe agoraphobia (see **Table 13.1**)

QUESTION 4: *"Can you tell me about Dr. Couch and others that are involved in your care, including emergency room doctors, chiropractors, counselors, etc.?"*

FOLLOW-UP QUESTIONS

4.1 "Primary care physician/nurse practitioner?"

4.2 "Medical specialists?"

4.3 "Mental health providers, e.g., psychiatrists, psychologists, social workers, nurses, etc.?"

4.4 "Other providers, e.g., chiropractors, naturopath, church counselor, etc.?"

4.5 "Can you tell me how you get along with your doctors?"

4.6 "How do those giving you care talk with each other and coordinate your treatment?"

4.7 "Do you have difficulty communicating with them?"

4.8 "Are their offices near each other and easy to get to?"

4.9 "Have you had conflicts or disagreements with any of your doctors/providers, your hospital/clinic, or your insurance company that have led to bad feelings or mistrust?"

Much has already been said about Dr. Couch but Robert fills in a number of other important items related to his care.

Notes

- Likes some of the emergency room doctors better than Dr. Couch, but Dr. Couch does not like them. Dr. Couch discontinues the treatments that emergency doctors recommend, such as fluoxetine for anxiety.
- Breathing treatment by Dr. Couch regimented to medications he likes. Dr. Couch ignores anxiety.
- Dr. Couch does not:
  - Take any time to talk with Robert other than about breathing problems
  - Refer him to other doctors
  - Believe in psychiatric illness; feels that mental health treatment, whether with medication or talk therapy, is both unnecessary and ineffective
  - Dislikes diazepam because of dependency and addiction concerns

EXHIBIT 13.1   Robert's Depression Symptoms Evaluation (Baseline)

The following are Robert's responses to the depression symptom evaluation questionnaire:
Over the last 2 weeks, how often have you been bothered by any of the following problems?

Response Key: Not at all = 0 Several days = 1 More than half the days = 2 Nearly every day = 3

1.	Little interest or pleasure in doing things	2
2.	Feeling down, depressed, or hopeless	0
3.	Trouble falling/staying asleep, or sleeping too much	0
4.	Feeling tired or having little energy	1
5.	Poor appetite or overeating	0
6.	Feeling bad about yourself, feeling that you are a failure, or feeling that you have let yourself or your family down	3
7.	Trouble concentrating on things, such as reading the newspaper or watching television	1
8.	Moving or speaking so slowly that other people could have noticed, or being so fidgety or restless that you have been moving around a lot more than usual	2
9.	Thinking that you would be better off dead or that you want to hurt yourself in some way	0
	Total Score for 1 to 9:	9

Scoring Key for PHQ-9: Minimal < 5; Mild 5–9; Moderate 10–14; Moderately severe 15–19; Severe > 19

Impairment: If you checked off any problem on this questionnaire so far, how difficult have these problems made it for you to do your work, take care of things at home, or get along with other people?   1

Response Key for Impairment Question: Not Difficult at All = 0; Somewhat Difficult = 1; Very Difficult = 2; Extremely Difficult = 3

TABLE 13.1   Robert's Anxiety Symptoms Evaluation (Baseline)

Over the last 2 weeks, how often have you been bothered by the following problems?	Not at all sure (Mark 0)	Several days (Mark 1)	Over half the days (Mark 2)	Nearly every day (Mark 3)
Feeling nervous, anxious, or on edge				3
Not being able to stop or control worrying				3
Worrying too much about different things				3
Trouble relaxing				3
Being so restless that it's hard to sit still			2	
Becoming easily annoyed or irritable			2	
Feeling afraid as if something awful might happen				3
Add the score for each column	0	0	4	15
Total Score (add column scores)[a]		19		

If you marked any problems, how difficult have these problems made it for you to do your work, take care of things at home, or get along with other people?

Not difficult at all	Somewhat difficult	Very difficult	Extremely difficult (Robert's response)

[a]*For case management purposes, use total scores of 10 and above as significant levels of anxiety.*

- Occasional chiropractor for back pain but no other providers than emergency room and inpatient doctors
- Dr. Couch does not get emergency room notes because his office is not connected to the hospital and he does not have privileges. He gets information about the emergency room visits from Robert, but Robert only tells Dr. Couch about some of them (e.g., when he needs disability papers filled out). Dr. Couch does not take calls after five in the afternoon.
- Robert would like to change from Dr. Couch but cannot afford it. Further, Dr. Couch's office is just down the street from his house.

Martin gets the distinct impression that Dr. Couch has not been good for Robert. While Robert describes no direct conflicts with Dr. Couch, it is apparent that Robert has little trust in what Dr. Couch does for him. Robert, however, has not taken steps to change.

Dr. Couch is biased against mental health problems and their treatment, which has limited Robert's access to treatments that have been shown effective for Robert's anxiety in the past. The situation, however, is complicated because the anxiety could also be related to alcohol withdrawal or drug seeking. There appears to be an alcohol problem, which was uncovered during discussion about Robert's headaches. Martin will discuss this with Robert in greater detail later.

QUESTION 5: *"Can you tell me about the insurance change that took place 3 years ago? It sounds like this really made it difficult to continue with your old doctors."*

FOLLOW-UP QUESTIONS
5.1 "What type of medical insurance do you have and does it cover the services you need?"
5.2 "Do you have trouble finding medical doctors who will accept you as a patient?"
5.3 "Do you need to go to separate clinics for mental health treatment?"
5.4 "Are there separate payment rules for mental health care?"
5.5 "Have you or your primary care physician had difficulty in finding a mental health provider for you?"
5.6 "How far do you live from the medical clinics and doctors you need to improve (control) your health?"
5.7 "Do you need a translator or someone from your culture to assist with health needs?"
5.8 "Can you afford your medical care, i.e., medications, needed tests, copays for appointments and hospital costs, needed medical equipment/devices, etc.?"
5.9 "Is transportation a problem in getting to your appointments?"
5.10 "Are there long waiting lists for the kind of care you need?"

Notes
- Problems began when Robert was forced to change his doctor 3 years ago because of a change in the health plan through which his company bought insurance.
  □ Limited in-network group of doctors with higher copay for out-of-network services (Robert's old doctor not part of new network).
  □ Robert thinks that mental health and substance abuse coverage is excluded. Independent high-cost mental health coverage could be purchased through several separate insurance companies recommended by the medical health plan (not by Robert's employer).
  □ High deductible plans (early and large out-of-pocket expenses amounting to $4,000 last year and $4,500 this year) in addition to premium, but still limited coverage for medication costs even after maximum deductible reached.
  □ Emergency room and inpatient coverage nearly 100% after maximum deductible has been reached (March last year; February this year).
- Robert worked well with his old doctor who collaborated with a psychiatrist to keep his anxiety under control. This is no longer possible.
- No trouble with transportation to and from clinic visits. Occasionally uses ambulance for emergency room visits.
- Medication recommendations are all mixed up since many come from the emergency room doctors, who focus on the "admission/no admission" question. When admission is unnecessary as is often the case, then target symptoms are treated but the need for long-term anxiety treatment is ignored.
- If Robert wants to get mental health care, he is on his own to find it as far as Dr. Couch is concerned.

QUESTION 6: *"What kind of person are you, e.g., outgoing, suspicious, tense, optimistic?"*

FOLLOW-UP QUESTIONS
6.1 "Do you smoke?"
6.2 "On average, how many alcoholic beverages do you drink a day (week), e.g., glasses of wine, beers, etc.?
6.3 "Do you use painkillers: how often, how long, more often than prescribed?
6.4 "Do you use cocaine, marijuana, or other recreational drugs?"
6.5 "Have you ever been treated for substance abuse problems?"
6.6 "How do you handle difficult situations?" (alcohol or drug use, talkative, silent, procrastinate?)
6.7 "What are your biggest health concerns at this time?"

6.8 "During the next 1 to 3 months, what about your health would you like to have under better control (clinical), e.g., have less foot pain, have no asthma attacks for a solid month, etc.?"

6.9 "What would you like to be able to do that you can't do now (functional), e.g., attend church regularly, participate in family events, return to work, etc.?"

During the discussion with Robert, Martin is convinced that Robert feels defeated and does not know how to get out of his dilemma. Robert anticipates that he will go on long-term disability in the next several months and that he will receive disability thereafter. He has not thought through how he would support himself on half his current salary, how he will get insurance once his current job is terminated, and what will be needed to remain on disability roles. He is worried about breaking the relationship with Dr. Couch since he has always been supportive in filling out disability claims, something that emergency room doctors refuse to do.

Dr. Couch has also apparently not given much thought to Robert's future since he readily approves Robert for continued short-term disability. He does little to document objective medical evidence or psychiatric symptoms that would support it, and his clinic notes are skimpy. Robert clearly has lung disease but physiologic parameters are better than for most who require disability because of lung disease. Anxiety could be considered a cause for the disability; however, it is currently untreated. If it is once again effectively treated, Robert will be looking for another job but with a poor recent work and health history. Few will be interested in hiring him even with the electrical skills that he brings.

Notes
- Used to be outgoing and a hard worker; now stays at home, drinks alcohol, and watches television
- Avoids confrontations and crowds; embarrassed about not working
- Uses alcohol more often now; drinking a six-pack daily and more three to four times a week to relieve tension (more than he admitted to initially); takes more to get the "buzz" he shoots for (tolerance?)
- Alcohol never kept him from working but now he does not even go drinking with friends
- Dr. Couch says that Robert's liver shows signs of "acting up," but has never talked with him about his alcohol intake (now in at least substance abuse category)
- Except for occasional diazepam and alcohol, states that there is no other recreational substance use

Martin has come to the end of the complexity assessment with the exception of baseline clinical, functional, and satisfaction measures. Robert also needs to define his personal clinical and functional goals. Martin asks Robert, "Are there any things that I have not asked about your health and current situation that you think are important for me to know about?" Robert tells Martin that he has enjoyed talking with him and says that no one for a long time has taken this much interest in the problems that he is having. However, he does not see how their conversation will lead to any change since his health is getting worse, he cannot work, and he is heading to long-term disability according to his doctor.

Martin shares the frustration about Robert's situation but indicates that he hopes that Robert is willing to work with him in an attempt to alter what seems to be inevitable. Robert indicates that he is willing to try.

At this point, Martin asks Robert about what he considers his personal level of function on a 10-point scale, with 1 being the worst. Robert says that he is at a 2. Martin already knows that Robert has not worked for the past 4 months and thus documents that the number of days missed in the past month is 24. Finally, Robert indicates that his satisfaction with the health care he has received in the past 6 months is 3 on a scale of 10, with 10 being the highest, and that he does not think that he had any "healthy days" during the previous month.

- Functional impairment on 10-point scale: 2 (with 1 being the worst)
- Missed work in past month: 24 days
- Satisfaction with health care: 3 (with 1 being the worst)
- Healthy days: 0 days

Martin now explains that he would like to make sure that as he works with Robert that Robert's personal goals are met. He would like Robert to pick out one goal related to his health and one related to the things that he would like to be able to do that he cannot do now. Robert chooses the following two goals:

- Clinical Goal—to stop having spells of shortness of breath and chest pain: estimated baseline is four major episodes (visits to Dr. Couch or the emergency room) and eight lesser episodes a month. (To change outcomes, it is necessary to understand more about the episodes and what has been helpful for them in the past. Martin listens to and documents Robert's story about how they come on and how they are treated. Martin plans to describe Robert's breathing difficulties to the medical director at the health plan as a part of the care plan. He anticipates that that medical director will in turn talk with Dr. Couch or Dr. Couch's replacement if Robert wishes. When Martin has additional information about the breathing problem and chest pain, the goal may need refining—for example, decrease the number of spells—but it will remain the goal.)

Functional Goal: go to sporting events with friends (has not gone to one in 6 months).

SUMMARY STATEMENT

Before closing the discussion, Martin asks Robert if he can summarize what he heard during their discussion so that he can be sure that he did not miss any important items. He says, *"Robert, it sounds as though you have been living alone for some time without much support and with pretty scary medical problems. It is obvious that breathing problems are a major issue but I am confused about how your lung problems relate to the anxiety you describe. Could anxiety be adding to symptoms that lead to your visits to Dr. Couch and the emergency room?"* Robert admits they may be related but says that he sure is short of breath when he goes to the emergency room. Further, they always treat him with oxygen, inhalers, and intravenous fluids, thus something must be wrong. Usually, but not always, they start him on an antibiotic. This, however, is confused by the fact that just as often the emergency room doctors put him on a medication for his "nerves."

"Thanks for the clarification. We will talk more about this later. Another thing that impressed me about your story is that your life has really changed in the past year or two. You tell me that you have not worked for nearly 4 months, but would really like to, and that you don't get to go out with friends as often, even to sporting events. That must be discouraging." Robert confirms that it makes him sad but shrugs that he does not feel he can do much about it.

"You had a medical doctor and psychiatrist you liked several years ago, however, you changed your insurance contract (through your company) to save money. When you did this, you were forced to get a new doctor at a different clinic or you would have to pay more money. Since being with your new doctor, your breathing situation has worsened and, as we discussed, your anxiety has been treated less consistently leading to more frequent use of alcohol. You tell me that you occasionally miss taking your breathing medications. You are also using the emergency room more for your breathing and other health concerns, such as chest pain.

You tell me that you don't trust Dr. Couch because he spends so little time with you and seems to ignore that anxiety may be playing a part in your current problems. He just stops medications you get in the emergency room, refills his own suggested prescriptions, and completes disability papers. He never asks for help from other doctors. It is my feeling that you consider yourself trapped and don't know what to do to change the situation."

Robert agrees and also says that he is afraid that he will lose his job unless things change. He is clearly concerned.

Martin and Robert discuss the fact that there may be a link between the lung and anxiety problem and that treatment for both may be necessary to control the number of breathing spells, which will ultimately allow Robert to get out of the house with his friends and even, down the line, back to work. Using motivational interviewing techniques, Martin allows Robert to work with him in developing an initial list of things to do, which includes:

- Reviewing the latest information about anxiety, chronic bronchitis, and heart disease and their treatment
- Getting information about what was used to control Robert's anxiety in the past
- Sorting out whether Robert wishes to stay with Dr. Couch, to go to his old doctors, or to find a new primary care doctor
- Finding out what mental health benefits are in Robert's current insurance contract

Martin makes an appointment with Robert in about 10 days. This will give Martin time to put his thoughts together and to discuss Robert's situation with his medical director. They can then work together on developing a plan that will allow Robert to get his breathing and anxiety under control and get back to a more normal social life. In the meantime, Martin tells Robert that he will send some information on anxiety and chronic bronchitis for him to review.

Martin also asks if it is okay for him or his medical director to contact Dr. Couch's clinic to get further information about Robert's care. Robert says that it will be fine and Martin makes sure that he has the correct releases of information signed by Robert. Finally, Martin indicates that he will be sending Robert a summary of his case management assessment. He asks if there is a confidential way to get the summary to Robert without others seeing it. Robert says that Martin can fax it or send it by mail to his home.

COMPLEXITY DOCUMENTATION, BASELINE RECORD OF OUTCOME MEASURES, CARE PLAN DEVELOPMENT

Based on the information available, Martin completes scoring of Robert's CAG (**Table 13.2**, see page i10 for color version). He edits and adds his notes related to the scored items into the software scoring template to help clarify for Robert the reason why each cell is represented by the color chosen (bottom of **Table 13.2**—see color template). Robert's total score is 45 (upper left

TABLE 13.2   Robert's IM-CAG (Baseline)

Baseline	HEALTH RISKS AND HEALTH NEEDS					
Robert	**HISTORICAL**		**CURRENT STATE**		**VULNERABILITY**	
Total Score = 46	Complexity Item	Score	Complexity Item	Score	Complexity Item	Score
Biological Domain	Chronicity **HB1**	3	Symptom Severity/Impairment **CB1**	2	Complications and Life Threat **VB**	2
	Diagnostic Dilemma **HB2**	1	Diagnostic/Therapeutic Challenge **CB2**	3		
Psychological Domain	Barriers to Coping **HP1**	2	Resistance to Treatment **CP1**	1	Mental Health Threat **VP**	3
	Mental Health History **HP2**	2	Mental Health Symptoms **CP2**	2		
Social Domain	Job and Leisure **HS1**	2	Residential Stability **CS1**	0	Social Vulnerability **VS**	3
	Relationships **HS2**	2	Social Support **CS2**	3		
Health System Domain	Access to Care **HHS1**	3	Getting Needed Services **CHS1**	3	Health System Impediments **VHS**	3
	Treatment Experience **HHS2**	3	Coordination of Care **CHS2**	3		

Comments	
HB1	Progressive history of chronic obstructive pulmonary disease (COPD) with moderate symptoms, no evidence of coronary artery disease (CAD) yet though at risk (lipids, family history)
HB2	Medical diagnoses straightforward
CB1	Chronic bronchitis with O_2 Sat of 94% and forced expiratory volume at one second (FEV1) of 65% predicted, nonspecific back pain, alcohol-related headaches
CB2	Anxiety complicating respiratory and cardiac symptoms leading to inconsistent treatment by multiple providers
VB	Persistent symptoms and emergency room use without change; need more information about COPD and chest pain; need to consider alternative caregiver
HP1	Alcohol abuse as adaptation technique; passive acceptance of situation
HP2	Family and personal history of treated anxiety with panic disorder
CP1	Wants to change but doesn't know how
CP2	Untreated severe anxiety; lots of medical complaints potentially related to anxiety; impaired because of alcohol abuse and perhaps dependence
VP	Needs psychiatric assessment and treatment for anxiety and likely at risk for drinking/substance abuse
HS1	Job at risk because of untreated anxiety exacerbating COPD, missed work, no social life at present
HS2	Poor family ties, child support requirements hard to meet, no clear relationships; close to social isolation
CS1	Apartment for several years
CS2	Nonexistent family or friend support when Robert is having medical or anxiety difficulties
VS	At risk for potential job loss, drinking buddies are not the best support
HHS1	Insurance limitations leading to frequent emergency room use, poor access to psychiatric services, alcohol problem never addressed, unknown mental health benefits
HHS2	Bad experience with current general practitioner (GP), good experience with prior docs before insurance change
CHS1	Forced to change GP because of change in insurance plan, no referral for needed mental health services, needs money for medications
CHS2	No communication among emergency room doctors and GP; GP needs to find and communicate with mental health professional who would treat Robert's anxiety
VHS	At risk for continued unwanted single provider, poor physician communication, limitations in access to mental health services

hand of **Table 13.2**). Martin prints a color copy of the scored IM-CAG and instructions about the purpose of the complexity grid and how it is scored. He mails this material to the address provided by Robert.

In addition to completion of Robert's IM-CAG, Martin also finishes filling in the baseline record of outcome measures (see **Table 13.3**). This provides a longitudinal way for Martin to confirm the assistance the he has given to Robert and the results that it has on health and functional outcomes. Robert is deceptively complex with significant impact of his health on his life. While impaired health is a primary concern, Robert is at risk of losing his job, his health insurance, and his stable living situation. He has few remaining life enjoyments and is without personal resources if a major change in his life occurs. Martin has his job cut out for him. Luckily, Robert appears motivated to alter his current situation, but it will not be easy.

As a last step before reconnecting with Robert, Martin creates a draft of a care plan from Martin's perspective (see **Table 13.4**). This will not be sent to Robert; however, it will inform the discussion that Robert and Martin have as they develop a plan to work through barriers to improvement. Since Robert's condition is so complex, there are many items on the complexity grid that are red (see color version) and a number that are related to each other. Goals associated with each combined barrier will be discussed using motivational interviewing skills. Actions for both Martin and Robert will be defined. Importantly, Robert will be a part of the decision-making process.

It is important not to overwhelm Robert. For instance, he will probably benefit from seeing a psychiatrist to assist with anti-anxiety medication choices in a person with chronic lung disease or a psychologist who does cognitive behavioral therapy with exposure for his anxiety, but it is first important for Robert to understand more about symptoms and treatments for all of his conditions and how they interact. It will also be important to clarify whether Robert will stay

---

TABLE 13.3   **Robert's Record of Outcome Measures (Baseline ROM)**

OUTCOME MEASURES	BASELINE	FOLLOW-UP ASSESSMENTS		
Time period recorded	Week 1			
Clinical measure (personal goal) *Fewer breathing episodes/chest pains*	4 to doctor; 8 other/month			
Functional measure (personal goal) *Go to sporting events*	None in 6 months			
Health-related quality of life *Number of days healthy/month*	0			
Patient satisfaction *(Scale: 0 low, 10 high)*	2			
CAG score *(Total for period)*	46			
Health care clinical measure *FEV1*	58%			
Health care clinical measure *Percent O$_2$ saturation*	91%			
Health care clinical measure *PHQ-9*	9			
Health care clinical measure *GAD-7*	19			
Health care functional measure *Level of function (scale 0–10)*	3			
Health care functional measure *Number of work days lost/24 days*	24			
Health Care Economic Measure *Annual cost of care*	$55,000			

TABLE 13.4   Robert's Care Plan Development (Baseline CD)*

BARRIERS	GOALS		ACTIONS
CAG items	Personal followed by health care		Prioritized
CB1, CB2, CP1, and VP	Short-term	Improve illness understanding; ensure adequate psychiatric and pulmonary/cardiac assessment for treatment to occur	1. MAIL AND GO OVER EDUCATIONAL MATERIALS AND ANSWER QUESTIONS; DISCUSS THE RELATIONSHIP OF POOR CONTROL TO ROBERT'S PERSONAL GOALS (BREATHING PROBLEM AND SOCIAL LIFE) 2. Clarify preference about which doctor will care for Robert in future 3. Get permission for health plan medical director to talk with Dr. Couch or alternative to clarify plan 4. REVIEW MEDICATIONS (DUPLICATIONS, DIFFICULTIES, COSTS); DISCUSS ILLNESS SEVERITY AND TREATMENT ALTERNATIVES WHEN ASSESSMENTS COMPLETE (MEDICAL DIRECTOR HELPS) 5. Work through steps on care plan to CONTROL COPD AND ADDRESS ANXIETY/CHEST PAIN as means to goals
	Ultimate	Participate in self-care; improved COPD, anxiety symptoms; no chest pain; few ER visits	1. CONFIRM THAT ROBERT HAS A COHERENT PLAN AND IS ADHERING TO TREATMENT 2. Problem solve crises with Robert when they arise; suggest support group as appropriate 3. Ensure adequate frequency of follow-up 4. Medical director to Robert's clinician contact to discuss plans for Robert and to MENTION POTENTIAL FOR PSYCHIATRIST/PULMONOLOGIST INVOLVEMENT
HHS1, HHS2, CHS1, CHS2, and VHS	Short-term	Overcome barriers to diagnoses and effective treatment; improve adherence	1. Review health coverage contract with Robert 2. Discuss his situation with medical and mental condition medical directors or other case managers (case conference) to better understand approaches to care that might work better for Robert 3. Medical director discussion with Dr. Couch or new doctor about plans for Robert and to ASK ABOUT THE NEED FOR PSYCHIATRIST/PULMONOLOGIST INVOLVEMENT 4. Discuss conversation with GP and help Robert initiate conversations related to care; if he chooses to return to prior GP, assist with record transfer and flex benefits 5. If more than one provider, set up communication network; coordinate intervention plan among providers
	Ultimate	Assist Robert in asking his doctor questions about changes in treatment that may help him; full adherence	1. IDENTIFY A CARE APPROACH THAT IS MUTUALLY ACCEPTABLE TO ROBERT AND HIS DOCTOR AND POTENTIALLY EFFECTIVE FOR ROBERT'S CONDITION, E.G., MORE FREQUENT DOCTOR VISITS, REFERRALS, TREATMENT OF ANXIETY, CONSOLIDATION OF MEDICATIONS 2. Monitor clinical decisions through medical director and clinician communication 3. Coordination of clinician care; communication
CS1	Short-term	Establish back-to-work plan	1. Check on restricted duty availability 2. Have Robert talk with human resources and employee assistance program (EAP) at work 3. Identify way to reintroduce Robert to the workplace
	Ultimate	Full-time employment	1. Support progression of work to full duties
CP2, HS1, HS2, CS2, and VS	Short-term	Get treatment for mental health issues, improve exercise tolerance and Robert's function	1. ASSURE REFERRAL AND ANXIETY ASSESSMENT BY MENTAL HEALTH PROFESSIONAL (COGNITIVE BEHAVIORAL THERAPIST OR PSYCHIATRIST) 2. Mention cutting back on smoking; brief intervention for alcohol abuse, formal alcohol Rx if necessary 3. Coordinate mental health with medical care. 4. DISCUSS WHEN IT WOULD BE POSSIBLE TO GO TO A SPORTING EVENT; SET GOAL DATE
	Ultimate	Controlled mental health symptoms, socially active. return to work	1. Check on adherence to diet and exercise, treatment plan

*Actions directly linked to Robert's personal goals are in small caps.

with Dr. Couch for future care. This will be influenced by benefits included in Robert's insurance policy and whether there is any latitude in flexing them to achieve better health control. Martin's experience as a case manager will help modulate the balance between achieving early health stabilization and overwhelming Robert with the number of things that need to be done.

CASE MANAGEMENT

CASE MANAGEMENT PROCESS

When Martin reaches Robert for the follow-up phone call, Robert expresses concern about the IM-CAG that he was sent. He looked at all the red boxes and was not sure whether he should be happy or upset. He skimmed the several-page explanation of the complexity grid but said that it was just too complicated. Further, he indicates that it looked like whatever would need to be done would take a lot of work. Robert is not sure that he is up to it. He also cannot understand where his personal goals will fit into this complicated complexity assessment.

Martin uses the first 15 minutes of their conversation to explain how the complexity assessment allows him to sort out the areas in Robert's life that led to his persistent health problems. The first thing that he will want to do is to go over the scoring with Robert to make sure that he, Martin, got it right. He explains that one of the nice things about the multicolored table is that it helps him to talk with people like Robert, who are having trouble figuring out where to start as they try to get their health under control.

For instance (Martin told Robert to look at the color chart), Robert has red bars in all of the boxes to the right of the domain labeled "Health System." This indicates that for Robert there are many things related to Robert's insurance and doctors that are making it difficult for Robert to get control of his health. These will be important to try to address as Martin starts to work with Robert. As examples, Martin talks about the requirement that Robert had to change his personal doctor because his employer changed insurance companies. As a result, Martin will want to clarify Robert's wishes regarding who he wants to give him health services in the future. Martin mentions that during the assessment, Robert had expressed displeasure about Dr. Couch since he does not recognize the importance of Robert's anxiety symptoms, does not take much time with him when Robert does have an appointment, and does not refer Robert to others for help when symptoms do not get better.

Robert starts to see how the complexity assessment and scoring sheet works but he does not know how it

will lead to his improvement. Martin describes how each score is associated with specific actions. He and Robert will draw from these as they initiate a joint plan designed to recapture health and reduce the impairment Robert is experiencing. Robert now understands that red and orange are the challenges, that yellow is a warning sign, and that green means there is no problem. Robert had only one green.

Martin cautions that he cannot fix all of Robert's reds and oranges. Using the guidance of the complexity assessment, however, they can likely figure out solutions to many of Robert's challenges. Robert starts accepting the potential value that working with Martin may bring and states that he is willing to give it a go.

After all of Robert's questions and concerns about the use of complexity as a point of departure, Martin and Robert discuss the various red and orange items (barriers to improvement, as Martin calls them) and their connection to each other, goals they may wish to set related to reversing the effect of these barriers on Robert's health, and the steps they will take to move toward these goals. Martin emphasizes that it is not what he will do for Robert but what they will do together that will make the difference. Ultimately, Martin tells Robert he hopes that Robert will get so good at fending for himself in a couple of months that he will no longer need Martin. Thus, expectations are set.

The care plan they develop together is remarkably similar to the one that Martin had created but not sent to Robert (**Table 13.4**). There is different wording in the various columns. The care plan is not quite as robust as Martin's original, but it identifies problems, goals, and solutions that Robert owns and is willing to work on with Martin. Importantly, Martin does not push Robert too hard as they create the template for the initial care plan. Martin knows that they will fill in the gaps during the next several months. They will address preventive measures, such as attempting to stop smoking, and stabilizing features, such as developing a social support system as Robert nears graduation. At the start, Robert needs doable goals with identifiable outcomes in high-need areas.

Launching into their mutually agreed-on care plan, Robert indicates that he would like to look for another doctor to help with his care. Martin describes the steps that he needs to take and helps him with the names of other doctors both within and outside of Robert's provider network. Martin also finds out about Robert's insurance benefits (i.e., what will and will not be covered as Robert changes). Robert chooses to return to his former family doctor, Dr. Ochoa, since he liked him. His health was in better control when Robert was under his care. Robert anticipates that it will mean that he will also be seeing his old psychiatrist,

Dr. Mitchell. Since Robert has already reached the maximum out-of-pocket he could pay for the year, going to his old doctor would not significantly affect his immediate health expenses. There is, however, a higher amount of copay. He is also gambling that recovering his health will lead to lower total health care and out-of-pocket expenses in the future, even if Dr. Ochoa was out-of-network.

Other early care plan activities included:

- Discussing information about illnesses; assessing caffeine intake (addressing items HB1, CB2, CB1, HP2)
- Reviewing prior treatments for anxiety and the providers who administered them along with their perceived response (addressing items CP2, HP2, CB2)
- Getting a better understanding of the regular and take as needed (PRN) medications Robert is taking—that is, the dosages, duplications, medication interactions, and the frequency of administration (addressing items CB1, CB2)
- Reviewing Robert's medical and mental health insurance benefits with him (addressing items HHS1, CHS1)
- Transitioning from Dr. Couch to Drs. Ochoa and Mitchell and talking with them about Robert's complexity assessment results (addressing item CHS2)
- Offering assistance in achieving adherence to Robert's new doctors treatment recommendations (addressing items HHS2, CHS2, HHS2)

Each of these measures is discussed in terms of Robert's personal goals. Within four weeks, he is on steady doses of breathing medications that have worked for his chronic lung problems in the past. Dr. Ochoa calls Dr. Sally Mitchell after Robert's first visit. Since she was familiar with Robert's pulmonary problems, she recommends that Dr. Ochoa start Robert on a new anti-anxiety medication, a serotonin reuptake inhibitor that has few respiratory side effects, and to gradually push the dose while Robert waits the several weeks needed to get an appointment with Dr. Mitchell.

After the appointment with Dr. Mitchell, Dr. Ochoa is cautioned against using additional diazepam because Robert has a history of alcohol abuse and is currently using more alcohol than is good for him. Dr. Mitchell mentions the possibility of a referral to a chemical dependence specialist if Robert's new anti-anxiety medication does not reverse Robert's use of alcohol. Further, there is a possibility that Robert may go into withdrawal. Dr. Mitchell also tells Robert (and Dr. Ochoa) that she will refer Robert to see a psychologist for cognitive behavioral therapy with exposure if his anxiety symptoms do not improve during the next month or two. Drs. Ochoa and Mitchell easily accessed each other's clinical notes through a common medical record in their clinic system.

In keeping with the prime focus on Robert's own goals, Martin had Robert track the number of breathing attacks he has using a health diary. Though not pushing to get Robert out of the house too early, Martin encourages Robert to re-initiate communication with his old workmates by phone and even with Charlene, his disability manager, to find out if restricted work might be available when his new doctors feel that he was ready.

FOLLOW-UP AND MEASUREMENT

Robert's breathing episodes start coming under control shortly after he returns to Dr. Ochoa. For the 3 weeks following Robert's transition of care, he has four breathing attacks. On one occasion, he goes to see Dr. Ochoa, who does a quick examination and oxygen saturation in his office, confirming no dangerous acute lung problem and a significant anxiety component. Robert is reassured that his symptoms will go away. Robert rests for a time in the office waiting room and returns home when his symptoms have subsided. No attacks require emergency room visits.

Martin suspects that Robert's improvement has as much to do with the trust he has in the clinical care of Dr. Ochoa and the weekly and then biweekly appointments as the changes in Robert's breathing medications. He also feels that the medication for anxiety is taking effect though it has been rocky when Robert stopped his alcohol intake. During the second 3 weeks of the first 6 weeks, Robert has no breathing episodes. He is on stable medications for the breathing problem. Other than the activating side effects common in the first weeks while using fluoxetine (the anti-anxiety medication), about which Robert had been warned, there are no other complications. Robert's dosage is increased as suggested by Dr. Mitchell. Martin makes sure that Robert is refilling his prescriptions and had money to pay for his medications.

Robert came to Martin's attention since Robert's disability manager, Charlene, was sharp enough to recognize the potential for case management to change Robert's march toward long-term disability, potential total unemployment, and all the indirect consequences of this. She had used case management services with other employees and had been impressed at the results. She is, therefore, not surprised to get a call from Robert, at Martin's encouragement, four weeks after her referral to case management asking if there is light duty possible at his worksite. When she checks about light duty, which is available, she also finds out from the occupational health nurse that there are also a number of fences to mend between Robert and his supervisor because of work performance issues.

When Charlene called Robert to inform him of the availability of restricted work, she also suggests that he contact the company employee assistance program to make sure that work reentry progresses smoothly. Robert knows that work performance was an issue. Prior to his departure for medical leave he had been placed on probation because of frequent absences. Robert's return, even to restricted activity, is not going to be a cakewalk. When he is at work, he will be expected to perform. Charlene encourages Robert to talk with his case manager about this problem as well.

When Robert explains his conversation with Charlene to Martin, Martin now knows what he had expected—that is, that Robert's reluctance to initiate finding out about return to work at an earlier date was at least in part due to his performance and the relationship with his supervisor. It was not just related to breathing spells and panic attacks. Robert's alcohol use has not helped either. Armed with this additional and important information, Martin encourages Robert to follow through on meeting with employee assistance but also suggests that Robert talk with Dr. Mitchell (and Dr. Ochoa) about the issue. Luckily, Robert has over 20 years of good work performance to draw on to support his retention despite the downward spiral at work for the last 2 years. Plus, it will cost his employer thousands of dollars to find and train a replacement. If he can get back to work, it will be a win for everyone.

In the fifth week, Robert is approved to return to 4 hours of work daily. By this time, he has had no breathing spells for nearly 2 weeks. Anxiety is present but there have been no recent panic spells and he has been instructed in how to manage these by Dr. Mitchell if they occur. Dr. Ochoa's disability form instructions indicate that, initially, Robert is not to be around dangerous machinery, climb ladders, or work with live wires.

The first week at work is not easy for Robert, but he is back and it is good to see his old work buddies. His supervisor is not enthusiastic about Robert's return but he is fair and respects the restrictions outlined for Robert. Plus, Robert is really trying to make this work. Working with employee assistance is helpful since it gives Robert someone to go to for suggestions in case conflicts arise.

Robert's return to work is in many ways a turning point for his improvement. Rekindling friendships with peers at work allows him to start doing things with friends again. He resumes his attendance when they gather at the sports bar. While he found it difficult at first, he now has no problem in being the only one to order soft drinks instead of beer. He accurately tells them that his doctors recommended against drinking because alcohol interacts with his medications. Dr. Mitchell has also cautioned him that alcohol aggravates the anxiety issues. In the long run, he should totally abstain until his breathing and anxiety symptoms are under good control.

At the end of the sixth week, Martin reassesses Robert's complexity (**Table 13.5**, see page i11 for color version). While there have been other unanticipated additional challenges, such as those uncovered as Robert reentered the workplace, so far they have not been insurmountable. Further, Robert is beginning to learn some tricks from Martin about breaking problems into parts and tackling them little by little. During the first 6 weeks, Robert's IM-CAG total score dropped by 12 points.

Several significant changes have occurred since Martin started working with Robert. Robert is back with two doctors he respects and trusts. It was a stroke of luck that Robert was willing to pay the extra price to return to their services. Even with the extra cost of Dr. Ochoa and Mitchell, Martin anticipates lower out-of-pocket expenses once Robert is no longer buying as many medications or visiting doctors or the emergency room as frequently. Importantly, breathing and anxiety symptoms are subsiding.

This is a difficult time because Robert is reentering a worksite in which he has not performed well for some time and is still on probation. Whether he does well will in part depend on the level of Robert's residual anxiety symptoms and in part on the attitude of his supervisor. Martin is monitoring the situation closely with Charlene, with whom Robert has given permission to talk.

Robert is now getting out of the house with friends, though not yet to a sporting event, and he is less anxious (**Table 13.6; GAD-7 from 19 to 9**). He is able to describe some quality days during the last month. His satisfaction with his health care has dramatically improved.

Reassessment of Robert's breathing during the most recent clinic visit to Dr. Ochoa suggests that his symptoms have stabilized. FEV1 was 65% of predicted and percent saturation was 94%. He has had no chest pain or emergency room visits in the past 6 weeks. Dr. Ochoa thinks that Robert is about halfway back to normal. The changes in Robert's condition are documented on a follow-up record of outcome measures (**Table 13.7**).

At 6 weeks, Robert has shown substantial improvement but he still has an IM-CAG score of 34 and a number of orange complexity components for which additional services will be helpful. Two red items remain, HHS1 and VHS. Martin is further investigating the possibility of ways to flex Robert's benefits. Robert has one of Martin's insurance company's less robust plans and little in the way of mental health benefits. Why Robert did not choose the plan with mental health benefits 3 years ago when he made the change is a mystery to Martin because Robert has such a long history

TABLE 13.5	Robert's IM-CAG (Week 6) Using Follow-Up Scoring Rules for Historical Items					
Week 6	**HEALTH RISKS AND HEALTH NEEDS**					
Robert	**HISTORICAL**		**CURRENT STATE**		**VULNERABILITY**	
Total Score = 34	Complexity Item	Score	Complexity Item	Score	Complexity Item	Score
Biological Domain	Chronicity **HB1**	2	Symptom Severity/Impairment **CB1**	2	Complications and Life Threat **VB**	1
	Diagnostic Dilemma **HB2**	1	Diagnostic/Therapeutic Challenge **CB2**	2		
Psychological Domain	Barriers to Coping **HP1**	1	Resistance to Treatment **CP1**	1	Mental Health Threat **VP**	2
	Mental Health History **HP2**	2	Mental Health Symptoms **CP2**	2		
Social Domain	Job and Leisure **HS1**	1	Residential Stability **CS1**	0	Social Vulnerability **VS**	2
	Relationships **HS2**	2	Social Support **CS2**	2		
Health System Domain	Access to Care **HHS1**	3	Getting Needed Services **CHS1**	2	Health System Impediments **VHS**	3
	Treatment Experience **HHS2**	2	Coordination of Care **CHS2**	1		

Comments	
HB1	Progressive history of COPD with moderate symptoms, no evidence of coronary artery disease (CAD) yet at risk (6 weeks: education about COPD and CAD and their treatment)
HB2	Medical diagnoses straightforward
CB1	Chronic bronchitis with O_2 Sat of 94% and forced expiratory volume at one second (FEV1) of 65% predicted, nonspecific back pain, alcohol-related headaches (6 weeks: symptom improvement but still occasional breathing spells)
CB2	Anxiety complicating respiratory and cardiac symptoms leading to inconsistent treatment by multiple providers (6 weeks: substantial improvement in response to consistent treatment; intervention for anxiety underway)
VB	Persistent symptoms and emergency room use without change; need more information about COPD and chest pain; need to consider alternative caregiver (6 weeks: previous care providers with better track record involved in care)
HP1	Alcohol abuse as adaptation technique; passive acceptance of situation (6 weeks: has stopped drinking for the time being)
HP2	Family and personal history of treated anxiety with panic disorder (6 weeks: anxiety and panic disorder and its treatment discussed, now in treatment)
CP1	Wants to change but doesn't know how (6 weeks: participating in change programs, adhering to medications and other treatments)
CP2	Untreated severe anxiety; lots of medical complaints potentially related to anxiety; impaired because of alcohol abuse and perhaps dependence (6 weeks: anxiety attacks decreasing with medication, still just starting to work and go out with friends, has psychiatrist involved)
VP	Needs psychiatric assessment and treatment for anxiety and likely at risk drinking/substance abuse (6 weeks: mental health professional supervising care but not out of the woods)
HS1	Job at risk because of untreated anxiety exacerbating COPD, missed work, no social life at present (6 weeks: starting to go out with friends but still to high-risk locations, e.g., sports bar; tenuous situation at work since on probation)
HS2	Poor family ties, child support requirements hard to meet, no clear relationships; close to social isolation
CS1	Apartment for several years
CS2	Nonexistent family or friend support when Robert is having medical or anxiety difficulties
VS	At risk for potential job loss, drinking buddies are not the best support (6 weeks: still at risk)
HHS1	Insurance limitations leading to frequent ER use, poor access to psychiatric services, alcohol problem never addressed, unknown mental health benefits (6 weeks: poor mental health coverage by Robert's plan, try to have Dr. Ochoa provide care and Dr. Mitchell supervise care, will try to flex benefits to pay for Dr. Mitchell's involvement)
HHS2	Bad experience with current GP, good experience with prior docs before insurance change (6 weeks: Dr. Couch no longer involved [Robert's decision], respects Drs. Ochoa and Mitchell)
CHS1	Forced to change GP due to change in insurance plan, no referral for needed mental health services, needs money for medications (6 weeks: trusted medical and mental health providers, affordable and limited number of medications, will need to keep an eye on finances)
CHS2	No communication among ER doctors and GP; GP needs to find and communicate with mental health professional who would treat Robert's anxiety (6 weeks: no ER visits, communication between GP and psychiatrist)
VHS	At risk for continued unwanted single provider, poor physician communication, limitations in access to mental health services (6 weeks: poor insurance benefits still a significant potential problem)

TABLE 13.6   Robert's Anxiety Symptoms Evaluation (Week 6)

Over the last 2 weeks, how often have you been bothered by the following problems?	Not at all sure (Mark 0)	Several days (Mark 1)	Over half the days (Mark 2)	Nearly every day (Mark 3)
Feeling nervous, anxious, or on edge			2	
Not being able to stop or control worrying		1		
Worrying too much about different things			2	
Trouble relaxing			2	
Being so restless that it's hard to sit still	0			
Becoming easily annoyed or irritable		1		
Feeling afraid as if something awful might happen		1		
Add the score for each column	0	3	6	0
Total score (add column scores)[a]			9	

If you marked any problems, how difficult have these problems made it for you to do your work, take care of things at home, or get along with other people?

Not difficult at all	Somewhat difficult (Robert's response)	Very difficult	Extremely difficult

[a]For case management purposes, use total scores of 10 and above as significant levels of anxiety.

TABLE 13.7   Robert's Record of Outcome Measures (Week 6 ROM)

OUTCOME MEASURES	BASELINE	FOLLOW-UP ASSESSEMENTS		
Time period recorded	Week 1	Week 6		
Clinical measure (personal goal) *Fewer breathing episodes/chest pains*	4 to doctor; 8 other/month	1 to doctor; 3 other/month		
Functional measure (personal goal) *Go to sporting events*	None in 6 months	Going to sports bar occasionally		
Health-related quality of life *Number of days healthy/month*	0	11		
Patient satisfaction *(Scale: 0 low, 10 high)*	2	8		
CAG score *(Total for period)*	46	34		
Health care clinical measure *FEV1*	58%	65%		
Health care clinical measure *Percent O$_2$ saturation*	91%	94%		
Health care clinical measure *PHQ-9*	9			
Health care clinical measure *GAD-7*	19	9		
Health care functional measure *Level of function (scale 0–10)*	3	5		
Health care functional measure *Number of work days lost/23 days*	24	20; 4 hours/day		
Health care economic measure *Annual cost of care*	$55,000			

of difficulties with anxiety and substance abuse. Martin hopes that the out-of-pocket expenses for Dr. Mitchell will not be too great and that Dr. Ochoa will be able to do most of Robert's mental health care when Robert's condition has stabilized. Luckily, Robert does not have a mental health condition that typically requires hospitalization. If he responds to fluoxetine, which is generic, a month supply is only about $40, compared to $350 per month for the name brand equivalent.

Martin anticipates that there will still be bumps in the road as Robert reenters the workplace. Not only has the marginal care given to Robert by Dr. Couch affected his health, it may also have indirectly affected his job. It will be hard for Robert to mend fences with his supervisor, who will have little sympathy for soft reasons for work nonattendance, such as nerves. Nonetheless, helping Robert retain his job and get back to normal work performance is a major goal of Martin.

Since the core health symptoms for Robert are coming under control, it is time for Martin to also start addressing less pressing yet important barriers to stable health for Robert (**Table 13.8**). For instance, Robert has been encouraged to reinitiate some of his out of the house interests, such as making and flying model airplanes, joining a health club, going to sporting events, or volunteering his time at a local charity. He may even want to consider going on a vacation with his kids or dating. Martin knows that health is fickle. It will improve and then get worse. Now is the time to develop personal relationships on which Robert can draw in times of need. Martin talks with Robert about the importance of this component of his personal life, especially since his family lives so far away.

Martin works with Robert for another 11 weeks. The frequency of contact decreases substantially during the last month, but Martin feels that it is necessary to maintain contact with Robert to provide support and reassurance during stabilization. Work reentry has not been easy. As expected, the supervisor harbored bad feelings about Robert's return. Several panic attacks occurred at work leading to several additional days of disability. It also took longer than anticipated to increase from 4 hours a day to full time and then to full activities related to his job. Things are still not perfect.

The company's employee assistance staff have become actively involved with both Robert and the supervisor, though using different personnel to work with each. It has also been necessary for Robert to augment his anti-anxiety medication with cognitive behavioral therapy. For this, Martin was able to persuade his insurance company to see if Robert's company would support the therapy even though it was not covered. They agreed (this once).

By the end of the 17th week, Robert's IM-CAG has dropped to 25 (**Table 13.9**, see page i12 for color version), his respiratory and anxiety symptoms are largely under control and he has had no panic attacks, even at work, for about 2 months. Several weeks before Martin ramped down active case management, Robert was finally working full duties at work and had gone to three baseball games with several workmates. His personal goals have been realized and his life is back together after a hiatus of 3 years.

TABLE 13.8   Additions to Robert's Care Plan Development (Week 6 CD)

BARRIERS		GOALS	ACTIONS
CAG items		Personal followed by health care	Prioritized
HS1, HS2, CS2, and VS	Short-term	Establish a personal support system	1. Assist Robert in contacting family, making new friendships, and using community resources 2. Explore availability of COPD and/or anxiety support groups
	Ultimate	Friendships and social support system when crises occur	1. Explore social activity options 2. Support constructive personal activities and social support system
HHS1 and VHS	Short-term	Consistent coverage for mental health and substance abuse treatment	1. Work out an arrangement between Dr. Ochoa and Dr. Mitchell 2. Try to have most of Robert's mental health treatment in primary care
	Ultimate	Parity coverage for both medical and mental health problems	1. Investigate other insurance coverage options with Robert

TABLE 13.9   Robert's IM-CAG (Week 17) Using Follow-Up Scoring Rules for Historical Items

Week 17	HEALTH RISKS AND HEALTH NEEDS					
Robert	**HISTORICAL**		**CURRENT STATE**		**VULNERABILITY**	
Total Score = 25	Complexity Item	Score	Complexity Item	Score	Complexity Item	Score
Biological Domain	Chronicity **HB1**	2	Symptom Severity/Impairment **CB1**	1	Complications and Life Threat **VB**	1
	Diagnostic Dilemma **HB2**	1	Diagnostic/Therapeutic Challenge **CB2**	1		
Psychological Domain	Barriers to Coping **HP1**	2	Resistance to Treatment **CP1**	0	Mental Health Threat **VP**	1
	Mental Health History **HP2**	2	Mental Health Symptoms **CP2**	1		
Social Domain	Job and Leisure **HS1**	1	Residential Stability **CS1**	0	Social Vulnerability **VS**	1
	Relationships **HS2**	2	Social Support **CS2**	1		
Health System Domain	Access to Care **HHS1**	3	Getting Needed Services **CHS1**	1	Health System Impediments **VHS**	2
	Treatment Experience **HHS2**	2	Coordination of Care **CHS2**	0		

Comments	
HB1	Progressive history of COPD with moderate symptoms, no evidence of coronary artery disease (CAD) yet, though at risk (6 weeks: education about COPD and CAD and their treatment)
HB2	Medical diagnoses straightforward
CB1	Chronic bronchitis with O_2 Sat of 94% and forced expiratory volume at one second (FEV1) of 65% predicted, nonspecific back pain, alcohol-related headaches (6 weeks: symptom improvement but still occasional breathing spells; 17 weeks: no breathing episodes or chest pain in 4 weeks)
CB2	Anxiety complicating respiratory and cardiac symptoms leading to inconsistent treatment by multiple providers (6 weeks: substantial improvement in response to consistent treatment; intervention for anxiety underway; 17 weeks: stable response to medications for the past 6 weeks)
VB	Persistent symptoms and emergency room use without change; need more information about COPD and chest pain; need to consider alternative caregiver (6 weeks: previous care providers with better track record involved in care; 17 weeks: chronic bronchitis stable and starting to decrease smoking)
HP1	Alcohol abuse as adaptation technique; passive acceptance of situation (6 weeks: has stopped drinking for the time being; 17 weeks: no alcohol use in 4 months)
HP2	Family and personal history of treated anxiety with panic disorder (6 weeks: anxiety and panic disorder and its treatment discussed, now in treatment)
CP1	Wants to change but doesn't know how (6 weeks: participating in change programs, adhering to medications and other treatments; 17 weeks: consistent adherence to medications, shows up for therapy sessions, exercising)
CP2	Untreated severe anxiety; lots of medical complaints potentially related to anxiety; impaired due to alcohol abuse and perhaps dependence (6 weeks: anxiety attacks decreasing with medication, still just starting to work and go out with friends, has psychiatrist involved; 17 weeks: still some situational anxiety but no panic attacks)
VP	Needs psychiatric assessment and treatment for anxiety and likely at risk drinking/substance abuse (6 weeks: mental health professional supervising care but not out of the woods; 17 weeks: fewer anxiety symptoms at work and home)
HS1	Job at risk due to untreated anxiety exacerbating COPD, missed work, no social life at present (6 weeks: starting to go out with friends but still to high risk locations, e.g., sports bar; tenuous situation at work since on probation; 17 weeks: supervisor and Robert issues controlled, Robert working full duties, three trips to baseball stadium with friends, joined exercise club)
HS2	Poor family ties, child support requirements hard to meet, no clear relationships; close to social isolation (17 weeks: Robert has called children twice, will visit them at holidays, doing more with workmates)
CS1	Apartment for several years
CS2	Nonexistent family or friend support when Robert is having medical or anxiety difficulties (17 weeks: still no ready help for crises, joined emphysema support group, thinking about volunteering at food bank through church)
VS	At risk for potential job loss, drinking buddies are not the best support (6 weeks: still at risk; 17 weeks: situation stable with no crisis, potential support in crisis through volunteer group at his church, Robert knows that this still needs work)

(Continued)

TABLE 13.9	**Robert's IM-CAG (Week 17) Using Follow-Up Scoring Rules for Historical Items (Continued)**
HHS1	Insurance limitations leading to frequent ER use, poor access to psychiatric services, alcohol problem never addressed, unknown mental health benefits (6 weeks: poor mental health coverage by Robert's plan, try to have Dr. Ochoa provide care and Dr. Mitchell supervise care, will try to flex benefits to pay for Dr. Mitchell's involvement; 17 weeks: poor mental health insurance is still a significant issue, stable now but small change could create crisis, Robert talking with human resources at work about new insurance options through company)
HHS2	Bad experience with current GP, good experience with prior docs before insurance change (6 weeks: Dr. Couch no longer involved [Robert's decision], respects Drs. Ochoa and Mitchell; 17 weeks: trust in existing doctors, problems with insurance being worked on)
CHS1	Forced to change GP because of change in insurance plan, no referral for needed mental health services, needs money for medications (6 weeks: trusted medical and mental health providers, affordable and limited number of medications, will need to keep an eye on finances; 17 weeks: pays for medication and shows up for appointments, special arrangement for therapist, some help through employee assistance)
CHS2	No communication among ER doctors and GP; GP needs to find and communicate with mental health professional who would treat Robert's anxiety (6 weeks: no ER visits, communication between GP and psychiatrist; 17 weeks: no ER use, doctors talk directly and through shared notes)
VHS	At risk for continued unwanted single provider, poor physician communication, limitations in access to mental health services (6 weeks: poor insurance benefits still a significant potential problem; 17 weeks: still significant risk of progress reversal if anxiety and panic problems resurface, change in insurance will take time, Robert aware and is looking into options)

Martin has been documenting outcomes related to barriers and goals on the care plan measurement of progress sheet as integrated case management milestones have been reached (**Table 13.10**). The primary goals related to Robert's immediate health and socialization needs had been met by the end of the third month. By the fourth month, there was some assurance that the improvements that Robert had experienced would not be short lived. Nonetheless, Robert's mental health coverage remains an unresolved barrier to long-term and consistent health.

Since Robert has a long history of anxiety disorder with panic, and other family members have also been affected, he is at high risk for future problems. He has also demonstrated that he turned to alcohol as a solution when others were not available. For this reason, Martin does not completely close Robert's case. He will continue to work with Robert on a monthly or bimonthly basis while trying to identify affordable ways that will allow him to have mental health coverage. Robert should really have a steady mental health professional that is involved in his care. Dr. Ochoa can cover during times of stable anxiety, but if Robert starts having more symptoms, he will soon exceed Dr. Ochoa's clinical competence and comfort. Dr. Mitchell and Robert's psychologist can become more involved, but they will need to be paid for their services. With Robert's current coverage, this will not be possible.

In addition to documenting Robert's IM-CAG and care plan outcomes, Martin also updates clinical and functional outcomes on the record of outcome measures that tracks patient, case manager, and case management performance (**Table 13.11**). From this it can easily be seen that Robert has achieved his personal goals and that his health and function have improved substantially. His complexity scores have significantly decreased from his original assessment, but Robert's situation still presents complicated problems for Dr. Ochoa, Dr. Mitchell, and Robert's therapist. A score of 25 is still complex. Robert will need to be followed relatively closely since small challenges can tip him. Further, he does have moderate to severe chronic bronchitis as indicated by his FEV1 and percent O_2 saturation. Though he is now stable, impaired lung function will progress, especially if Robert cannot discontinue smoking.

At this point, Martin is only in contact with Robert about once a month or less. They respect each other and have had mutual success. Not all cases turn out like Robert's, but success feels good. In fact, Martin now likes to call and talk with Robert, and Robert likes to hear from him. Nevertheless, this is the point at which it is time for Robert to take responsibility for his future health and for Martin to transition Robert back to standard care. While Martin will continue to look into the insurance situation, it is up to Robert to maintain his health, work with his doctors, remain productive at work, use preventive services, and continue to improve his social situation. For both, it will be hard and sad to wind down the relationship and eventually end it in the next several months.

It would be easy for Robert to rationalize that he needs Martin to maintain his health and for Martin to reason that Robert will not succeed unless he remains

TABLE 13.10	Robert's Measurement of Progress (Week 17 MP3)		
	GOAL	**ACTION**	**OUTCOME**
Barrier CHS1 and CHS2	Getting appropriate services and coordination of medical and mental health care	1. Review past effective treatments 2. Clarify who will be treating clinicians 3. Coordinate actions of clinicians	Return to prior family doctor and mental health professional before insurance change; implementation of effective treatments
Barrier CB1, CB2, and CP2	Understands chronic bronchitis and anxiety; participation in treatment	1. Education about illnesses 2. Confirm consistent evidence-based medical and mental health treatment 3. Document adherence	Participating in appropriate COPD and anxiety assessment and treatment, adherence to stabilized pulmonary medications and mental health treatments
Barrier CB1 and CB2	Stabilized respiratory symptoms	1. Support clinician's interventions 2. Decrease cost barriers 3. Monitor clinical outcomes with doctor	Taking consistent and affordable medications regularly with good follow-up and symptom control; no ER visits and lessened likelihood of admission
Barrier CB1 and HS1	Exercise program	1. Discuss graded exercise 2. Assist in finding suitable health club	Gradually increasing exercise each day; joins health club in week 11
Barrier CP2 and CHS2	Effective treatment of anxiety	1. Assist in involving mental health professionals 2. Confirm initiation and follow-up of treatment 3. Monitor symptoms with clinicians	Psychiatrist supervised anxiety medication; cognitive behavioral therapy with exposure with functional outcomes
Barrier HS1, HS2, and CS2	Going to sporting events with colleagues; return to work	1. Help renew contacts with friends 2. Monitor health improvement 3. Support exercise 4. Facilitate socialization 5. Check on restricted work potential	Socializing with friends in week 4; partial work started in week 5 (with stutter start); full duties at 13 weeks; first baseball game with friends during month 3
Barrier HHS1 and HHS2	Consistent way to pay for needed health care	1. Review health contracts and benefits 2. Try to flex benefits 3. Coordinate health services 4. Explore other insurance product	Insurance still inadequate; on low-cost medications and getting major mental health services from Dr. Ochoa (goal not achieved)
Barrier CS2	Social support network to help in crisis	1. Reinitiate contact with kids 2. Support socialization at work 3. Encourage volunteering	Building friendships and entering situations in which help could be solicited (still needs work)
Barrier CB1	Healthy behavior	1. Educate about illnesses 2. Encourage treatment adherence 3. Review preventive measures	Considering stopping smoking, plans to get flu shots, allergy appointment made

involved. These impulses must be resisted, otherwise the last and perhaps most important growth experience will not occur—that is, that Robert takes ownership of his health and well-being. Further, Martin must close cases in order to open others.

While Martin will not close contact with Robert for several months, he initiates the steps that will allow Dr. Ochoa and Robert's other practitioners to resume the major responsibility for Robert's health needs. As a part of this process, Martin copies and sends the baseline and final IM-CAG, the latest care plan measurement of progress, and the record of outcome measures for Robert to Dr. Ochoa, Dr. Mitchell, and Robert's therapist. In addition, Martin writes a summary statement about Robert's progress, both successes and failures; continued issues of concern related to Robert's complex health situation, such as the need for an expanded support system and better mental health insurance coverage; and what the clinicians may wish to consider as they continue to provide Robert's care. Martin includes his contact information so that they can call if there are questions.

Martin tells Robert that he will be calling no more than once every month or two for the next several

TABLE 13.11	Robert's Record of Outcome Measurement (Week 17 ROM)			
OUTCOME MEASURES	**BASELINE**	**FOLLOW-UP ASSESSMENTS**		
Time period recorded	Week 1	Week 6	Week 17	
Clinical measure (personal goal) *Fewer breathing episodes/chest pains*	4 to doctor; 8 other/month	1 to doctor; 3 other/month	0	
Functional measure (personal goal) *Go to sporting events*	None in 6 months	Going to sports bar occasionally	3 baseball games	
Health-related quality of life *Number of days healthy/month*	0	11	24	
Patient satisfaction *(Scale: 0 low, 10 high)*	2	8	8	
CAG score *(Total for period)*	46	34	25	
Health care clinical measure *FEV1*	58%	65%	64%	
Health care clinical measure *Percent O2 saturation*	91%	94%	94%	
Health care clinical measure *PHQ-9*	9		6	
Health care clinical measure *GAD-7*	19	9	7	
Health care functional measure *Level of function (scale 0–10)*	3	5	8	
Health care functional measure *Number of work days lost/23 days*	24	20; 4 hours/day	0; full duty	
Health care economic measure *Annual cost of care*	$55,000			

months but that he should continue with the activities that they started together. He encourages Robert to take the complexity grid and the care plan record of outcome measures to Dr. Ochoa and his other clinicians so that they can ask Robert to explain questions they may have about the materials that they were sent.

By now, Robert is pretty familiar with integrated case management lingo and the approach that has been taken to help him get back to normal. Since Martin will continue to talk with Robert during the next several months, it will also allow Martin to see how Robert does on his own.

CHAPTER 14

Assisting Paul: Thirteen-Year-Old With Congenital Heart Disease, Family Anxiety, and School Nonattendance

OBJECTIVES

- To illustrate the use of integrated case management assessment and intervention in a child of 13
- To highlight unique issues faced in working with children/youth and caregivers/parents in the pediatric setting
- To use The Pediatric INTERMED Complexity Assessment Grid (PIM-CAG) findings to develop a care plan
- To measure health and function outcomes in children/youth using a record of outcome measures and integrated case management success using a care plan measurement of progress
- To demonstrate how to move a child/youth and his/her caregivers/parents toward case management graduation

PAUL'S STORY

Paul is a 13-year-old male with truncus arteriosis, a congenital heart condition, for which he is currently receiving symptomatic care. The reason for the cardiology clinic visit was to evaluate high levels of fatigue, which significantly affect his ability to attend school. Consistently for the past 9 months, Paul's oxygen saturation levels have been running between 85% and 89% (pO$_2$ 50–55), a dangerously low range, and are slowly becoming progressively worse. His extremities have a blue/purple tint, and there is significant clubbing of his fingers.

Paul has very limited daily activities. He becomes easily fatigued when he goes out, and he has not attended middle school since the beginning of the academic year (nearly 6 months). Despite nonattendance at his school, he receives no tutoring or home schooling and is far behind in the special program provided by his middle school teachers.

Medical management consists of water pills and heart strengthening medications. His cardiologist also recommends the use of oxygen while sleeping. However, Paul is very anxious about wearing an oxygen mask or even nasal prongs. His parents have not followed through to arrange for this and are not pushing him. As a result, Paul has been to the emergency room six times in the last 2 months for water pill adjustments and oxygen supplementation. He has never been admitted to the hospital, though it was encouraged on three occasions.

Paul's cardiologist recommends cardiac catheterization to determine the status of his heart condition. Paul and his parents, however, are very fearful about his undergoing this procedure. Paul underwent several surgeries during his first few years of life to correct his cardiac defect. Paul's doctors feel that given the physical deterioration observed in him, he will likely require further corrective surgery. Both parents are fearful that surgery will kill Paul or that it would provide little benefit to their son's quality of life.

TRIAGE STAFF INTERACTION

Paul and his family are identified as potentially benefiting from a referral for integrated case management by his cardiologist, Dr. Sarah Davis, because of several factors. First, Paul's health status has been clinically deteriorating, especially in the last 9 months. His oxygen saturation is decreasing, and he is experiencing increasing fatigue, breathlessness, dizziness, and poor sleep. Second, he is now significantly impaired, spending most of his time at home with no schooling or age-appropriate peer interactions. Any activity is quite limited by his physical symptoms. Third, his family is reluctant to move forward even with basic clinical cardiac investigations.

Dr. Davis feels handicapped. She cannot proceed with optimal care, which, due to procrastination by Paul's parents, would entail a now high-risk cardiac catheterization. Regardless of catheterization findings, it is likely that cardiac surgery will be needed to replace Paul's pulmonary artery conduit. Paul's parents were unwilling to even discuss their son's medical condition openly in front of him. According to Dr. Davis, they are overly concerned that catheterization may lead to a recommendation for further surgery, something they wish to avoid, seemingly at all cost. Further, during clinic visits with Dr. Davis, Paul has appeared overwhelmed. He will often break down and cry.

Dr. Davis feels she can wait no longer. It is important to take the next steps because Paul is at a critical age and has progressive symptoms. No action predicts deterioration and potential, if not likely, death. This is why she refers Paul and his family to case management. In the back of her mind, she thinks that the alternative will eventually be a ruling by a child protective agency since Paul's condition is life threatening and Paul's parents are obstructing care.

Paul's parents, Imee and Ray, are hesitant about making an appointment with Debbie, the hospital and clinic's case management triage staff (enrollment specialist), but agreed to find out more about the program. Debbie suspects that she would not have succeeded in making contact with them at all had Dr. Davis not walked them to Debbie's office after their clinic visit. Debbie has been prewarned by Dr. Davis of her intentions earlier in the week and has set aside time. When they arrive, they tell Debbie that they prefer to talk with Debbie without Paul knowing about their visit. Whenever possible, they protect Paul from information about his health, noting that he becomes very anxious when issues related to his medical condition are discussed. While Debbie explains the program, they also indicate that new situations and acquaintances worry Paul.

Paul's parents have many questions about the new case management program at Children's Hospital and Clinics. They know that things are not going well with Paul and that Dr. Davis is showing increasing concern about Paul's condition. Their experience with the medical care that Paul has received in the past, however, make them reluctant to trust advice from doctors and agree to invasive medical procedures. Debbie explains that the case management program has been created to help patients such as Paul, who are having difficulty in optimizing their health status because of the complicated nature of their illnesses, and to assist families in gathering the information they need to make serious decisions related to their child's health. She also points out that the case manager's primary responsibility is to Paul and the family, not to the doctors.

During the meeting with Debbie, Paul's parents share that there are a number of factors in Paul's situation that lead them to feel immobilized and unable to proceed with decisions about Paul's medical care. They are aware that not doing anything can potentially affect his future health and function but note their own concerns about "acting too soon," negative experiences they had with doctors in the past, and the fragile emotional state of Paul as reasons for their delay.

Debbie's review of Dr. Davis's referral message and her office clinic notes suggest that Paul was at a moderate (Level III) to high (Level IV) stratification level (Table 3.3; Appendix A, see www.springerpub.com/kathol). Paul has a serious and potentially reversible condition with concurrent and untreated mental health components. Further, he has demonstrated symptom progression and increased service use.

Paul's parents are aware of the gravity of the situation but are paralyzed by their own anxiety about potential consequences despite Paul's withdrawal from normal activities as a 13-year-old. They know that something is needed and are willing, though reluctant, to explore options (Appendix B, "Readiness for Change," 6 on a scale of 10 for importance, see www.springerpub.com/kathol) but have little confidence that the advice the doctors are giving would improve the situation (Appendix B, "Readiness for Change," 2 on a scale of 10 for confidence). Since Paul is a long-term patient in the Children's Hospital system, there will be no difficulty in communicating with Paul and his parents. Paul is also new to integrated case management, if he and his parents agree to participate. These factors identify Paul and his parents as high-priority candidates for the new case management service (Table 3.4; Appendix A, see www.springerpub.com/).

Although somewhat hesitant, the parents agree to initiate case management for Paul. Debbie obtains baseline administrative information and has Paul's parents sign needed consent forms so that the assigned case manager can communicate with those involved in Paul's care. During the conversation with Debbie, Paul's parents indicate that they will speak with Paul about their discussion with Debbie and their decision to try case management. Rather than wait to schedule an appointment later, Debbie introduces Paul's parents to Rachel, the pediatric nurse case manager who will be working with them and Paul.

INITIAL INTERVIEW BETWEEN RACHEL AND PAUL'S PARENTS

Rachel tells Paul's parents a little about her background and how she will be working with them during the next several months. She notes that much of what she does with them can be done over the phone since they live so far from the medical center. She answers questions and concerns about the integrated case management process but says that she needs to understand more about Paul's health problems before she can be more specific about suggestions.

After exchanging contact information, she and Paul's parents set up a face-to-face meeting 2 days later in Rachel's office at the Children's Hospital Clinic. Rachel indicates that the total assessment will likely take several hours. Paul's parents insist that they talk with Rachel first, without Paul. After their first official meeting with Rachel, they will decide whether it will be in Paul's interest to participate in the assessment. While this is not Rachel's preferred approach, she knows that establishing rapport and gaining their trust is an important first step in the case management process.

Prior to the initial meeting with Paul's parents, Rachel reviews Paul's medical records and talks with the advance practice nurse in the pediatric clinic because Dr. Davis is not available. This preliminary review gives Rachel a general picture of Paul's situation and the concerns of his practitioners. It does not provide detailed information about Paul's early management and treatment because Paul's parents moved to their current residence 3 years ago from another Canadian province. It will be necessary to obtain records from the health facilities that have been involved in Paul's care since his birth.

INTEGRATED CASE MANAGEMENT ASSESSMENT

Paul's parents show up on time for their appointment with Rachel. Paul sits in the waiting room with a book and magazines as his parents are ushered into Rachel's office. As expected, they have additional questions and concerns about the case management process. Rachel indicates that there is no obligation to participate; however, she feels that it may be of significant benefit to Paul and to them if they do. She says that she has reviewed information about Paul's condition and has talked with the staff in Dr. Davis's office in an attempt to better understand issues of concern for Paul. Rachel summarizes what she has found, including information about Paul's heart condition; his personal reaction to health concerns (i.e., anxiety) and the limitations in his personal activities, including school nonattendance.

Rachel allows Paul's parents to fill in additional information related to her summary. She jots down notes while they talk since many of their comments cover content related to the complexity assessment that she will more formally pursue later in their discussion. When Paul's parents are comfortable with Rachel's understanding of Paul's current situation from their perspective, Rachel asks to review some basics of the case management process. Paul's parents already know that Rachel will be working to improve Paul's health, but it will also be important for them to know how both they and Paul will be involved, the degree to which the information that they share with Rachel will be shared with Paul and vice versa, and that it will be helpful to have information from Paul's prior health providers.

Considerable time is spent talking about the degree to which Paul understands his heart condition and about Paul's parents' comfort with discussions related to it. Rachel notes that she will respect the parents' wishes about how much she shares with Paul. It is too early in Rachel's relationship with Paul's parents to express concerns about trying to hide things from a 13-year-old. Further, it is better for Rachel to meet and find out about Paul's needs and strengths before deciding whether sharing information about Paul's illness is a good or bad idea.

This discussion is a natural segue into a description about Rachel's requirements as a health professional regarding the limits of confidentiality. She tells Paul's parents that she is obliged to report to child protection authorities any specific information or suspicions of abuse or neglect. In addition, confidentiality can be broken if she has any concerns about Paul's or his parents' safety, particularly with regard to suicidal or homicidal thoughts. If Paul is considered to be dangerous to himself or others, she notes that she will inform them immediately. When she meets Paul, she will tell him about the limits of confidentiality as well.

Following a few clarifying questions, Rachel reinforces that she will not share information with Paul that they are uncomfortable with him hearing. She tells them that the reverse will also be true unless concerns with regard to his safety are disclosed. This will allow her to talk with both the parents and with Paul without either having to be careful in what they say. Paul's parents are relieved to know that Rachel will respect their protection of Paul from his health information. They do not think that Paul is hiding things from them.

By this time, Paul's parents remain somewhat guarded in their responses to Rachel; however, they are starting to gain an appreciation that Rachel really wants to make it easier for them to help Paul. Rachel now starts the complexity assessment process with the question, *"Is it okay to ask some questions to get to know about you and Paul better before we focus on Paul's health situation?"* They are fine with this so Rachel asks, *"Can you tell me a little about yourselves and Paul, such as where you live, who your friends and Paul's friends are, what you and Paul like to do together (hobbies/interests, extracurricular activities), what Paul likes to do when you aren't around?"*

This question elicits a flood of information about which Paul's parents have not had a chance to talk with Dr. Davis or her team. The initial question naturally leads to others concerning Paul, his parents, and their current life situation. By the completion of their general discussion, much information has been recorded related to Paul's home, school, and social life. Most listed caregiver/parent follow-up questions that Rachel uses to ensure that she did not miss any important content areas (see Exhibit 10.2; Appendix F, Question 1, www.springerpub.com/kathol) are unnecessary. Several, however, require attention (**Exhibit 14.1**).

Notes

- Lives with parents, older sister, Dalisay (age 14), and cocker spaniel named Piddle in small town several hours drive from Children's Hospital
- Mother is originally from the Philippines, father is Canadian; married 18 years
- Paul was born in the Philippines while his father worked for a company with international contracts and received his initial medical care there
- Gets along well with Dalisay, who is quite independent and has good grades; band and choir; Paul looks to her for support
- Seventh grade; modified home study program (not doing any school work at home); 2 weeks total

attendance during the first 6 months of the school year; no seventh grade classes completed; parents less concerned about Paul's schooling and socialization than Paul's health limitations (school not a priority)
- Average grades but with modifications and accommodations to his academic program; better than average in art; few school friends; no disciplinary problems
- Age 6 to 10 guitar lessons and school choir (not for past year); no sports except badminton but unable to play now because of fatigue; one-time attendance at computer club in seventh grade
- One childhood friend, who he sees monthly; spends most of his time at home with parents and sister
- Paul enjoys playing games on the computer, watching television
- Parents do not encourage Paul to engage in activities, such as doing things with friends or going to school; occasionally outings with family (e.g., movies); Paul's handicaps significantly limit family social life; family largely isolated
- Mother not currently working; 8 years on disability because of chronic pain condition, fibromyalgia; anxiety with panic attacks since Paul's birth and surgeries (highly traumatic events); anxiety less of a problem when Paul is home with her
- Father has a part-time job as a finish carpenter (makes cabinets and custom furniture); works mainly from home; financial resources for food and basics but have to budget; no money for crises; no disability insurance
- Father "nervous" but never treated; back problems
- Father's family lives 300 kilometers away; support available during crises from family acquaintances (mainly Dalisay's friends' families), but this is inconsistent

When talking about Paul's school attendance, a number of issues related to Paul's heart condition come out. For this reason, it is not necessary to specifically ask about how Paul feels physically (see Exhibit 10.2; Appendix F, Question 2). Rather, Paul's parents are asked for clarification about the level of current symptoms and how they have progressed in the past year.

EXHIBIT 14.1 **Follow-Up Questions After Initial Discussion**

- "Can you tell me about current stresses or changes in your family situation that are worrying you about the future?"
- "Can you tell me about any physical or mental conditions or disability that either of you have?"
- "Who helps you when a crisis arises?"
- "How does Paul's health situation affect your family?"

Notes

- Paul's parents indicate that Paul is tired much of the time, can't catch his breath, complains of headaches, and has too little energy to even pick up his room; turns "blue" with small exertion; feet swollen
- Food sensitivities, such as to meatloaf, pizza, and casseroles, which are commonly served at school; stomachaches common complaint when going to school
- Paul doesn't ask questions about why he takes daily heart medications and goes to doctors; no memory of surgery at age 5
- Heart surgery as a baby and heart specialist follow-ups; water and heart pills not working as well; frequent visits to emergency room and cardiologist in past 6 months (turns blue, feet swell, and cannot breathe; oxygen and medication helps)
- Doctors have been recommending for the past year that Paul undergo a heart catheterization but both parents are afraid to have it done, citing the fact that Paul's arsenic levels are currently elevated; they bypass Paul's appointments to avoid pushy doctors but show up in the local emergency room
- Parents don't understand about Paul's heart condition (e.g., physiology and treatment); don't remember anyone explaining it to them

Paul's parents downplay the degree to which they worry about Paul's heart condition. They suggest that the problem is with the doctors being too pushy rather than them being too resistant. This is at odds with clinical information described in Dr. Davis's cardiology notes. She considers Paul's parents' emotional state a significant contributor to both Paul's physical condition and his emotional reactions. Dr. Davis indicates that she and her team have tried to broach this subject with them but they then do not show up for appointments. She thinks that they know how serious Paul's condition is and that this is what scares them.

While Paul's parents declare that Paul is a very sensitive boy, they indicate little about the symptoms he has that make them describe him as such (see Exhibit 10.2; Appendix F, Question 3). Both, however, feel that he would not handle knowing the severity of his heart condition well and assiduously avoid talking about it with him. Whenever they see Dr. Davis, they always have Paul leave when there is a discussion about diagnosis and treatment. Both indicate that Dr. Davis has become more insistent about doing something. They like her and think that she cares about Paul but are too nervous to approve of a heart catheterization for Paul. Approaching age 14, Paul would also have to consent, but he does not even know what kind of heart condition he has, or so the parents' think.

Rachel asks them how Paul feels about his heart condition. They have never asked him but say that he worries a lot just like they do. Follow-up questions about Paul's and Paul's mother's emotional condition (see Exhibit 10.2; Appendix F, Question 3) provide additional information from his parents' perspective.

Notes

- Learning difficulties at school, likely resulting from the impact of Paul's cardiac condition on central nervous system (CNS) function; special assistance needed at school but no school disruption
- No traumatic life events other than surgery as an infant and young child
- Seen by a psychiatrist in the local children's hospital at the age of 6; psychotherapy recommended but parents did not think that Paul needed it
- History of anxiety with sleep difficulties since preschool, including phobias of thunderstorms, attending medical appointments, and undergoing medical procedures, such as getting shots or having blood drawn; no prior or current treatment
- Paul currently worried about perceptions by his peers and embarrassed about academic performance
- Family history of anxiety and depression (especially mother); long-term treatment *only* by general practitioner for Paul's mother with medication (inconsistent adherence) and counseling (none for years); father says medication helps when mother takes it consistently; father not treated though "nervous"

Several times during the conversation with Paul's parents, they state that they do not trust doctors. Rachel has already identified that Paul's primary physician is Dr. Davis, a cardiologist, though he sees a pediatrician in his hometown as well. Dr. Davis has been seeing Paul for nearly 2 years and communicates regularly with his pediatrician, but Rachel needs to know more about why Paul's parents are so reluctant to follow through with Dr. Davis's recommendations. She asks them, "Can you tell me about your experience with doctors, including Dr. Davis?" After Rachel reassures Paul's parents that she will not discuss issues they wish to avoid sharing with Dr. Davis, Paul's parents recount their experiences during Paul's two earlier surgeries, one at birth and one at age 5. While the surgery at birth was lifesaving, the surgery at age 5 was more problematic.

Paul had many symptoms at age 4, similar to the ones that he has currently. Paul's parents indicated that they did not want Paul to have surgery then, but the doctors insisted. They had only been back in Canada for about a year and felt unfamiliar with the health system and the doctors. Paul's parents still harbor anger and frustration at what happened. During the surgery, Paul's heart stopped for several minutes. Though he was brought back to life, the doctors said he might have brain damage from the incident. In fact, that appears to be the case, because neuropsychological testing when Paul was 8 led to a diagnosis of a learning disability with weaknesses in nonverbal processing skills. Attentional difficulties are also present. The presumption is that these deficits are related to his surgical event. Ever since then, Paul's parents have not trusted doctors and have been set against further surgery.

Paul's parents indicate that they like Dr. Davis, think she is a good doctor, and want to continue to work with her. They, however, do not want to be forced into doing things for Paul with which they do not agree. Currently, they are feeling her pressure.

Rachel talks with Paul's parents about other experiences that they have personally had with health professionals and more about other care that Paul and they have received (see Exhibit 10.2; Appendix F, follow-up questions for Question 4). Rachel notes the following:

Notes
- All clinical contact notes from the cardiologist are sent to Paul's pediatrician in the community and vice versa; emergency room notes do not always reach Dr. Davis
- Paul adheres to heart medications at insistence of parents but does not use oxygen (due to anxiety, according to parents); parents support no oxygen use
- Paul also seeing naturopath who has little communication with other providers; herbal remedies for heart problems; naturopath suspicious of interventions recommended by mainstream health professionals; suggests that "high arsenic levels" from his blood tests contribute to Paul's clinical symptoms; herbal remedies for this
- Paul sees pediatrician for stomach complaints, headaches; no food allergy testing
- No mental health intervention for Paul since it may mean that he would be told of the seriousness of his heart disease; Paul's anxiety is "understandable" given his heart problems according to his parents
- Paul's mother sees many different doctors for pain; complains about their noncooperation with her medication and disability application needs

- Paul's father describes anxiety symptoms but has not been treated; back problems stable

Rachel confirms that the Canadian health system has been working well for Paul and his parents (see Exhibit 10.2; Appendix F, Question 5). They have had no difficulty in getting needed medical services from Dr. Davis, other than long waits between appointments. Payment for care is covered by their provincial health insurance plan. Travel to and from Dr. Davis's appointments at Children's Hospital, however, is expensive, time consuming, and difficult to arrange since they have only one car. This is one of the reasons they use the local emergency room so often. It does not help that Paul's father has to miss work. Medications are also expensive.

Paul's parents consider themselves lucky to have found a pediatrician, naturopath, cardiologist, and social worker whom they like since they have no real choice in selection of Paul's providers. They like all of these professionals. Their experience with the emergency room doctors and the cardiac surgeon, on the other hand, have been less satisfactory.

There is a waiting list for procedures, such as cardiac catheterization, and for inpatient beds for elective services. If heart surgery should be recommended, Dr. Davis tells Paul's parents that Paul's condition is getting serious enough that she should be able to get Paul in quickly, but there are no guarantees. Knowing this is both comforting and disconcerting for Paul's parents.

Rachel has now been with Paul's parents for nearly an hour. She has taken her time during the assessment, making sure that she has answered Paul's parents' questions to their satisfaction. It is apparent that they have little medical sophistication despite a long history of interaction with Paul's heart specialists. She now feels more comfortable in asking Paul's parents to describe Paul, as a person: "What kind of person is Paul?" (see Exhibit 10.2; Appendix F, Question 6). She already has an appreciation for what the parents are like from her conversation with them; however, she pursues additional and somewhat sensitive questions (**Exhibit 14.2**).

EXHIBIT 14.2   Personal Questions About Paul and His Parents

- "How does Paul get through difficult situations?"
- "How would each of you describe yourself?"
- "How is your marriage?"
- "Do either of you or Paul smoke?"
- "Do either of you use alcohol or recreational drugs?"
- "Do you use prescription medications, such as pain medications, more than recommended?"
- "Do you think that Paul or his sister use alcohol or drugs?"

Notes

- Parents see Paul as caring and good natured but shy, stoic, sensitive, and withdrawn with few friends; lonely and bored because of lack of activities; difficult to read how he is feeling
- Paul relies on parents and sister when health and other difficulties occur; lets others take over
- Parents see themselves as caring parents appropriately protective of their sick child; rely on each other when crises occur; little friend or extended family involvement
- Marriage rocky, with disagreements and fights, mainly due to finances and Paul's health needs; no plans for divorce or separation
- No smoking or drinking in the entire household; Paul's mother uses many pills; often has to go to multiple doctors to get enough pills for pain

Rachel ended the interview with her usual final question: "Are there things that I didn't ask you that you think are important?" Both parents say that the assessment was very thorough but that they are not sure how the discussion will alter Paul's care or outcomes. Rachel reinforces that she is trying to uncover the things that make it difficult for Paul to get better. When the assessment is complete (i.e., after she has input from Paul), she will summarize what she has found out with them. They, together, will develop goals and actions that may be of assistance to Paul. Paul's parents are satisfied with this explanation and indicate that they do not have additional information to share.

Rachel asks if it is okay to visit with Paul now. She explains that she will discuss a number of the same questions with Paul that she has discussed with them. For part of the interview, both the parents and Paul will be present. For part, Rachel will speak to Paul alone. She explains that it is important for Paul to have an opportunity to talk with her alone. This will help her determine if there were things that he feels uncomfortable discussing when they are present. The parents look at each other and say in unison that it is all right. Paul's mother retrieves Paul from the waiting room.

INTERVIEW WITH PAUL AND HIS PARENTS

Paul's parents tell Paul about their conversation with Rachel and how she is going to try to help them with his health. To further clarify the situation for Paul, Rachel asks the parents to describe what they thought was important from their discussion thus far. This will allow them to indicate the areas of content that they are comfortable discussing as well as help Rachel understand the message that they have received during the dialogue and the general information that they have remembered.

Paul's father recounts that they have talked about the family's personal and living situation, the doctors that Paul is seeing, and the treatments that Paul receives from Dr. Davis. He also indicates that there was discussion about Paul's school situation and the limits that he is experiencing related to physical activity. Paul's mother also mentions that she has discussed a concern about Paul's reaction to doctors and all the tests that he has to go through.

Rachel accepts these summary comments and says that she would now like to have a better understanding about some of the same issues but from Paul's perspective. Before asking him questions, however, she wants him to know how she will handle the things that he tells her. At this point, she reiterates what she has told Paul's parents about her professional reporting requirements and the degree to which what Paul tells her will be kept confidential. Both Paul's parents and Paul now have a clear understanding of privacy rules and limits. Paul is also told that Rachel will ask some questions while both he and his parents are present and some when she and Paul talk alone.

After breaking the ice with questions about Paul's likes and dislikes (e.g., computer games, television programs, music genres, etc.), Rachel covers many of the same content areas that she has with Paul's parents. She starts with Paul's personal and family life, including his perception of the things that keep him from going to school, making friendships, and doing things with others. This is followed by questions about his perception of his past and current health and his emotional reaction to his personal limitations and the health care he is receiving. Rachel follows this with questions about how he gets along with his doctors and the treatments that they are giving him. When this is discussed, Paul talks a bit about his visits to the emergency room and how scared these incidents made him. He really did feel that he was going to die when his parents took him to the emergency room.

Rachel records the following.

Notes

- Likes action (Harry Potter) and sports (NBA) video games; favorite television program, *Friends, Seinfeld*; "independent rock" music
- Any exercise makes him weak, short of breath, tired; misses doing things
- Confirms parent's information about living situation and interaction with sister; gets along with parents (not much said)
- Sorry that he is not attending school but knows that he could not make it through a full day because of his fatigue, exercise intolerance, and shortness of breath; would like to do band and computer club;

cannot get into studying at home due to fatigue; nervous around peers at school

- Never had a chance to make friends at school since starting middle school; childhood friends at other schools
- Parents monitor adherence to heart medications; few discussions about the type of heart problem he has but knows that his parents take it seriously; likes Dr. Davis but misses some appointments for unknown reasons; aware of prior surgery but knows little of what was done
- Admits to worries about being suffocated if the oxygen mask is used at night; anxious, like mom, in new situations and when having to come to the hospital for his appointments
- (Rachel notes Paul's appearance during the interview) rapid breathing, slow to do things, finger clubbing, bluish/purple lips and fingers

During the initial conversation with Paul and his parents, Paul demonstrates considerable anxiety. His answers are short or delayed so that his parents will try to fill the silence. Rachel emphasizes the need to find out Paul's feelings and impressions of his situation and thus directs the questions back to Paul. After a short while, Paul becomes more responsive and eventually shares spontaneous answers to Rachel's questions resulting in the preceding notes.

Paul's interview in the presence of his parents takes much less time than the interview with his parents since he is unaware, as a 13-year-old, of many factors related to his family and health (e.g., the family's financial situation, his parents' social support system, historical information about his and his parents' health, etc.). Within 20 minutes, Rachel is ready to talk with Paul in an independent conversation. She asks the parents if it will be okay if they step out while she and Paul spend a couple of minutes together. They agree.

By now, Paul is more comfortable with Rachel; nevertheless, she indicates that she realizes that he may be a little nervous talking with her alone. She notes that most kids his age would be. Paul says that he is, but then goes on to talk with Rachel about the closeness of his family, how he spends his days, what he would like to do in the future if he wasn't hampered by a heart problem, and his concerns that he will never get better.

Paul tells Rachel that he knows more about his heart disease than his parents think. He has heard Dr. Davis talk about the kind of heart abnormality that he has. With the help of Dalisay, he has looked it up on the Internet and read about it. He knows that surgery was important in correcting symptoms but his parents never want to talk about it. He also says that whenever he tries to talk about it, his mother becomes very

nervous and starts talking about how pushy and self-centered doctors are. He feels that his parents are over-protective of him.

Rachel is able to document the following during her discussion with Paul.

Notes
- Lonely at home without friends but loves all of family; does not know how to act with others, withdraws
- Wants to return to school but does not know how he would be able to do so with his current symptoms; trouble concentrating; fatigues easily; is concerned that he is so far behind
- Nervous about using oxygen at night but mainly because his mother and father are; does not like needles and unusual tests; new doctors scare him
- Is aware that surgery would likely be necessary for him to feel better and get back to more normal life after researching his problem with Dalisay
- No alcohol or drug use
- Symptom scale score compatible with moderate anxiety

Rachel is impressed with the candor with which Paul has shared his thoughts with her. She has had just as many patients who have been much more guarded in what they say, particularly when there are mental health symptoms present, such as anxiety. Rachel indicates that she has asked all of the questions that she has but wonders if there are things that Paul thinks are important that they have not discussed. It looks like Paul wanted to add something but then thinks better of it. He says "no." At this point, Rachel asks that Paul's parents join Paul and her so that she can summarize her conversation with them to make sure that she has understood correctly what their situation is. She then wants to ask them one last, but important, question.

Speaking to Paul's parents, Rachel shares, "From our conversation, it is clear how much you both care about your son and want to make sure that you are making the best decisions for him regarding his health care. You have been through some very difficult experiences related to Paul's past heart surgeries, which worry you. For this reason, I see that you want to make sure that things go well in the future."

Rachel now looks at both Paul and Paul's parents. "Both Paul and the two of you recognize that Paul's health is creating some real problems for him. He frequently has to go to the emergency room at the hospital to stabilize symptoms. The level of symptoms he experiences, such as feeling drained all the time, having trouble sleeping, experiencing headaches and always being short of breath, prevents him from doing things that normal 13-year-olds do, such as going to school, participating in school and extracurricular activities, and getting out and just having fun with friends. Both of you indicate that he was able to do much more prior to this year. Importantly, Paul seems to be getting worse on his current medications.

Another thing that seems to be influencing Paul's situation are emotional factors. For instance, Paul is afraid to use oxygen at night because he worries that the mask might suffocate him. He also becomes nervous about new doctors and medical procedures. In addition, all three of you are very worried about whether Dr. Davis is giving you the right treatment. Plus, your naturopath indicates that high arsenic levels may be contributing to Paul's symptoms." Rachel pauses and then says, "Can you tell me if I am on the right track?"

Rachel has been treading a fine line. She wants to hit the high points of the assessment but knows that she cannot divulge the recommendations that Dr. Davis has been giving to Paul's parent. Nor can she tell the parents that Paul knows more about his illness than they are aware. In fact, he knows that it is likely that he will have to have heart surgery. Of course, this scares Paul, thus he just wants to leave those kinds of decisions to his parents. They will know what is best.

Paul's dad agrees with the summary that Rachel has given but is not sure that emotional factors play as large a role as Rachel has suggested. He agrees that they are worried, but "There was good reason to worry! Further, none of the heart doctors ever gave serious consideration that arsenic was a concern." Paul's mother also highlights Paul's many strengths in coping with restrictions in his life, noting his kind heart, eagerness to learn and help others, courage, and caring nature.

Rachel now tells the three of them that she is working for them. Since she is, it is important for her to know what personal goals they would like to accomplish while she helps them. She indicates that she is interested in identifying one goal related to Paul's health that they would like changed and one goal that will allow Paul to do something that he cannot do now. Rachel indicates that she would prefer the goals to be Paul's but that Paul's parents may have different ones.

The three of them talk it over and decide that they wish to pursue the following:

Clinical Goal: fewer "breathing spells." This was translated after discussion to a reduced number of trips to the emergency room. Baseline: occurrence two to three times a day; ER three times a month.

Functional Goal: "being able to get out and actually do something with Paul's childhood buddy" This was translated into the number of times out of the house with a friend. Baseline: none.

Rachel also confirms that Paul's parents' satisfaction with the health care that Paul has received could be rated as a 4 on a scale of 10, with 10 being the highest. Paul and his parents indicate that there have been no days in the past month in which it could be said that Paul had a "healthy day."

CLOSING THE COMPLEXITY ASSESSMENT

It was now time to put the information together. Rachel thanks Paul and his parents for their willingness to spend nearly two and a half hours with her. She tells them that she has many notes from their discussion. She now has to put that information together in a format in which she can start working with them on Paul's behalf. She says that this will take about a week. She does not want them to have to drive back to Children's Hospital so she asks if there is a number that she can call so that she can go over her findings and discuss what actions can be taken to improve Paul's health. They indicate that the following Tuesday in the afternoon will work.

In the meantime, Rachel asks if she can send them some information about Paul's heart condition. She indicates that she will try to find something that is written in understandable English, perhaps with pictures. Rachel also asks if it is okay for her to send information about anxiety and its treatment. Though Paul's father does not think that it is a significant problem, it won't hurt to see if there are some things that might help Paul and Paul's mom to get through this difficult time.

Between now and next Tuesday, Rachel says that she will be talking with Dr. Davis, the naturopath (to clarify the arsenic concern), and her medical director to help her give them the best assistance. With Paul's parents' permission, she will also connect with the social worker in cardiology and send for Paul's health records from before they started working with Dr. Davis and his current pediatrician. Outside information from prior doctors may help all of Paul's clinicians to better understand Paul's health problems.

Paul and Paul's parents are agreeable to all this. Rachel has much to do. She encourages Paul and his parents to make a list of Paul's medications and herbal remedies and to send a copy of the list to her. She also requests that Paul's parent have the naturopath send her a copy of his clinical notes. This way she can share them with Dr. Davis and Paul's pediatrician.

COMPLEXITY DOCUMENTATION, BASELINE RECORD OF OUTCOME MEASURES, CARE PLAN DEVELOPMENT

Based on the information provided by Paul and his parents, Rachel scores the items in the PIM-CAG

(**Table 14.1**, see page i13 for color version). Paul's total score is 52, well into the high complexity range. Not only is Paul's situation complex, but there is also growing danger to Paul with further delay in evaluation and adjustment in treatment. Dr. Davis's personal delivery of Paul's parents to Debbie's office, rather than through one of her nurses, highlights her concern. It is also evident that Paul is more aware of the nature of his cardiac condition than his parents realize.

In addition to completing the PIM-CAG, Rachel fills out the baseline record of outcome measures (**Table 14.2**) and created a draft care plan (**Table 14.3**) that will be used to discuss next steps with Paul's parents. It remains to be determined what Paul's parents (first), and then hopefully Paul, would be comfortable in pursuing as a part of Paul's care plan. Targeted items, identified in the PIM-CAG as having high complexity levels, are logical starting points. CB1, CB2, and VB triggered the referral to case management; however, the level of complexity in these areas is influenced by Paul's parents' prior experiences with doctors (HHS2). This has contributed to their inability to follow through on Dr. Davis's recommendations (CP1). Dissonance is also introduced by the naturopath's suggestion that "arsenic" may be contributing to Paul's symptoms. Neither Dr. Davis nor Paul's pediatrician are aware that this is even an issue (CHS2), though Paul's dad has mentioned it to both. Finally the role of the parents' (HS3) and Paul's (CP2) anxiety adds to their resistance. It also needs to be addressed.

Rachel agrees with Paul's parents that the issues related to school are of secondary importance in light of his current medical status; however, she notes that addressing school issues will be important for Paul's long-term development and effective functioning, as well as for his quality of life. Paul's heart condition may make school nonattendance and lack of socialization skills a nonissue if he dies or becomes permanently disabled. Correction of the school problem is directly related to Paul's health condition.

Rachel recognizes that implementing the care plan will be tricky. Part of it will entail helping Dr. Davis, Paul's pediatrician, and others involved in Paul's care understand the past experiences of Paul's parents and the effect of those experiences on the parents' decision making. She will also need to clarify the issue related to the arsenic. After talking with her medical director, it does not appear that arsenic intoxication, acute or chronic, would lead to the level of fatigue symptoms that Paul is experiencing; however, Rachel needs to confirm the levels and the naturopath's interpretation of them. Rachel's medical director will talk with him the first of next week if Paul's pediatrician cannot. Perhaps the greatest challenge, however, will be in attempting to help Paul and Paul's mother initiate treatment for anxiety.

Rachel sends a copy of Paul's PIM-CAG, instructions on how to interpret the PIM-CAG, and information about Paul's heart condition and anxiety to Paul's parents' home address. She sends them by express post. Rachel wants them to have time to look at the information before their scheduled phone call.

CASE MANAGEMENT

CASE MANAGEMENT PROCESS

Rachel calls at the appointment time. Paul's mother answers and Paul's father picks up an extension. They sound cold and upset as they exchange pleasantries. The parents indicate that Paul will not be in on the conversation. Rachel has expected this. Rachel asks if they have received the materials that she has sent. They have, but they state that they have spent so much time trying to figure out Paul's PIM-CAG that they didn't have time to read about Paul's heart condition or anxiety. Of the two, Paul's mom is audibly more upset.

Paul's mother is overwhelmed by the scored PIM-CAG. It has so many red and orange bars. Further, as she says, it is too confusing, inaccurate, and personally disparaging. It is as if Paul's mother has only seen the caregiver/parent health and function item (HS3), which is red ("bad" according to her) and that the notes talked about her anxiety. She perceives this as a personal indictment.

Rachel had suspected that this item might become a focus of discussion. She also knows that it is one creating a major challenge to Paul's health. While she would have preferred to discuss several other issues first, it is time to listen, to remain nonjudgmental, and to "roll with resistance," as motivational interviewing language calls it. When (and if) the time comes, Rachel can share her message—that is, that she feels it is important to decrease the family's emotional suffering so that it does not interfere with the added stress related to addressing the needs of a child with a serious health problem.

Paul's father is a bit more balanced in his reaction to the PIM-CAG but he too is confused about how it will lead to a plan to help Paul. This is Rachel's cue to open the discussion about how the PIM-CAG works and what the scores related to Paul's situation mean. She starts with the seriousness of Paul's cardiac condition (i.e., CB1, CB2, and VB) and how the red scores indicate a need for them to work together to alter these barriers to Paul's improvement. Only by doing so will Paul's breathing spells improve and will he be able to play with friends (their personal clinical and functional goals for Paul).

Rachel explains that this means that the three of them need to better understand how Paul's cardiac condition contributes to his fatigue and breathing

TABLE 14.1   Paul's PIM-CAG (Baseline)

Baseline	HEALTH RISKS AND HEALTH NEEDS						
Paul	**HISTORICAL**		**CURRENT STATE**		**VULNERABILITY**	
Total Score = 52	Complexity Item	Score	Complexity Item	Score	Complexity Item	Score
Biological Domain	Chronicity **HB1**	2	Symptom Severity/Impairment **CB1**	3	Complications and Life Threat **VB**	
	Diagnostic Dilemma **HB2**	1	Diagnostic/Therapeutic Challenge **CB2**	3		
Psychological Domain	Barriers to Coping **HP1**	2	Resistance to Treatment **CP1**	3	Learning and/or Mental Health Threat **VP**	2
	Mental Health History **HP2**	2	Mental Health Symptoms **CP2**	2		
	Cognitive Development **HP3**	1				
	Adverse Developmental Events **HP4**	2				
Social Domain	School Functioning **HS1**	3	Residential Stability **CS1**	1	Family/School/Social System Vulnerability **VS**	2
	Family and Social Relationships **HS2**	2	Child/Youth Support **CS2**	0		
	Caregiver/Parent Health and Function **HS3**	3	Caregiver/Family Support **CS3**	2		
			School and Community Participation **CS4**	3		
Health System Domain	Access to Care **HHS1**	0	Getting Needed Services **CHS1**	2	Health System Impediments **VHS**	
	Treatment Experience **HHS2**	3	Coordination of Care **CHS2**	2		

Comments	
HB1	Congenital heart disease (truncus arteriosis) with multiple complications
HB2	Known congenital heart defect with symptoms consistent with cardiac compromise; some uncertainty about current hemodynamic status
CB1	Fatigue and shortness of breath, dizziness, discoloration of extremities, abdominal pain, all of which impact functioning significantly
CB2	Need for invasive tests to clarify current medical status to facilitate decision-making, Paul's and parents' anxiety about procedures interfere with this, difficulty complying with assessments and treatments (nocturnal oxygen supplementation)
VB	Imminent risk of cardiac failure (event) with status quo, high risk associated with possible future interventions, such as surgery or heart transplant
HP1	Anxiety; withdrawal/avoidance and dependency on parents
HP2	Presumed long-standing anxiety disorder though never formally evaluated or treated
HP3	Documented learning disability; no recent assessment to document change in cognitive functioning
HP4	Complications during surgery in first year of life, cardiac arrest—near death experience
CP1	Paul's and parents' anxiety and parents' mistrust of doctors interfere with adherence to assessment and intervention recommendations
CP2	Significant symptoms of anxiety, easily overwhelmed
VP	Risk of persistent or worsening anxiety, decreased functioning, and further cognitive effects from medical condition

(Continued)

TABLE 14.1   Paul's PIM-CAG (Baseline) (Continued)

HS1	Good school adjustment until past year; in past year essentially non-attendance; no completed courses; minimal peer contact
HS2	Positive family relationships, very limited peer relationships
HS3	Mother on long-term leave due to chronic coping difficulties/anxiety, father anxious but never evaluated or treated; provide parental support for Paul but find it difficult to take next steps related to heart condition
CS1	Stable housing, able to meet Paul's needs
CS2	Good support from parents and sibling
CS3	Quite isolated family; few supports in the region
CS4	School non-attendance in past month, no community activities
VS	Risk of increased social isolation and school non-attendance; change needed
HHS1	No access difficulties
HHS2	Distrust of health professionals due to Paul's early traumatic health complications; anxiety/avoidance with regard to medical interventions
CHS1	Frequent cancellations of some appointments due to transportation difficulties, Paul's health (too tired); no mental health intervention despite need
CHS2	Generally good coordination and communication of pediatrician and cardiologist; conflicting alternative medicine provider; recommendations to cardiologist and family physician; no mental health intervention for parents or Paul
VHS	Significant risk of poor outcome unless consensus reached about needed care and distrust of doctors is resolved/addressed

TABLE 14.2   Paul's Record of Outcome Measures (Baseline ROM)

OUTCOME MEASURES		BASELINE	FOLLOW-UP ASSESSMENT		
	Time period recorded	Week 1			
Clinical measure (personal goal) *Breathing spell #*		2–3/day			
Functional measure (personal goal) *Out of house with friends*		0			
Health-related quality of life *Number of days healthy/month*		0			
Patient satisfaction *(Scale: 0 low, 10 high)*		4			
CAG score *(Total for period)*		52			
Health care clinical measure *Percent O_2 saturation*		86%			
Health care clinical measure *Anxiety scale score*		32 (high)			
Health care functional measure *Level of function (scale 0–10)*		3			
Health care functional measure *Number of school days missed in last month*		all			
Health care economic measure *Number of emergency room visits*		3/month			

TABLE 14.3   Paul's Care Plan Development (Baseline CD)*

BARRIERS		GOALS		ACTIONS
CAG items		Personal followed by health care		Prioritized
HHS2, CP1	Short-term	Understanding of Paul's parents' concerns by Dr. Davis		1. Set up dialogue between Paul's parents and Dr. Davis (and pediatrician) so Paul's parents can tell about their experience before Paul's last surgery 2. Discuss options considered viable by Paul's parents in working with Dr. Davis 3. Allow Dr. Davis to express her concerns about Paul's condition (connect with educational session below)
	Ultimate	Collaboration between Paul's parents and Dr. Davis		1. LISTEN TO CONSENSUS RECOMMENDATIONS ABOUT PAUL'S CARE BY PROVIDERS 2. WORK WITH PAUL'S PARENTS TO IMPLEMENT INTERVENTIONS
CP2, HS3	Short-term	Facilitate referral for anxiety in Paul and his mom (this is touchy and may require Paul's pediatrician's input)		1. Discuss concerns about role of anxiety in decision making (motivational interviewing techniques) 2. Check options considered viable by Paul's parents for treatment of Paul and Paul's mom (and dad?); connect to support for getting through Paul's cardiac needs 3. Ask pediatrician to assist in referral to mental health specialist
	Ultimate	Control of anxiety		1. Ensure initiation of treatment by mental health clinician for mom and Paul 2. Monitor adherence and symptoms 3. Confirm symptom improvement/resolution
CB1, CB2, VB, CHS2	Short-term	Paul's parents (and Paul) understand Paul's health condition and its relation to symptoms		1. CLARIFY PAUL'S PARENTS' UNDERSTANDING OF BREATHING SYMPTOMS AND HEART PROBLEM 2. DETERMINE ROLE OF ARSENIC IN PAUL'S SYMPTOMS; TALK WITH NATUROPATH 3. DISCUSS HEART DISEASE AND POTENTIAL ARSENIC TOXICITY IN CONFERENCE CALL WITH STAKEHOLDERS AND PAUL'S PARENTS
	Ultimate	Coordinated heart disease and anxiety treatment		1. LISTEN TO CONSENSUS RECOMMENDATIONS ABOUT PAUL'S CARE BY PROVIDERS 2. WORK WITH PAUL'S PARENTS TO IMPLEMENT INTERVENTIONS 3. ENSURE ADHERENCE TO RECOMMENDATIONS
HS1, CS4	Short-term	Reinitiation of academic-level-appropriate education (start only after above three goals are being pursued)		1. Clarify parents' attitude about educational activities 2. Work with parents to review educational options with middle school; personnel initiate home school program 3. INVESTIGATE MIDDLE SCHOOL CLASSMATE AVAILABILITY TO HOME TUTOR PAUL
	Ultimate	Back to school with full participation		1. Create home schooling plan based on health and function 2. Develop school reentry plan when health issues are resolved 3. Assist Paul with the aid of school counselor and parents with resocialization at school 4. Gradually assist in participation with extracurricular activities
HS2, CS2, CS3	Short-term	Increased contact with peers		1. ORGANIZE VISIT OF FRIEND THROUGH PARENTS 2. INVESTIGATE TUTORING BY CLASSMATES
	Ultimate	Age-appropriate peer interaction		WHEN HEALTH ALLOWS, PARTICIPATION IN SCHOOL AND NON-SCHOOL AGE-APPROPRIATE EXTRACURRICULAR ACTIVITIES

*Actions directly linked to Paul's personal goals are in small caps.

problems and what Paul and they can do to address these symptoms. As a part of this plan, Rachel explains that it is important to include a better understanding of the reported high arsenic levels since there is poor communication among Paul's doctors (CHS2) as well as of Paul's known congenital health condition. The first order of business is to really comprehend Paul's health situation. She asks how they might do this. After some discussion, they agree to have Rachel's medical director talk with the naturopath and to set up an appointment to have Dr. Davis go over in detail the material she has given to Rachel to give to Paul's parents. Rachel indicates that she will follow through on their decisions.

As a part of this process, Rachel indicates that she scored the "Treatment Experience" item (HHS2) as red because she thinks that Dr. Davis and Paul's pediatrician need to know the problems that the parents have experienced in the past related to Paul's care. From her perspective, this is another barrier to Paul's improvement. If the parents cannot trust Paul's doctors, how can they feel comfortable about making a decision in favor of what the doctors suggest? Rachel feels that it will be helpful for the parents to tell their story of mistrust and the difficulties experienced during Paul's last surgery to his current doctors. Both Paul's mother and father are reluctant but say they will talk it over.

Finally, Rachel mentions that though Paul's "Mental Health Symptoms" (CP2) are only scored as orange because the level of anxiety-type symptoms are insufficient to fall into the red category. Nevertheless, Paul's anxiety is affecting his ability to undergo even less-invasive treatments, such as using oxygen at night. Rachel wants to open discussion about the potential to help Paul with his anxiety as a way of improving his capacity to cope with his medical care. After some discussion, Paul's parents see the rationality of this and say that they will talk with Paul's pediatrician about potential treatment. Since Paul is seriously medically ill, Rachel suggests that it may be good to consider involvement of a mental health professional through referral by the pediatrician to make sure that Paul gets the best and least risky treatment. Rachel says, "Therapy may be better than medication with Paul's heart condition. Doctors who deal with anxiety more often, such as a child psychiatrist and child psychologist, may have more options and better suggestions." Rachel asks if she can share the PIM-CAG with the pediatrician and Dr. Davis. Paul's parents agree.

While Rachel would have liked to return to address the mother's anxiety (HS3), she senses that that discussion is best pursued at another time. If she is able to help Paul get mental health support, perhaps in the process, working through the pediatrician and Dr. Davis, treatment for the mother can be initiated as well. She will have her medical director talk with

Dr. Davis and the pediatrician after they have seen the PIM-CAG for Paul.

Rachel recaps the initial discussion with Paul's parents. She notes that they have not completed the discussion of other areas of concern (i.e., red and orange items) on the PIM-CAG; however, they cannot do everything at once. The most important issue right now is reversing Paul's current physical symptoms. Once that is underway they will start with other items of concern on the PIM-CAG, such as helping Paul get together with friends and return to school. Rachel emphasizes that during the entire process the parents and Paul will be in control. The three of them can switch directions or change priorities.

Paul's parents and Rachel review their assignments. Rachel will request clinical notes from the naturopath's office, have her medical director talk with the naturopath about the actual arsenic levels, and set up a discussion with the pediatrician and Dr. Davis. She says that she will send a copy of Paul's PIM-CAG with scoring instructions to the pediatrician and Dr. Davis. She will follow this with a call about what the results of the PIM-CAG mean. Paul's parents are asked to send a copy of all Paul's medications, including those from the naturopath, and to review the information on Paul's heart disease in preparation for the discussion with Dr. Davis or her staff. They are also encouraged to make an appointment with Paul's pediatrician so that a referral to a mental health specialist can be made. The sooner that this happens, the sooner it will be possible for Paul to feel comfortable using the oxygen he requires during the night.

Paul's parents and Rachel indicate that they will connect by phone later in the week to update progress on their respective assignments. Rachel suggests that Paul's parents keep Paul in the loop about what they will be doing on his behalf. Paul is 13 and inquisitive, Rachel notes. She suggests that he may be more interested in what is going on than his parents realize. The conversation ends on a positive note, with the parents being much more engaged in and open to the ongoing case management process.

Over the next several weeks, Rachel is busy with a number of the assignments related to Paul. She has intermittent conversations with Paul's parents and Paul's doctors. After she sends Paul's PIM-CAG to Dr. Davis and Paul's pediatrician along with instructions about how to interpret the score and grid, she sets up a conference call between them and her medical director. Included with the PIM-CAG are the office visit notes of Paul's naturopath. In the conference call, Rachel's medical director briefly explains the concept, use, and scoring of the complexity grid, using Paul's CAG as an example of how it is scored. Both doctors pick up on the concept and scoring quickly since they are already very familiar with Paul and the challenges they have faced in taking care of him.

During the conference call, both doctors express the frustrations they have experienced in working with Paul and his parents. Both also express the need to move forward relatively quickly with his care. Rachel and Rachel's medical director indicate that they consider reconciling the dissonance related to naturopathic treatment and the treatment of anxiety in the mother and Paul as key ingredients on the path to intervention for Paul's heart condition. Rachel shares that Paul's parents like the pediatrician and Dr. Davis but do not trust doctors in general. She requests that they consider allowing Paul's parents to tell them about their experience before and during Paul's surgery at age 5. Both agree to do this at the time of the educational session with Paul's parents. Rachel hopes that Paul's parents will agree to share the story. Paul's pediatrician indicates that he will conference in on the meeting that will take place at Children's Hospital.

In the meantime, the pediatrician indicates that he knows the naturopath and will talk with him about the arsenic levels and the homeopathic dilutions that he is administering to Paul. The naturopath has suggested chelation therapy, but, as with cardiac catheterization, Paul's parents have refused since it seems risky for Paul. The pediatrician also knows of a child psychologist who might be able to fit Paul into her schedule relatively soon. The pediatrician will talk about this with Paul's parents at a clinic visit early next week. Since the difficulties of Paul's mother are also a part of the PIM-CAG report, he will also be able to gingerly explore family problems with anxiety and treatments that may have been effective in the past. It is not, however, his role to suggest treatment for Paul's mother.

The meeting between Paul's parents, Rachel, and Dr. Davis occurs 3 weeks after completion of the PIM-CAG in Dr. Davis's office. Paul's pediatrician is present for the first half hour by conference phone. During this period, Paul's parents talk about difficulties related to Paul's surgery at age 5. Following this there is a dialogue between Dr. Davis and Paul's parents about the best way that they can work together, given their bad experience with doctors. Just airing the problem eases tensions.

The pediatrician indicates that Paul's first visit with the child psychologist has been last week and shares that his understanding after a conversation with the naturopath is that the naturopath has not intended to convey that Paul's overwhelming fatigue and breathing difficulties are related to arsenic and that he will support the treatment of Paul's heart condition proposed by the cardiology team if it is needed. Paul's parents are encouraged to confirm this with the naturopath.

The pediatrician signs off the call after the first half hour since he already knows about the type of cardiac difficulty that Paul has. During the second half hour, Dr. Davis does a splendid job of describing Paul's heart condition, using pictures to illustrate the back up of blood that is likely causing Paul's fatigue and breathing difficulty. She shares the stepwise procedures that are typically needed to correct the problem and why catheterization and surgery are commonly necessary. The educational session is very difficult for Paul's mom, who continues to argue that Paul's heart condition is not "as bad as all that." Nonetheless, both parents cannot remember anyone taking the time to describe Paul's condition in such detail. Both appreciate it but neither is ready to move to the next step (i.e., catheterization). They need time to think.

Finally, Dr. Davis indicates to them that the oxygen that has been recommended provides more than symptom relief. It also delays the progression of damage to Paul's heart by decreasing the stress placed on it. She encourages them to work with Paul's therapist to help Paul feel more comfortable with the nighttime oxygen. If needed, Dr. Davis is sure that Paul's pediatrician will be willing to help them find a mask that is not too confining for Paul. They can even start with nasal prongs and work up.

This is all very difficult for Paul's mother. Things are moving too fast. She does not feel in control but she now knows that Paul's condition is serious and that he will likely need surgery. She confirms that the naturopath has talked with the pediatrician. While he does not generally agree with exclusive traditional medical care, he is in agreement that Paul's heart condition is likely the cause of most of Paul's symptoms. He still recommends the preparations that he has been giving them but does not think that they will solve all of Paul's problems.

At Paul's father's suggestion, Paul's mother seeks additional assistance for her anxiety from her general practitioner at this "time of stress." During one of the now numerous telephone calls between Paul's parents and Rachel, Paul's mother mentions that she has been placed back on medication for anxiety. Since Paul's mother's anxiety is still prominent, Rachel asks whether she has considered seeing a psychiatrist and psychologist to get better symptom control and to obtain psychotherapeutic support in order to decrease her discomfort. Paul's mother indicates that she will talk with her family doctor about it.

FOLLOW-UP AND MEASUREMENT

By 6 weeks, Paul is using supplemental oxygen at night. While it does not change his overall health, it retards progression of his heart damage and makes his breathing difficulties at night more bearable. The nighttime visits to the emergency room have stopped, but symptom control is still difficult during the day. As a result, the pediatrician and Dr. Davis have obtained agreement to schedule a catheterization for Paul. As a part of the approval process, they have discussed that surgery will likely be considered the only option to alleviate Paul's symptoms and impairment. With both Paul and Paul's mother receiving treatment for their anxiety, it is easier for them to accept.

Paul confesses to his mother and father that he and Dalisay had looked up information about Paul's heart condition on the Internet when he was told by them that they were seriously considering a heart catheterization for him. They are surprised by his industriousness and secrecy. Once this cat is out of the bag, it makes it easier for Rachel to work with both Paul and his parents as they deal with the seriousness of the procedure and the potential for follow-up surgery. Paul's mother is back on antianxiety medication, and both she and Paul are receiving psychotherapy. While it is a difficult time, both are managing.

Now that the trust issues between Paul's parents and his doctors have substantially improved and the dissonance created by the naturopath has been resolved, it is possible for Rachel to turn her attention to other complexity items uncovered by the PIM-CAG. In a sense, doing so distracts Paul and his family from ruminating about the upcoming procedures and their potential consequences. Further, it allows them to focus on the future rather than the present.

Paul and Paul's mother visit Paul's school and meet with Paul's special education resource teacher and his homeroom teacher. They discuss what Paul has missed during his seventh-grade year and define a process through which he can begin to catch up. Paul's mother notes that Paul's symptoms continue but that steps are being taken to correct the problem. She does not want to push Paul too much but wants to have a plan for school reentry when he starts to feel better.

They create a step-wise reentry plan, with ongoing academic supports at school for Paul. The resource teacher also indicates that there is a group of students in his class that has volunteered to help classmates who are unable to attend school because of illness. Paul likes this idea, and indicates that he is receptive to their involvement. It is also felt that it will be helpful to have an updated assessment of Paul's learning strengths and weaknesses, in light of the ongoing progression of his cardiac condition. Rachel indicates that she will facilitate a referral for an updated neuropsychological assessment, through Paul's cardiologist, as he qualifies for this service at the Children's Hospital because of his chronic medical condition.

It is not possible to alter Paul's level of activity until after his catheterization and surgery. The catheterization is performed 8 weeks after Rachel started working with Paul, and the surgery is performed a week

after that. Recovery from surgery, unlike at age 5, is uneventful but it is helpful for Paul's mom to have a therapist, Rachel, and the professionals on the cardiology team to support her through the ordeal.

Convalescence from the surgery takes about 2 months. During that time, Paul receives home-based tutoring provided by the school and is making friends with a number of his classmates who have volunteered to help Paul with his lessons. This opens the door to making new friends and feeling more comfortable socially when he finally does return to his school toward the end of the school year.

Paul is amazed at the difference the surgery makes in his ability to do things. He is told that he still has a large heart related to all the stress that it has been under but that he should be able to get back to relatively normal teenage activity. He has missed much school, thus he will need to retake some classes missed during seventh grade. He is given a slightly reduced coarse load, with resource periods integrated into this, to ensure that he does not feel overwhelmed, particularly in light of his learning difficulties.

During the summer after surgery, Paul gets together with his grade school friend every other week. He has also made friends with a couple of peers who have volunteered to help him with his home study. His social life is taking on characteristics more consistent with a that of an average seventh grader. Paul is even demonstrating age-appropriate disagreements with the restrictions imposed on his social life by his parents.

STEPS TO GRADUATION

Rachel has now been working with Paul, Imee, and Ray—as they liked Rachel to call them—for 5 months. However, she has only been in contact with them once a month during the past 2 months. This was mainly a time of consolidation of gains, stabilization, and follow-through with regard to the school situation and Paul's social development.

The total score on Paul's PIM-CAG (**Table 14.4**, see page i14 for color version) is 23 at Week 22. Progress in each of the item areas has been noted on the PIM-CAG scoring sheet related to the approximate week that an item barrier has been addressed or changed (see bottom notes in **Table 14.4**). The only area in the current state that suggests a need for continued work relates to the support system for Paul's parents. Imee and Ray are not socially inclined. However, since both Paul and Dalisay are now active at school and their worries about Paul's health have decreased, they anticipate that they will now become more involved in their children's daily lives. Hopefully, this will help them establish community connections and friendships.

TABLE 14.4 Paul's Graduation PIM-CAG Using Follow-Up Scoring Rules for Historical Items (Week 22)

Week 22	HEALTH RISKS AND HEALTH NEEDS					
Paul	**HISTORICAL**		**CURRENT STATE**		**VULNERABILITY**	
Total Score = 23	Complexity Item	Score	Complexity Item	Score	Complexity Item	Score
Biological Domain	Chronicity **HB1**	2	Symptom Severity/Impairment **CB1**	1	Complications and Life Threat **VB**	1
	Diagnostic Dilemma **HB2**	1	Diagnostic/Therapeutic Challenge **CB2**	1		
Psychological Domain	Barriers to Coping **HP1**	1	Resistance to Treatment **CP1**	0	Learning and/or Mental Health Threat **VP**	1
	Mental Health History **HP2**	1	Mental Health Symptoms **CP2**	1		
	Cognitive Development **HP3**	1				
	Adverse Developmental Events **HP4**	1				
Social Domain	School Functioning **HS1**	2	Residential Stability **CS1**	1	Family/School/Social System Vulnerability **VS**	1
	Family and Social Relationships **HS2**	1	Child/Youth Support **CS2**	0		
	Caregiver/Parent Health and Function **HS3**	2	Caregiver/Family Support **CS3**	2		
			School and Community Participation **CS4**	0		
Health System Domain	Access to Care **HHS1**	0	Getting Needed Services **CHS1**	0	Health System Impediments **VHS**	0
	Treatment Experience **HHS2**	2	Coordination of Care **CHS2**	0		

Comments	
HB1	Congenital heart disease (truncus arteriosis) with multiple complications; (4 weeks: education about illness)
HB2	Known congenital heart defect with symptoms consistent with cardiac compromise; some uncertainty about current hemodynamic status; (8 weeks: cardiac catheterization)
CB1	Fatigue and shortness of breath, dizziness, discoloration of extremities, abdominal pain, all of which impact functioning significantly (4 weeks: oxygen at night; 9 weeks: cardiac surgery; 15 weeks: completion of formal cardiac rehabilitation)
CB2	Need for invasive tests to clarify current medical status to facilitate decision-making, Paul's and parents' anxiety about procedures interfere with this, difficulty complying with assessments and treatments (3 to 4 weeks: treatment of Paul's anxiety, "arsenic" problem excluded; 6 weeks: treatment of Paul's mother's anxiety, nocturnal oxygen supplementation improving breathing; 8 weeks: clarification of Paul's cardiac pathology with catheterization; 9 weeks: correction of Paul's cardiac pathology; 15 weeks: normal exercise tolerance for Paul with cautions not to overdo)
VB	Imminent risk of cardiac failure (event) with status quo, high risk associated with possible future interventions, such as surgery or heart transplant (9 weeks: correction of cardiac lesion, cooperation and participation in cardiac support by parents; 15 weeks: confirmation of surgical success with normal hemodynamics; 22 weeks: good exercise tolerance, few physical symptoms)
HP1	Anxiety; withdrawal/avoidance and dependency on parents
HP2	Presumed longstanding anxiety disorder though never formally evaluated or treated (2 weeks: education about anxiety)
HP3	Documented learning disability; no recent assessment to document change in cognitive functioning (7 weeks: repeat neuropsychological testing)
HP4	Complications during surgery in first year of life, cardiac arrest—near death experience (12 weeks: discussion with parents about supporting Paul, recognizing anoxic event at age 5 years)
CP1	Paul's and parents' anxiety and parents' mistrust of doctors interfere with adherence to assessment and intervention recommendations (2 to 4 weeks: clarification of arsenic relation to symptoms, discussion of parent experience at Paul's prior surgery; 8 weeks: close communication between parents and Dr. Davis around catheterization and surgery)

(Continued)

TABLE 14.4   **Paul's Graduation PIM-CAG Using Follow-Up Scoring Rules for Historical Items (Week 22) (Continued)**

CP2	*Significant symptoms of anxiety, easily overwhelmed (4 weeks: evaluation and treatment for anxiety with cognitive behavioral therapy; 8 weeks: significant improvement in anxiety symptoms using therapy techniques; 12 weeks: monthly CBT maintenance therapy)*
VP	*Risk of persistent or worsening anxiety, decreased functioning, and further cognitive effects from medical condition (22 weeks: evidence that maintenance is controlling anxiety symptoms)*
HS1	*Good school adjustment until past year; in past year essentially non-attendance; no completed courses; minimal peer contact (6 weeks: discussion about prior school performance)*
HS2	*Positive family relationships, very limited peer relationships (8 weeks: tutoring by peers, developing friendships; 11 to 20 weeks: increasing social activities with childhood friend and school tutors)*
HS3	*Mother on long-term leave due to chronic coping difficulties/anxiety, father anxious but never evaluated or treated; provide parental support for Paul but find it difficult to take next steps related to heart condition (5 weeks: mother restarted on antianxiety medication; 6 weeks: mother starts treatment with mental health professional; 8 to 12 weeks: mother has close therapeutic support for anxiety during Paul's catheterization, surgery, and postoperative period; 15 weeks: mother has persistent residual anxiety but is coping)*
CS1	*Stable housing, able to meet Paul's needs*
CS2	*Good support from parents and sibling (12 weeks: less reliance on parents and sister for support)*
CS3	*Quite isolated family; few supports in the region (22 weeks: still concentrate on immediate first degree family interactions, starting involvement in Paul and Dalisay's school functions)*
CS4	*School nonattendance in past month, no community activities (6 weeks: academic plan for Paul reviewed with middle school personnel; 7 to 8 weeks: tutoring by classmates at Paul's home; 11 weeks: return to school part time; 12 weeks: return to school full time; 14 to 20 weeks: remedial summer school tutoring; 21 weeks: return to full time school at "repeat" seventh grade level)*
VS	*Risk of increased social isolation and school non-attendance; change needed (22 weeks: Paul's socialization improving, mother's anxiety controlled though still present, return to full school, but held back a year)*
HHS1	*No access difficulties*
HHS2	*Distrust of health professionals due to Paul's early traumatic health complications; anxiety/avoidance with regard to medical interventions (2 weeks: doctors informed of parent trust issues; 3 to 4 weeks: discussion between doctors and Paul's parents with venting of Paul's prior health events; 7 weeks: collaboration between parents and doctors related to Paul's health condition; 15 weeks: trust by parents in current doctors)*
CHS1	*Frequent cancellations of some appointments due to transportation difficulties, Paul's health (too tired); no mental health intervention despite need (3 weeks: coordination of long range doctor visits, resolution of nathuropath dilemma; 7 weeks: improvement of doctor trust issues, better communication, decreased use of emergency room in home town)*
CHS2	*Generally good coordination and communication of pediatrician and cardiologist; conflicting alternative medicine provider; recommendations to cardiologist and family physician; no mental health intervention for parents or Paul (3 weeks: communication established among Paul's pediatrician, cardiologist, and mental health professional)*
VHS	*Significant risk of poor outcome unless consensus reached about needed care and distrust of doctors is resolved/addressed (22 weeks: trust and communication issues resolved)*

Paul's record of outcome measures (**Table 14.5**) demonstrates that positive value and change have occurred through the assistance provided by Rachel. The primary value appeared during the first 6 weeks despite the fact that the majority of drop in total score of Paul's PIM-CAG took place between week 6 and week 22. If it had not been for Rachel's involvement in resolving trust issues between Imee and Ray and Paul's doctors, the addressing of the dissonance created by the naturopath, and promoting treatment of both Paul's and Imee's anxiety, Paul's dramatic clinical and functional improvement as a result of his undergoing surgery might not have occurred. Worse, Paul could have died of progressive heart failure from the inadequate conduit placed at age 5, which was now insufficient for Paul's growth and oxygenation needs. A third possibility would have been that Dr. Davis and Paul's pediatrician would have been required to notify child protective services since the anxiety of the parents prevented them from agreeing to the medical care that Paul needed. In that situation, lifelong hostility of the parents toward the health care system might have resulted. Rachel has provided a truly important service to Paul, his parents, and Paul's doctors because Paul's prognosis for a full

TABLE 14.5   **Paul's Record of Outcome Measures (Week 22 ROM)**

OUTCOME MEASURES	BASELINE		FOLLOW-UP ASSESSMENTS	
Time period recorded	Week 1	Week 6	Week 12	Week 22
Clinical measure (personal goal) Breathing spell #	2–3/day	1-2/day	0/day	0/day
Clinical measure (personal goal) Exercise tolerance			Walks to school (5 blocks)	Jogs one mile with parent
Functional measure (personal goal) Out of house with friends	0	0	Daily	Daily
Functional measure (personal goal) School extracurricular activities				Computer club
Health-related quality of life Number of days healthy/month	0	0	25	30
Patient satisfaction (Scale: 0 low, 10 high)	4	8	9	10
CAG score (Total for period)	52	44	33	23
Health care clinical measure Percent O_2 saturation	86%	87%	96%	96%
Health care clinical measure Anxiety scale score	32	25	12	12
Health care functional measure Level of function (scale 0–10)	3	4	9	10
Health care functional measure Number of school days missed in last month	All	All	School break	0
Health care economic measure Number of emergency room visits	3/month	1/month	0	0

and unhampered life after surgical correction for his congenital heart problem is nearly 90%.

CASE MANAGEMENT GRADUATION

When Rachel started working with Paul, Imee, and Ray, Paul was essentially confined to home and nearly bedridden. Five months later he is a typical 14-year-old. He is looking forward to a new school year in which he can do things with friends, participate in computer club, and, yes, attend classes regularly. In addition to new friends at school, he has also become quite close to Rachel. This is also true for Imee and Ray. The four of them have gotten through some very difficult times and have experienced significant success. Of course, it was Paul's doctors who are the heroes, but Rachel feels pride in having contributed a small part to Paul's transformation.

Paul and his family are now ready to return to standard care. Vulnerability in all four domains has returned to 0 or 1. In fact, Rachel has probably retained Paul among her active, near-closure caseload a month longer than necessary. She will miss the chewy coconut cookies that Imee brought to her when Paul had a follow-up visits with Dr. Davis, but she knows that it is time.

The transition back to standard care is much easier with Paul than many of her other cases. By now, both Dr. Davis and Paul's pediatrician are very familiar with the PIM-CAG and outcome templates that Rachel used. They have also been actively engaged in Paul's care plan activities, so next steps are familiar to them. Finally, while Paul came to her with a chronic problem, his surgery is expected to return him to a full and active life. Rachel cannot say the same for her cystic fibrosis patients. Perhaps the hardest part of closing Paul's case is losing contact with people for whom she now cares. Nonetheless, this happens every day in her line of work. She takes consolation in knowing that each day she has opportunities to build new relationships, ones that will change lives.

Integrated Case Management Team Formation and Training

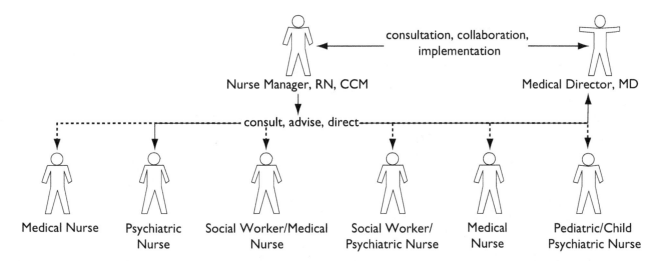

Skills
- Manager (RN, CCM)—preferably with background in general medical and mental health nursing, otherwise cross-training (CCM; certificate—integrated CM, motivational interviewing)
- Medical Director, MD—this is either a physician having comfort with assessment and treatment of physical and mental health problems or a collaborative team including a primary care physician and psychiatrist.
- Staff (CCM or working toward CCM; certificate—integrated CM with basic cross-training in the discipline from which they do not come); team size can vary by 1 or 2 either way

Cross-Training—basics started in integrated CM manual and onsite training (extra training required for child/youth integrated CM)
- Three weeks didactics in cross-discipline
- Three weeks direct mentoring in cross-discipline
- Case management vignettes
- Special integrated case management issues—legal, documentation standards, care coordination; emergency procedures (medical, psychiatric, and pediatric)

Shift Work
- During the first 4 months, there will always be staff from both disciplines available for consultation
- Team composition ratios adjusted based on clinical needs of the population served

Case Responsibility
- Full indirect, nonclinical assistance for patient needs (physical and mental condition care coordination, authorization, etc.) with advice from cross-trained teammates when needed
- Initial assignment should take into account the CM's case load composite IM-CAG or PIM-CAG-based health complexity level
- Few handoffs

Continuing Educational Enhancement
- Integrated CM grand rounds; complicated case reviews; news and views handouts on common problems, member outcomes, obstacles, successes; consultation with medical director (special arrangements for child/youth CM)

Expert Backup
- Team member collaboration
- Medical directors—general medical, psychiatric, pediatric
- Expert consultant specialists

Cross-Disciplinary Integrated Case Manager Training

Case Manager Training

All Trainees (use integrated care vignettes, e.g., diabetic crises, suicidal, medically compromised eating disorder)
- Case Management Standards (see CMSA Standards of Practice, Chapter 1 and www.cmsa.org), e.g., assessment, planning, facilitation, advocacy
- Standards of care, e.g., identification of patient's need for CM services; problem identification; planning; monitoring; evaluating; outcomes measurement; case closure
- Interpersonal skills, coping skills training
- Interviewing techniques, e.g., developing a relationship, use of open-ended questions, when and how to share personal information, motivational interviewing techniques
- Assessment of physical and mental condition insurance coverage limitations and exclusions
- Documentation processes, e.g., check sheet for opening and closing cases, use of scripts, use of computer, here and now entry
- Follow-up, e.g., how often should the patient be seen, how to work through prioritized actions
- Legal concerns, e.g., HIPAA; privacy; physical, mental health, and child/youth consents; approach to confidentiality; objective documentation techniques
- Closing cases, e.g., proper graduation processes with the patient/client; handling of medical records received, etc.
- Use of internet, e.g., educational sites and social service and community resource links

From Psychiatric Background
- General medical disorders/problems update, e.g., diabetes, hypertension, back pain, asthma, enuresis, congestive heart failure, emphysema, ischemic heart disease, dementia, head injury
- Community resources available for medically ill
- Basics on medical emergencies, medical admissions, placement, durable medical equipment procurment and use in the medical setting

From Medical Background
- General psychiatric disorders/problems update, e.g., affective disorders, anxiety, eating disorders, schizophrenia, autism, delirium, somatoform disorders, chemical dependence
- Community resources available for psychiatrically ill
- Basics on psychiatric emergencies, admissions, placement; payment issues in the psychiatric setting, levels of care (residential, partial hospitalization, intensive outpatient, etc.)

Pediatric Case Management
- Pediatric Management Practices, e.g., working with parents/caregivers and children/youth
- Cross-disciplinary updates, e.g., child psychiatry for those with medical backgrounds and medical for those with psychiatric backgrounds
- Pediatric Resources and Procedures, e.g., foster homes, abuse reporting, guardianship

Integrated Case Manager Care Plan: Triggering and Triage

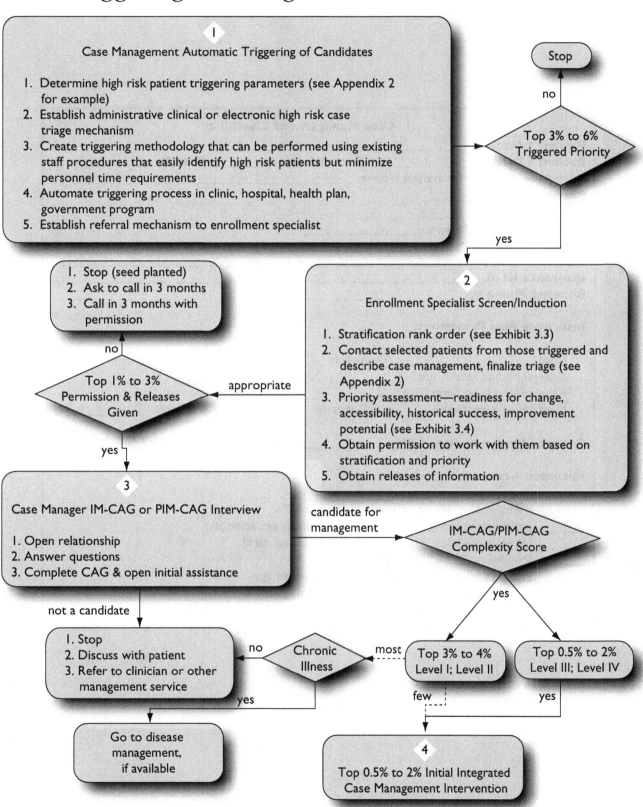

1

Case Management Automatic Triggering of Candidates

1. Determine high risk patient triggering parameters (see Appendix 2 for example)
2. Establish administrative clinical or electronic high risk case triage mechanism
3. Create triggering methodology that can be performed using existing staff procedures that easily identify high risk patients but minimize personnel time requirements
4. Automate triggering process in clinic, hospital, health plan, government program
5. Establish referral mechanism to enrollment specialist

Stop

no

Top 3% to 6% Triggered Priority

yes

2

Enrollment Specialist Screen/Induction

1. Stratification rank order (see Exhibit 3.3)
2. Contact selected patients from those triggered and describe case management, finalize triage (see Appendix 2)
3. Priority assessment—readiness for change, accessibility, historical success, improvement potential (see Exhibit 3.4)
4. Obtain permission to work with them based on stratification and priority
5. Obtain releases of information

1. Stop (seed planted)
2. Ask to call in 3 months
3. Call in 3 months with permission

no

Top 1% to 3% Permission & Releases Given

appropriate

yes

3

Case Manager IM-CAG or PIM-CAG Interview

1. Open relationship
2. Answer questions
3. Complete CAG & open initial assistance

candidate for management

IM-CAG/PIM-CAG Complexity Score

yes

not a candidate

1. Stop
2. Discuss with patient
3. Refer to clinician or other management service

no

Chronic Illness

most

Top 3% to 4% Level I; Level II

Top 0.5% to 2% Level III; Level IV

yes

few

yes

Go to disease management, if available

4

Top 0.5% to 2% Initial Integrated Case Management Intervention

Integrated Case Management Checklist

Case Management Checklist

Patient's Name: _____

Patient's DOB: _____ **Patient's Sex:** _____ **Case #** _____

Caregiver/Parent/Guardian Name: _____

Phone: _____

Email: _____

Primary Clinician Name: _____

Primary Clinician Phone: _____

Insurance Company: _____

Insurance ID #: _____

Benefits Phone #: _____

Insurance Plan Provisions:

Copay _____; Deductible _____

General Medical Health Inpatient _____; Outpatient _____

Residential or Long Term Care _____

Mental Health Inpatient _____; Outpatient _____; Day Treatment _____

Covered Licensure (e.g., LPN): _____

Initiation Activities:

_____ Verbal and written consents obtained and on file

_____ Introductory phone call to patient made (document attempts)

_____ Introductory letter to patient sent (with business card)

_____ IM-CAG or PIM-CAG completed

_____ Primary clinician(s) offices contacted by case manager

_____ Family contact information on file (if consents given)

_____ Patient added to case management log

Integrated Case Manager Care Plan: Initial and Iterative Intervention

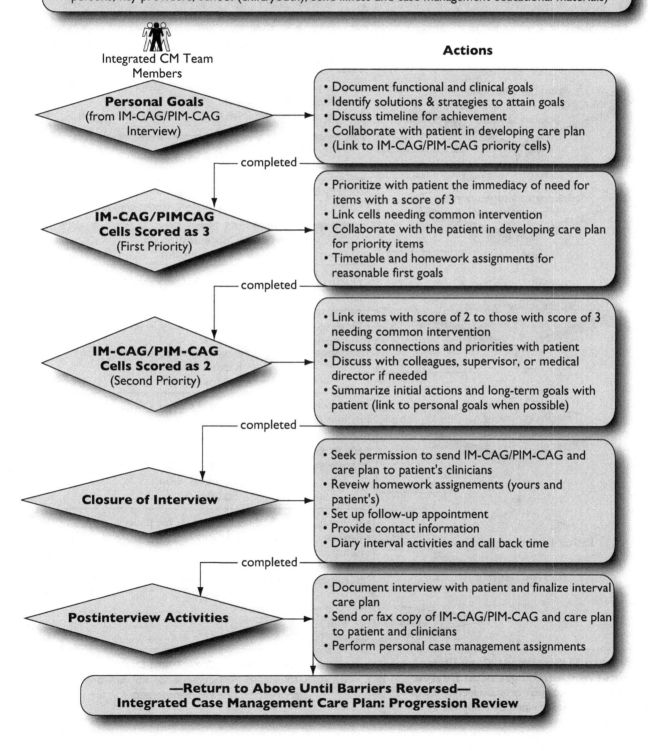

Initial & Iterative Case Management Intervention
(develop relationship and, with informed consent, share assessment results with patient, primary support persons, key providers, school (child/youth); send illness and case management educational materials)

Integrated CM Team Members

Actions

Personal Goals
(from IM-CAG/PIM-CAG Interview)

- Document functional and clinical goals
- Identify solutions & strategies to attain goals
- Discuss timeline for achievement
- Collaborate with patient in developing care plan
- (Link to IM-CAG/PIM-CAG priority cells)

completed

IM-CAG/PIMCAG Cells Scored as 3
(First Priority)

- Prioritize with patient the immediacy of need for items with a score of 3
- Link cells needing common intervention
- Collaborate with the patient in developing care plan for priority items
- Timetable and homework assignments for reasonable first goals

completed

IM-CAG/PIM-CAG Cells Scored as 2
(Second Priority)

- Link items with score of 2 to those with score of 3 needing common intervention
- Discuss connections and priorities with patient
- Discuss with colleagues, supervisor, or medical director if needed
- Summarize initial actions and long-term goals with patient (link to personal goals when possible)

completed

Closure of Interview

- Seek permission to send IM-CAG/PIM-CAG and care plan to patient's clinicians
- Reveiw homework assignements (yours and patient's)
- Set up follow-up appointment
- Provide contact information
- Diary interval activities and call back time

completed

Postinterview Activities

- Document interview with patient and finalize interval care plan
- Send or fax copy of IM-CAG/PIM-CAG and care plan to patient and clinicians
- Perform personal case management assignments

—Return to Above Until Barriers Reversed—
Integrated Case Management Care Plan: Progression Review

Integrated Case Manager Care Plan: Progression Review

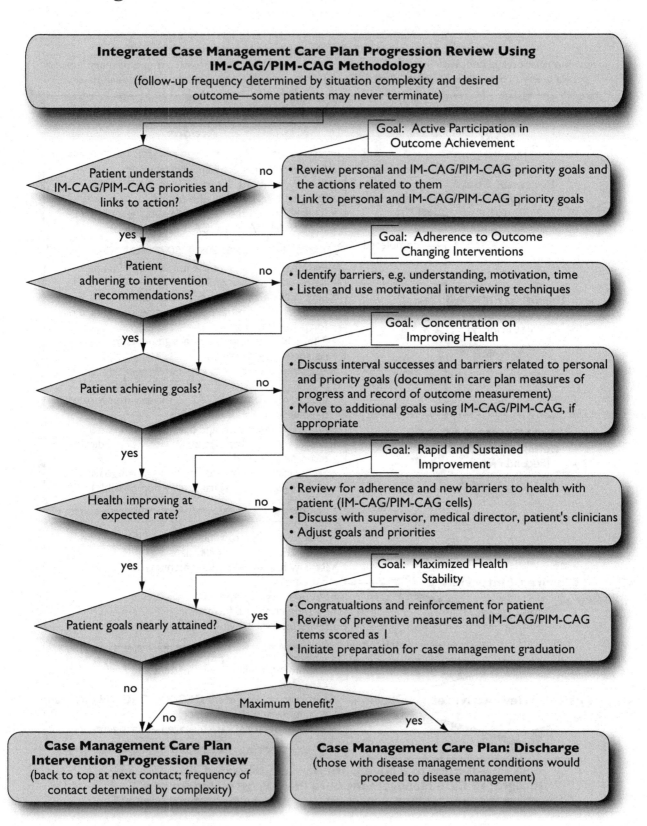

Integrated Case Manager Care Plan: Discharge

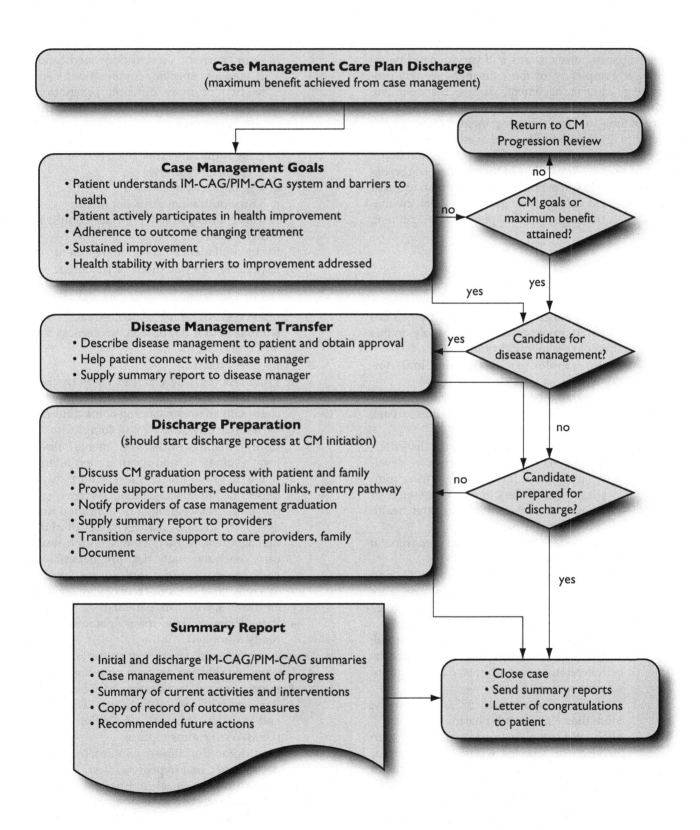

Case Management Care Plan Discharge
(maximum benefit achieved from case management)

Return to CM Progression Review

Case Management Goals
- Patient understands IM-CAG/PIM-CAG system and barriers to health
- Patient actively participates in health improvement
- Adherence to outcome changing treatment
- Sustained improvement
- Health stability with barriers to improvement addressed

no — CM goals or maximum benefit attained?

Disease Management Transfer
- Describe disease management to patient and obtain approval
- Help patient connect with disease manager
- Supply summary report to disease manager

yes — Candidate for disease management?

Discharge Preparation
(should start discharge process at CM initiation)

- Discuss CM graduation process with patient and family
- Provide support numbers, educational links, reentry pathway
- Notify providers of case management graduation
- Supply summary report to providers
- Transition service support to care providers, family
- Document

no — Candidate prepared for discharge?

Summary Report

- Initial and discharge IM-CAG/PIM-CAG summaries
- Case management measurement of progress
- Summary of current activities and interventions
- Copy of record of outcome measures
- Recommended future actions

- Close case
- Send summary reports
- Letter of congratulations to patient

Triage Guidelines with Examples of Case Management Triggers

Note: Triggering mechanisms will vary depending on the target complexity of the care management program (e.g., case management, disease management, disability management, health coaching), the availability of tools to uncover management candidates, the number of anticipated managers available to manage the population, and the goals of the organization doing the management. Regardless of these issues, triggering processes should uncover candidates for management as precisely and efficiently as possible so that the majority of case manager time is spent in management, not in triage.

I. Case management triggering: example
   A. From claims, care delivery system, and/or clinical data
   (Keep in mind claims data frequently is a *late* identifier. It is not possible to rely solely on this method of case identification.)
   1. Illness complexity with a longitudinal component
      a. General medical (e.g., migraines, brain injury, diabetes, renal failure, back pain)
      b. Mental health (e.g., eating disorders; chronic schizophrenia; pervasive developmental disorders, such as autism; somatization disorders; major depression or bipolar illness; combined mental health and substance use disorders)
      c. Concurrent *active* physical *and* mental conditions
   2. Child inpatient admission: age 12 and younger for psychiatric diagnosis, or more than three emergency room admissions (e.g., for asthma) in a 12-month period
   3. Readmissions and long stays in hospital: three inpatient admissions within 12 months or two admissions within 60 days; length of stay more than 15 days
   4. High dollar: more than $25,000 annually; more than $200/month pharmacy
   5. High utilization for outpatient: more than 20 visits or sessions within 12 months or less; more than 3 emergency room visits in 3 months
   6. Greater than:
      a. Four treating doctors in a given year
      b. Four current prescription medications (Consider specific combinations, such as two or more different psychotropic classes, medical and psychiatric drug combinations.)
      c. One drug being taken from the same class at the same time (e.g., two serotonin reuptake inhibitors)
      d. Use of three pharmacies
      e. Three outpatient visits per month
      f. Three unexplained physical complaints in 6 months
   7. Residential mental condition treatment
   8. Experimental evaluations or treatment: surgeries, total body computed tomography (CT) scans, medications, psychoanalysis, electroencephalographic neurofeedback, vagal stimulation for depression, wilderness therapy, and so forth
   B. From direct referral:
   1. Providers: already complex cases or those with strong potential, especially from clinicians with an understanding of the difference between acuity/severity and complexity
   2. Courts: distinguish between mental illness, legal evaluation, and incarceration alternative with or without medical comorbidity
   3. Other health management services (employee assistance programs, utilization management, disease management, disability management, workers' compensation, health care coaching, high risk pregnancy, etc.): early recognition of complex cases (encourage referral of chronic, recurrent, or complex employees, enrollees, patients)
   4. Patient/family: use triage parameters already described
II. Disease management triggering: example
   A. Uncovering selected diseases from claims
   1. International Classification of Disease, 9th Revision (ICD-9), ICD-10, or Diagnostic and Statistical Manual, 4th Edition Revised (DSM-IV-R) claims capture
   2. Medication for illness capture (e.g., antidepressants, oral hypoglycemics)
   3. Procedures for illness capture
   B. Uncovering selected diseases from care delivery electronic record system: ICD-9 or ICD-10

diagnostic capture, Current Procedural Terminology (CPT) coding

C. Uncovering selected diseases from direct clinician referral, such as clinic visit and hospital-based admission identification through health plan/care delivery system/clinician collaboration

III. Health coaching: example
   A. Predictive modeling tools or claims reviews
   B. Health risk assessments
   C. Other health manager referrals
   D. Clinical staff referral

IV. Other triggers, such as disability, workers' compensation, employee assistance, and so forth

Universal Consent Form*

TEMPLATE FOR CLINICAL CONSENT FORM

CLINICAL CONSENT FORM FOR *(NAME OF COMPANY)* PARTICIPANTS

I want to participate in the Integrated Case Management Program provided by representatives affiliated with the *(name of company, hospital, etc.)*. I authorize the release of my protected health information for the purposes of collaboration and consultation among my health care team for the development and implementation of an integrated case management plan focused on achieving optimal improvement and a return to a healthy productive life.

The information to be released includes the following:

☐ Physical and mental health care provider notes, records, reports
☐ Substance use disorder treatment notes
☐ Case/disease management notes
☐ Consultation reports
☐ Radiology and lab reports
☐ Other notes and reports

☐ Other
_____
_____
_____
_____
_____
_____

This information is to be released to the following:
(Check all that apply)

(Insurance Company Divisions/Subcontractors)
☐ Disease management clinicians
☐ Case management clinicians
☐ Healthy start clinicians
☐ Nurse line

Employer/Public Program Subcontractors
☐ Disability management clinicians
☐ Employee assistance program
☐ Health risk management clinicians
☐ Safety

Workers Compensation
☐ Comprehensive managed care

Health Providers
☐ Clinicians providing my care

I have been informed that:
• Information will be disclosed/requested only when necessary for collaboration and consultation relative to health care and management services.
• I have a right to request a copy of any information disclosed.
• I am not legally obligated to provide this informed authorization. However, declining to do so may hinder my health care team members from providing health services that are most likely to help me.
• I understand that the integrated case management program is voluntary and I may revoke this consent in writing at any time. This release form expires automatically one year after signing or upon termination of health services related to *(name of company, hospital, etc.)*.
• I understand that treatment and payment may not be conditioned on this authorization.
• Information disclosed may be subject to redisclosure by recipient and may no longer be protected by federal privacy laws.
• If I so choose, I may designate a representative for my health care team to work with on my behalf. I designate
_____ *(print)* as my representative _____ *(relationship to patient/client)*.

Patient's Printed First and Last Name _____

Patient Signature _____

Date _____

Date of Birth _____

Health Plan, Hospital, or Clinic Identification Number _____

Note: *This consent form was designed to be useful for numerous situations with a variety of organizations, such as hospitals, clinics, health plans, case management companies, government agencies, employee assistance programs, or other health care organizations providing health services to an individual.*

IM-CAG Scoring Sheet

See page i17 for color version.

Date	HEALTH RISKS AND HEALTH NEEDS					
Name	**HISTORICAL**		**CURRENT STATE**		**VULNERABILITY**	
Total score =	Complexity Item	Score	Complexity Item	Score	Complexity Item	Score
Biological Domain	Chronicity **HB1**		Symptom Severity/Impairment **CB1**		Complications and Life Threat **VB**	
	Diagnostic Dilemma **HB2**		Diagnostic/Therapeutic Challenge **CB2**			
Psychological Domain	Barriers to Coping **HP1**		Resistance to Treatment **CP1**		Mental Health Threat **VP**	
	Mental Health History **HP2**		Mental Health Symptoms **CP2**			
Social Domain	Job and Leisure **HS1**		Residential Stability **CS1**		Social Vulnerability **VS**	
	Relationships **HS2**		Social Support **CS2**			
Health System Domain	Access to Care **HHS1**		Getting Needed Services **CHS1**		Health System Impediments **VHS**	
	Treatment Experience **HHS2**		Coordination of Care **CHS2**			

Comments
(Enter pertinent information about the reason for the score of each complexity item here. For example, poor patient adherence, death in family with stress to patient, non-evidence-based treatment of migraine, etc.)

Scoring System

Green	0	= no vulnerability or need to act
Yellow	1	= mild vulnerability and need for monitoring or prevention
Orange	2	= moderate vulnerability and need for action or development of intervention plan
Red	3	= severe vulnerability and need for immediate action or immediate intervention plan

Biological Domain Items

HB1	Physical illness chronicity
HB2	Historic problems in diagnosing the physical illness
CB1	Physical illness symptom severity and impairment
CB2	Current difficulties in diagnosis and/or treatment
VB	Risk of physical complications and life threat if case management assistance is stopped

Psychological Domain Items

HP1	Problems handling stress and/or problem solving
HP2	Prior mental condition difficulties
CP1	Resistance to treatment; nonadherence
CP2	Current mental condition symptom severity
VP	Risk of persistent personal barriers or poor mental condition care if case management assistance is stopped

Social Domain Items

HS1	Personal productivity and leisure activities
HS2	Relationship difficulties
CS1	Residential stability or suitability
CS2	Availability of social support
VS	Risk of work, home, and relational support needs if case management assistance is stopped

Health System Domain Items

HHS1	Health system related access to appropriate care
HHS2	Experiences with doctors or the health system
CHS1	Logistical ability to get needed care at service delivery level
CHS2	Communication among providers and coordination of care
VHS	Risk of persistent poor access to and/or coordination of services if case management assistance is stopped

PIM-CAG Scoring Sheet

See page i18 for color version.

Date	HEALTH RISKS AND HEALTH NEEDS					
Name	**HISTORICAL**		**CURRENT STATE**		**VULNERABILITY**	
Total score =	Complexity Item	Score	Complexity Item	Score	Complexity Item	Score
Biological Domain	Chronicity **HB1**		Symptom Severity/Impairment **CB1**		Complications and Life Threat **VB**	
	Diagnostic Dilemma **HB2**		Diagnostic/Therapeutic Challenge **CB2**			
Psychological Domain	Barriers to Coping **HP1**		Resistance to Treatment **CP1**		Learning and/or Mental Health Threat **VP**	
	Mental Health History **HP2**		Mental Health Symptoms **CP2**			
	Cognitive Development **HP3**					
	Adverse Developmental Events **HP4**					
Social Domain	School Functioning **HS1**		Residential Stability **CS1**		Family/School/Social System Vulnerability **VS**	
	Family and Social Relationships **HS2**		Child/Youth Support **CS2**			
	Caregiver/Parent Health and Function **HS3**		Caregiver/Family Support **CS3**			
			School and Community Participation **CS4**			
Health System Domain	Access to Care **HHS1**		Getting Needed Services **CHS1**		Health System Impediments **VHS**	
	Treatment Experience **HHS2**		Coordination of Care **CHS2**			

Comments

(Enter pertinent information about the reason for the score of each complexity item here. For example, poor patient adherence, death in family with stress to child/youth, non-evidence-based treatment of celiac disease, etc.)

Scoring System

Green	0	=	no vulnerability or need to act
Yellow	1	=	mild vulnerability and need for monitoring or prevention
Orange	2	=	moderate vulnerability and need for action or development of intervention plan
Red	3	=	severe vulnerability and need for immediate action or immediate intervention plan

Biological Domain Items		**Psychological Domain Items**	
HB1	*Physical illness chronicity*	**HP1**	*Problems handling stress or engaging in problem solving*
		HP2	*Prior mental condition difficulties*
HB2	*Physical health diagnostic dilemma, prenatal exposures*	**HP3**	*Cognitive level and capabilities*
		HP4	*Early adverse physical and mental health events*
CB1	*Physical illness symptom severity and impairment*	**CP1**	*Resistance to treatment; nonadherence*
CB2	*Current difficulties in diagnosis and/or treatment*	**CP2**	*Current mental conditions symptom severity*
VB	*Risk of physical complications and life threat if case management is stopped*	**VP**	*Risk of persistent personal barriers or poor mental condition care if case management is stopped*

(Continued)

Social Domain Items		Health System Domain Items	
HS1	*Aptitude-correlated academic and social success*	**HHS1**	*Health system causes for poor access to appropriate care*
HS2	*Child/youth living environment and interactions*		
HS3	*Caregiver/parent physical and mental health condition and function*	**HHS2**	*Mistrust of doctors or the health system*
CS1	*Food and housing situation*	**CHS1**	*Ability to get and ease of getting needed services*
CS2	*Child/youth support system*		
CS3	*Caregiver/parent support system*	**CHS2**	*Coordination of and transitioning to age-appropriate care as requested*
CS4	*Attendance, achievement and behavior at school*		
VS	*Risk for home/school support or supervision needs if case management is stopped*	**VHS**	*Risk of persistent poor access to and/or coordination of services if case management is stopped*

IM-CAG Complexity Items and Anchor Points

The INTERMED-Complexity Assessment Grid (IM-CAG) evaluates complexity in adults. It provides the case manager with a rapid yet comprehensive assessment of adults presenting for health care that can be used: (a) to identify patient needs, (b) to initiate individual care plan development, and (c) to support stabilization or return patients to health through case management activities. The IM-CAG adopts a lifespan perspective in the assessment of barriers to improvement within the concept of health complexity. The instrument was developed to uncover actionable circumstances related to historical/developmental antecedents, their current life situation, and anticipated future vulnerabilities. *"Vulnerabilities" in the context of the IM-CAG specifically relates to the risk of barrier persistence and worsening domain-specific problems in the future if individualized care through case management is withdrawn.*

Instructions for scoring items:

1. Complexity is defined as the interference in standard care by biological, psychological, social, and health system factors, which require a shift from standard care to individualized care (case management) in order for patients to overcome barriers to improvement. Each complexity item (also called a "cell") on the IM-CAG is rated using four anchor points in a Likert-type scale. Each anchor point is designed to reflect a level of need, which in turn leads to specific actions to be taken by the case manager on behalf of the patient.
   Whenever a complexity item is rated, in addition to the clinical anchor points as defined later in this appendix, one should keep the following question in mind: "Will the situation recorded for this complexity item interfere with health outcomes if standard medical care is given?" Another important consideration, particularly when there is debate between two anchor point levels for an individual item (e.g., scoring a 1 vs. a 2 or a 2 vs. a 3), is to consider the immediacy of need for action on behalf of the patient. The time frame for action can inform the final decision.

2. All "Historical" complexity items refer to the last 5 years. The two exceptions are the cells labeled "Mental Health History" and "Access to Care." "Mental Health History" (HP2) relates to the patient's entire life and "Access to Care" (HHS1) relates to the preceding 6 months.

3. All "Current" complexity items refer to the 30-day period prior to the date that the IM-CAG assessment is completed.

4. All "Vulnerability" complexity items refer to the 3- to 6-month period after the date that the IM-CAG assessment is completed, based on the difference from an estimate of the natural history of the patient's health state when given standard medical care.

5. Actions corresponding to anchor point scores: 0 = no action; 1 = need for monitoring and/or prevention; 2 = need for intervention plan and action *soon*; 3 = need for *immediate* intervention plan and action

6. Several items in the complexity grid contain more than one content component that could be creating barriers to improvement (e.g., symptom severity or impairment in CB1, job or leisure problems in HS1, etc.). When scoring each item, the content component with the greatest potential for creating a barrier to improvement should direct the score, rather than the average of the item components. For instance, for "Coordination of Care" (CHS2), if there is excellent communication between a family physician and a patient's surgeon but no attempt by the family physician to find or communicate with a needed mental health specialist for the same patient, the anchor point score would be 3.

| TABLE A6.1 | INTERMED—Complexity Assessment Grid Summary Form |

ID Number _____ **Age** _____ **Gender** _____

Date	HEALTH RISKS AND HEALTH NEEDS					
Name	**HISTORICAL**		**CURRENT STATE**		**VULNERABILITY**	
Total score =	Complexity Item	Score	Complexity Item	Score	Complexity Item	Score
Biological Domain	Chronicity HB1		Symptom Severity/Impairment CB1		Complications and Life Threat VB	
	Diagnostic Dilemma HB2		Diagnostic/Therapeutic Challenge CB2			
Psychological Domain	Barriers to Coping HP1		Resistance to Treatment CP1		Mental Health Threat VP	
	Mental Health History HP2		Mental Health Symptoms CP2			
Social Domain	Job and Leisure HS1		Residential Stability CS1		Social Vulnerability VS	
	Relationships HS2		Social Support CS2			
Health System Domain	Access to Care HHS1		Getting Needed Services CHS1		Health System Impediments VHS	
	Treatment Experience HHS2		Coordination of Care CHS2			

Comments
(Enter pertinent information about the reason for the score of each complexity item here. For example, poor patient adherence, death in family with stress to patient, non-evidence-based treatment of migraine, etc.)

BIOLOGICAL DOMAIN

Items in the biological domain address how factors associated with physical conditions and their symptoms create barriers to the patient's optimal health.

In all situations except anchor point 3 for "Diagnostic/Therapeutic Complexity" (CB2), these items refer specifically to physical health issues. For CB2, anchor point 3 includes the potential for nonphysical factors, such as somatic preoccupation, a mental health contributor to physical symptoms, or cross-disciplinary (physical and mental health) treatment to contribute to complexity. This is a common source of anchor point scoring confusion.

HB1	Chronicity
0	Less than 3 months of physical symptoms/dysfunction; acute health condition
1	More than 3 months of physical symptoms/dysfunction or several periods of less than 3 months
2	A chronic disease
3	Several chronic diseases
HB2	**Diagnostic dilemma**
0	No period of diagnostic complexity
1	Diagnosis was clarified quickly
2	Diagnostic dilemma solved but only with considerable diagnostic effort
3	Diagnostic dilemma not solved despite considerable diagnostic effort

CBI	Symptom severity/impairment
0	No physical symptoms or symptoms resolve with treatment
I	Mild symptoms, which do not interfere with current functioning
2	Moderate symptoms, which interfere with current functioning
3	Severe symptoms leading to inability to perform many functional activities
CB2	Diagnostic/therapeutic challenge
0	Clear diagnoses and/or uncomplicated treatments
I	Clear differential diagnoses and/or diagnosis expected with clear treatments
2	Difficult to diagnose and treat; physical cause/origin and treatment expected
3	Difficult to diagnose or treat; other issues than physical causes interfering with diagnostic and therapeutic process
VB	Complications and life threat
0	Little or no risk of premature physical complications or limitations in activities of daily living
I	Mild risk of premature physical complications or limitations in activities of daily living
2	Moderate risk of premature physical complications or permanent and/or substantial limitations of activities in daily living
3	Severe risk of physical complications associated with serious permanent functional deficits and/or dying

PSYCHOLOGICAL DOMAIN

Items in the psychological domain address how factors associated with health behaviors, coping styles, and mental health conditions (which includes mental health and substance use disorders), create barriers to a patient's optimal health.

HPI	Barriers to coping
0	Ability to manage stresses/life and health circumstances, such as through seeking support or hobbies
I	Restricted coping skills, such as a need for control, illness denial, or irritability
2	Impaired coping skills, such as nonproductive complaining or substance abuse but without serious impact on medical condition, mental health, or social situation
3	Minimal coping skills manifested by destructive behaviors, such as substance dependence, psychiatric illness, self-mutilation, or attempted suicide
HP2	Mental health history
0	No history of mental health problems or conditions
I	Mental health problems or conditions, but resolved or without clear effects on daily function
2	Mental health conditions with clear effects on daily function, needing therapy, medication, day treatment, partial program, and so forth
3	Psychiatric admissions and/or persistent effects on daily function
CPI	Resistance to treatment
0	Interested in receiving treatment and willing to cooperate actively
I	Some ambivalence though willing to cooperate with treatment
2	Considerable resistance with nonadherence; hostility or indifference toward health care professionals and/or treatments
3	Active resistance to important medical care

CP2	Mental health symptoms
0	No mental health symptoms
1	Mild mental health symptoms, such as problems with concentration or feeling tense, which do not interfere with current functioning
2	Moderate mental health symptoms, such as an anxiety, depression, or mild cognitive impairment, which interfere with current functioning
3	Severe psychiatric symptoms and/or behavioral disturbances, such as violence, self-inflicted harm, delirium, criminal behavior, psychosis, or mania
VP	**Mental health threat**
0	No mental health concerns
1	Risk of mild worsening of mental health *symptoms*, such as stress, anxiety, feeling blue, substance abuse or cognitive disturbance with limited impact on function; mild risk of treatment resistance (ambivalence)
2	Moderate risk of mental health *disorder* requiring additional mental health care; moderate risk of treatment resistance
3	Severe risk of psychiatric disorder requiring frequent emergency room visits and/or hospital admissions; risk of treatment refusal for serious disorder

SOCIAL DOMAIN

Items in the social domain address how relationships; social connectedness and support; living arrangements; and function in a community, in the job setting, and with coworkers create barriers to a patient's optimal health.

HS1	Job and leisure
0	A job (including housekeeping, retirement, studying) and having leisure activities
1	A job (including housekeeping, retirement, studying) without leisure activities
2	Unemployed now and for at least 6 months with leisure activities
3	Unemployed now and for at least 6 months without leisure activities
HS2	**Relationships**
0	No social disruption
1	Mild social dysfunction; interpersonal problems
2	Moderate social dysfunction, such as inability to initiate or maintain social relations
3	Severe social dysfunction, such as involvement in disruptive social relations or social isolation
CS1	**Residential stability**
0	Stable housing; fully capable of independent living
1	Stable housing with support of others (e.g., family, home care, or an institutional setting)
2	Unstable housing (e.g., no support at home or living in a shelter; change of current living situation is required)
3	No current satisfactory housing (e.g., transient housing or dangerous environment; immediate change is necessary)
CS2	**Social support**
0	Assistance readily available from family, friends, and/or acquaintances, such as work colleagues, at all times
1	Assistance generally available from family, friends, and/or acquaintances, such as work colleagues, but possible delays
2	Limited assistance available from family, friends, and/or acquaintances, such as work colleagues
3	No assistance readily available from family, friends, and/or acquaintances, such as work colleagues, at any time

VS	Social vulnerability
0	No risk of need for changes in the living situation, social relationships and support, or employment
1	Mild risk of need for changes in the living situation (e.g., home health care), social relationships and support, or employment
2	Risk of need for social augmentation/support, financial/employment assistance, or living situation change in the foreseeable future
3	Risk of need for social augmentation/support, financial/employment assistance, or living situation change now

HEALTH SYSTEM DOMAIN

Items in the health system domain address how access, availability, and coordination of care and how the patient's experiences with his or her providers create barriers to the patient's optimal health.

Some find the distinction between "Access to Care" (HHS1) and "Getting Needed Services" (CHS1) confusing. HHS1 is intended to assess whether services have been available to patients for their health problems during the last 6 months. For instance, even if patients live in a clinician-rich community, they may still have had little access if they have no insurance or speak a foreign language when there are no interpreters. "Access to Care" limitations under HHS1 are not restricted to practitioners. For instance, if patients are underinsured, medications, medical devices, and ancillary treatments, such as physical therapy, may become out-of-pocket expenses. Often this is beyond the patient's ability to pay, thus it is essentially inaccessible. CHS1, on the other hand, assesses the current facility with which the patient can attend appointments with one or more practitioners, access needed health services through referral, and other service delivery-level challenges to getting needed services. For instance, if a patient has limited transportation capabilities and/or no phone, it may become logistically impossible to attend appointments or call in medication refills.

Lack of "Coordination of Care" (CHS2) is a major contributor to persistent health complexity. In order for coordination among clinicians to occur, it is necessary that those involved in a patient's treatment know who else is giving care and for what. While this is most often thought of in terms of direct written or verbal communication among practitioners, it also, and importantly, includes access by all providers to a patient's health records, which document assessments and treatment. This is particularly important in patients who have both physical and mental health contributors to complexity since general medical and mental health record systems are often disconnected. Record sharing is also a problem when patients transition from outpatient to inpatient care and vice versa. If noncommunicating health record systems contribute to a lack of awareness by any of the practitioners about contributing health problems and/or treatments, then this would influence higher anchor point scores for CHS2.

HHS1	Access to care
0	Adequate access to care
1	Some limitations in access to care due to financial/insurance problems, geographic reasons, family issues, language, or cultural barriers
2	Difficulties in accessing care due to financial/insurance problems, geographic reasons, family issues, language, or cultural barriers
3	No adequate access to care due to financial/insurance problems, geographic reasons, family issues, language, or cultural barriers
HHS2	Treatment experience
0	No problems with health care professionals
1	Negative experience with health care professionals (patient or relatives)
2	Dissatisfaction with or distrust of doctors; multiple providers for the same health problem; trouble keeping consistent and/or preferred provider(s)
3	Repeated major conflicts with or distrust of doctors, frequent emergency room visits or involuntary admissions; forced to stay with undesirable provider because of cost, provider network options, or other reasons

CHS1	Getting needed services
0	Easily available treating practitioners and health care settings (general medical or mental health care); money for medications and medical equipment
1	Some difficulties in getting to appointments or needed services
2	Routine difficulties in coordinating and/or getting to appointments or needed services
3	Inability to coordinate and/or get to appointments or needed services
CHS2	**Coordination of care**
0	Complete practitioner communication with good coordination of care
1	Limited practitioner communication and coordination of care; primary care physician coordinates medical and mental health services
2	Poor communication and coordination of care among practitioners; no routine primary care physician
3	No communication and coordination of care among practitioners; primary emergency room use to meet nonemergent health needs
VHS	**Health system impediments**
0	No risk of impediments to coordinated physical and mental health care
1	Mild risk of impediments to care, such as insurance restrictions, distant service access, and limited provider communication and/or care coordination
2	Moderate risk of impediments to care, such as potential insurance loss, inconsistent practitioners, communication barriers, poor care coordination
3	Severe risk of impediments to care, such as little or no insurance, resistance to communication and/or disruptive work processes that lead to poor coordination

PIM-CAG Complexity Items and Anchor Points

The Pediatric INTERMED-Complexity Assessment Grid (PIM-CAG) assesses complexity in children and adolescents, known together as children/youth. It provides the case manager with a rapid yet comprehensive assessment of the child/youth presenting for health care that can be used: (a) to identify patient and family needs, (b) to initiate individual care plan development, and (c) to support stabilization or return patients to health through case management activities. The PIM-CAG adopts a lifespan perspective in the assessment of barriers to improvement within the concept of health complexity. The instrument was developed to uncover actionable circumstances related to historical/developmental antecedents, the child/youth's current life situation, and anticipated future vulnerabilities. *"Vulnerabilities" in the context of the PIM-CAG specifically relate to the risk of barrier persistence or worsening domain-specific problems in the future if individualized care through case management is withdrawn.*

Children and adolescents with health complexity require a complementary yet augmented assessment, which includes the family unit, peer relationships, and school situation. In the case of children, for whom the specialized PIM-CAG has been developed, case management activities are just as likely to be directed toward assistance to family members/caregivers as to the child/youth since barrier reversal may only be possible when caregiver/parent problems are addressed.

In some situations, family members or caregivers may present with personal health-related complexity affecting the child/youth complexity such that a social services referral or adult integrated case management program, independent of the child/youth, should be considered. Whether the same case manager as the one working with the child/youth becomes involved in this or it is turned over to other health professionals will depend on the child's/youth's circumstances and the organization of the case management operation.

Instructions for scoring items:

1. Complexity is defined as the interference in standard care by biological, psychological, family/social, and health system factors, which require a shift from standard care to individualized care (in this situation, case management) in order for the child/youth to overcome barriers to improvement. Each complexity item (also called a "cell") on the PIM-CAG is rated using four anchor points in a Likert-type scale. Each anchor point is designed to reflect a level of need, which in turn leads to specific actions to be taken by the case manager on behalf of the patient or family.

   Whenever a complexity item is rated, in addition to the clinical anchor points as defined in this appendix, one should keep the following question in mind: "Will the situation recorded for this complexity item interfere with health outcomes if standard medical care is given?" Another important consideration, particularly when there is debate between two anchor point levels for an individual item (e.g., scoring a 1 vs. a 2 or a 2 vs. a 3), is to consider the immediacy of need for action on behalf of the child/youth. The time frame for action can inform the final decision.

2. All "Historical" complexity items refer to the child/youth's entire life with special attention to the year before assessment. The exception is the cell labeled "Access to Care." "Access to Care" (HHS1) relates to the preceding 6 months.

3. All "Current" complexity items refer to the 30-day period prior to the date that the PIM-CAG assessment is completed.

4. All "Vulnerability" complexity items refer to the 3- to 6-month period after the date that the PIM-CAG vulnerability scoring is performed, based on the difference from an estimate of the natural history of the child/youth's health state when given standard medical care.

5. Actions corresponding to anchor point scores: 0—no action; 1—need for monitoring and/or prevention; 2—need for intervention plan and action *soon*; 3—need for *immediate* intervention plan and action.

6. Several items in the complexity grid contain more than one content component that could be creating barriers to improvement (e.g., symptom severity or impairment in CB1, practitioner availability or clinic accessibility in CHS1, etc.). When scoring each item, the content component with the *greatest* potential for creating a barrier to improvement should direct the score, rather than the average of the item components. For instance, for "Coordination of Care" (CHS2), if there is excellent communication between a pediatrician and a child's/youth's neurologist but no attempt by the pediatrician to find or communicate with a needed mental health specialist for the same child/youth, the anchor point score would be 3.

TABLE A7.1   **Pediatric INTERMED—Complexity Assessment Grid Summary Form**

ID Number _____ Age _____ Gender _____

Date	HEALTH RISKS AND HEALTH NEEDS					
Name	**HISTORICAL**		**CURRENT STATE**		**VULNERABILITY**	
Total score =	Complexity Item	Score	Complexity Item	Score	Complexity Item	Score
Biological Domain	Chronicity HB1		Symptom Severity/Impairment CB1		Complications and Life Threat VB	
	Diagnostic Dilemma HB2		Diagnostic/Therapeutic Challenge CB2			
Psychological Domain	Barriers to Coping HP1		Resistance to Treatment CP1		Learning and/or Mental Health Threat VP	
	Mental Health History HP2		Mental Health Symptoms CP2			
	Cognitive Development HP3					
	Adverse Developmental Events HP3					
Social Domain	School Functioning HS1		Residential Stability CS1		Family/School/Social System Vulnerability VS	
	Family and Social Relationships HS2		Child/Youth Support CS2			
	Caregiver/Parent Health and Function HS3		Caregiver/Family Support CS3			
			School and Community Participation CS4			
Health System Domain	Access to Care HHS1		Getting Needed Services CHS1		Health System Impediments (VHS)	
	Treatment Experience HHS2		Coordination of Care CHS2			
Comments						
(Enter pertinent information about the reason for the score of each complexity item here. For example, poor patient adherence, death in family with stress to child/youth, non-evidence-based treatment of celiac disease, etc.)						

BIOLOGICAL DOMAIN

Items in the biological domain address how factors associated with physical conditions and their symptoms create barriers to the child/youth's optimal health.

In all situations except anchor point 3 for "Diagnostic/Therapeutic Complexity" (CB2), these items refer specifically to physical health issues. For CB2, anchor point 3 includes the potential for nonphysical factors, such as somatic preoccupation, a mental health cause for physical symptoms, or cross-disciplinary (physical and mental health) treatment to contribute to complexity. This is a common source of anchor point scoring confusion.

HB1	Chronicity
0	Less than 3 months of physical symptoms/dysfunction; acute health condition
1	More than 3 months of physical symptoms/dysfunction or several periods of less than 3 months
2	A chronic condition
3	Several chronic conditions
HB2	**Diagnostic dilemma**
0	No period of diagnostic complexity
1	Diagnosis was clarified quickly
2	Diagnostic dilemma solved but only with considerable diagnostic effort
3	Diagnostic dilemma not solved despite considerable diagnostic effort
CB1	**Symptom severity/impairment**
0	No physical symptoms or symptoms resolve with treatment
1	Mild symptoms, which do not interfere with current functioning
2	Moderate symptoms, which interfere with current functioning
3	Severe symptoms leading to inability to perform many functional activities
CB2	**Diagnostic/therapeutic challenge**
0	Uncomplicated diagnosis; treatment with few unpleasant side effects or risks
1	Clear differential diagnoses and/or diagnosis expected; noninvasive treatment with multiple components and/or minor but tolerable side effects
2	Difficult to diagnose but physical cause/origin expected; invasive treatment and/or multiple components with some risks and unpleasant side effects
3	Difficult to diagnose with interfering factors other than physical cause/origin; daily, complex, invasive, and/or cross-disciplinary treatment; potentially serious risks and toxic side effects
VB	**Complications and life threat**
0	Little or no risk of premature physical complications or limitations in activities of daily living
1	Mild risk of premature physical complications or limitations in activities of daily living
2	Moderate risk of premature physical complications or permanent and/or substantial limitations of activities in daily living
3	Severe risk of physical complications associated with serious permanent functional deficits and/or dying

PSYCHOLOGICAL DOMAIN

Items in the psychological domain address how factors associated with health behaviors, coping styles, mental health conditions (which includes mental health and substance use disorders), cognitive function, and early life exposures create barriers to a child's/youth's optimal health.

Among historical items, "Cognitive Development" (HP3) is separated from "Mental Health History" (HP2) since it is commonly associated with barriers to health improvement in children/youth and often requires home-based and education-related intervention. Among current items on the other hand, active cognitive difficulties are included under "Mental Health Symptoms" (CP2). Each may require focused intervention.

While "Adverse Developmental Events" (HP4) can result from mental health (e.g., sexual abuse) and physical (e.g., fetal alcohol syndrome, lead exposure) causes, they are included in the psychological domain since symptoms associated with them are typically cognitive or behavioral in nature. When exposure to toxic injuries leads to active physical symptoms or impairments, they would be scored under "Symptom Severity/Impairment" (CB1) in the biological domain. Unrecognized "Adverse Developmental Events" can make it difficult to determine the etiology of symptoms (HB2).

"Resistance to Treatment" (CP1) can occur as a result of caregiver/parent issues, child/youth issues, or a combination of both. Regardless of the etiology, attention to the child/youth and the caregiver will be necessary in order to ensure future adherence. In rare, life-threatening health situations of a child/youth (e.g., parental refusal of life saving chemotherapy for the child/youth), it may be necessary to involve child protective services in order to ensure safety and appropriate care.

HP1	Barriers to coping
0	Ability to adapt to stresses/life and health circumstances, such as through talking with parents/peers, sports, clubs, or hobbies
1	Restricted coping skills, such as acting out with authority figures, dependency, or irritability; no anticipated long-term difficulties
2	Impaired coping skills, such as frequent conflicts with parents/teachers or substance abuse but without serious impact on medical condition, mental health, or family/social situation; potential long-term difficulties
3	Minimal coping skills, manifest by destructive behaviors, withdrawal, and social isolation, such as substance dependence, mental illness, self-inflicted harm, or illegal behavior
HP2	Mental health history
0	No history of mental health problems or conditions
1	Mental health problems or conditions, but resolved or without clear effects on daily function
2	Mental health conditions with clear effects on daily function, needing therapy, medication, day treatment, partial program, etc.
3	Psychiatric admissions and/or persistent effects on daily function
HP3	Cognitive development
0	No cognitive impairment
1	Possible developmental delay or immaturity; low IQ
2	Delayed development; mild or moderate cognitive impairment
3	Severe and pervasive developmental delays or profound cognitive impairment
HP4	Adverse developmental events
0	No identified developmental traumas or injuries, e.g., physical or sexual abuse, meningitis, lead exposure, etc.
1	Traumatic prior experiences or injuries with no apparent or stated impact on child/youth
2	Traumatic prior experiences or injuries with potential relationship to impairment in child/youth
3	Traumatic prior experiences with apparent and significant direct relationship to impairment in child/youth
CP1	Resistance to treatment
0	Parent/caregiver and/or child/youth are interested in receiving treatment and willing to cooperate actively
1	Some parent/caregiver and/or child/youth ambivalence though willing to cooperate with treatment
2	Considerable parent/caregiver and/or child/youth resistance with nonadherence; hostility or indifference toward health care professionals and/or treatments
3	Active parent/caregiver and/or child/youth resistance to important medical care
CP2	Mental health symptoms
0	No mental health symptoms
1	Mild mental health symptoms, such as problems with risky behaviors or acting out, sadness, oppositionality, which do not interfere with current functioning
2	Moderate mental health symptoms, such as isolating, death preoccupation, defiance, or cognitive impairment, which interfere with current functioning
3	Severe psychiatric symptoms and/or behavioral disturbances, such as violence, self-inflicted harm, criminal behavior, severe autistic behaviors, psychosis, or mania
VP	Learning and/or mental health threat
0	No mental health or intellectual deterioration concerns
1	Risk of mild worsening mental health or cognitive *symptoms*, such as home or school conflict, anxiety, feeling blue, substance abuse or cognitive disturbance with limited impact on function; mild risk of treatment resistance (ambivalence)
2	Moderate risk of mental health *disorder* or impaired cognitive functioning requiring additional mental health care; moderate risk of treatment resistance
3	Severe risk of psychiatric disorder or cognitive impairment requiring frequent emergency room visits, hospital admissions, and/or specialized schooling; risk of treatment refusal for serious disorder

FAMILY/SOCIAL DOMAIN

Items in the family/social domain address how relationships, social connectedness and support, living arrangements, and function in the community, in the school setting, and with peers create barriers to a child/youth's optimal health. They also address the child's/youth's primary caregivers'/parents' health and function (HS3) as well as their support system (CS3), since deficits in either can create barriers to optimal health for the child/youth.

The focus of the family/social domain is on ensuring the optimal health and well-being of the child/youth, though it includes the assessment of complexity issues related to the caregiver/parent. To the extent that the child/youth case manager can address the caregiver/parent contributions to barriers to improvement within a reasonable time frame, they should be included in the assisting actions of the case manager. There are, however, some situations in which the needs of the caregiver/parent are of such a severe nature or are in excess of the time available for the case manager to effect change that the caregiver/parent should be encouraged or assisted in finding his or her own case manager or connected with community resources in an effort to obtain needed assistance. Since this is not always possible, consideration of involvement by child protective services for the child/youth may be necessary.

"School Functioning" (HS1) is intended to target how the child/youth is performing socially, behaviorally, and academically in school related to his or her cognitive abilities, whereas "School and Community Participation" (CS4) is more concerned with school attendance. "Family and Social Relationships" (HS2) have to do with factors that affect the ability to form and sustain relationships within and outside of the home (CS4). While "Residential Stability" (CS1) is nearly entirely associated with the housing itself in adults, it also includes the nutritional health needs for children/youth.

HS1	School functioning
0	Performing well in school with good achievement, attendance, and behavior
1	Performing adequately in school although some achievement, attendance, and behavior problems (e.g., missed classes, pranks)
2	Experiencing moderate problems with school achievement, attendance, and/or behavior (e.g., school disciplinary action, few school-related peer relationships, academic probation)
3	Experiencing severe problems with school achievement, attendance, and/or behavior (e.g., home-bound education, school suspension, violence, illegal activities at school, academic failure, school dropout, disruptive peer group activity)
HS2	Family and social relationships
0	Stable nurturing home, good social and peer relationships
1	Mild family problems, minor problems with social and peer relationships (e.g., parent-child conflict, frequent fights, marital discord, lacking close friends)
2	Moderate level of family problems, inability to initiate and maintain social and peer relationships (e.g., parental neglect, difficult separation/divorce, alcohol abuse, hostile caregiver, difficulties in maintaining same-age peer relationships)
3	Severe family problems with disruptive social and peer relationships (e.g., significant abuse, hostile child custody battles, addiction issues, parental criminality, complete social isolation, little or no association with peers)
HS3	Caregiver/parent health and function
0	All caregivers healthy
1	Physical and/or mental health issues, including poor coping skills, and/or permanent disability, present in one or more caregiver, which do not impact parenting
2	Physical and/or mental health conditions, including disrupted coping resources, and/or permanent disability, present in one or more caregiver, which interfere with parenting
3	Physical and/or mental health conditions, including disrupted coping styles, and/or permanent disability, present in one or more caregiver, which prevent effective parenting and/or create a dangerous situation for the child/youth
CS1	Residential stability
0	Stable housing and financial support for personal growth needs
1	Mild stress with multiple moves, school changes, financial issues

2	Moderate stress with unstable housing and/or living situation support (e.g., living in shelter, poor nutrition); change of current living situation is required
3	Severe stress with no current satisfactory housing (e.g., homelessness, transient housing, child/youth malnourished, or dangerous environment); immediate change is necessary
CS2	**Child/youth support**
0	Supervision and/or assistance readily available from family/caregiver, friends/peers, teachers, and/or community social networks (e.g., spiritual/religious groups) at all times
I	Supervision and/or assistance generally available from family/caregiver, friends/peers, teachers, and/or community social networks, but possible delays
2	Limited supervision and/or assistance available from family/caregiver, friends/peers, teachers, and/or community social networks
3	No effective supervision and/or assistance available from family/caregiver, friends/peers, teachers, and/or community social networks at any time
CS3	**Caregiver/family support**
0	Assistance readily available from family, friends, and/or acquaintances, such as work colleagues/employer, at all times
I	Assistance generally available from family, friends, and/or acquaintances, such as work colleagues/employer, but possible delays
2	Limited assistance available from family, friends, and/or acquaintances, such as work colleagues/employer
3	No assistance available from family, friends, and/or acquaintances, such as work colleagues/employer at any time
CS4	**School and community participation**
0	Attending school regularly, achieving and participating well, and actively engaged in extracurricular school or community activities (e.g., sports, clubs, hobbies, religious groups)
I	Average of one day of school missed/week and/or minor disruptions in achievement and behavior with few extracurricular activities
2	Average of 2 days or more of school missed/week and/or moderate disruption in achievement or behavior with resistance to extracurricular activities
3	Truant or school nonattendance with no extracurricular activities and no community connections
VS	**Family/school/social system vulnerability**
0	No risk from living situation; adequate social, personal, and developmental support; caregiver health and function
I	Risk of need for additional living situation stability, social or school support, and/or family/caregiver intervention
2	Risk of need for temporary or permanent alteration in home, school, and/or family/caregiver/social environment in the foreseeable future
3	Risk of need for immediate temporary or permanent alteration in home, school, and/or family/caregiver/social environment (e.g., assist with foster home placement, referral to child protective services)

HEALTH SYSTEM DOMAIN

Items in the health system domain address issues related to access, ability to get needed care, and the coordination of services among the child's/youth's treating clinicians. They also assess the child's/youth's and/or the caregiver's/parent's experiences with providers that create barriers to the child's/youth's optimal health, such as personality conflicts, loss of trust, or forced doctor-patient relationships due to insurance, geographic, or other factors.

Some find the distinction between "Access to Care" (HHS1) and "Getting Needed Services" (CHS1) confusing. HHS1 is intended to assess whether services are available to the child/youth for his or her health problems at a system level. For instance, even if the children/youth live in a clinician-rich community, they may have had little access to needed services because of lack of or poor insurance coverage, the paucity of interpreters, or culturally naïve practitioners. Limitations in "Access to Care" under HHS1 may not be just restricted to the child's/youth's available and appropriate practitioners. If the child/youth's parents are uninsured or transients, then medications, medical devices, and/or ancillary treatments, such as respiratory therapy, may become out-of-pocket expenses. If these costs are beyond the parent's ability to pay, such treatment needs are essentially inaccessible.

Unlike HHS1, "Getting Needed Services" (CHS1) is more concerned with the child's/youth's ability to actually attend appointments with one or more practitioners and/or to adhere to treatments recommended. For instance, if a child/youth and/or the child's/youth's family have limited transportation capabilities and/or no phone, it may become logistically impossible to show up for appointments or to renew prescriptions. If the child/youth and/or family have limited resources, it may be difficult or impossible to cover copays or medication costs. Thus, CHS1 has more to do with the mechanics of getting the care than health system issues that limit access to providers or services.

Lack of "Coordination of Care" (CHS2) is a major contributor to persistent health complexity. In order for coordination among clinicians to occur, it is necessary that those involved in a child's/youth's treatment know who else is giving care and for what. While this is most often thought of in terms of direct written or verbal communication among practitioners, it also, and importantly, includes access by all providers to a child's/youth's health records, which document assessments and treatment. This is particularly important in children/youth who have both physical and mental health contributions to complexity since general medical and mental health record systems are often disconnected. Thus, if noncommunicating health record systems contribute to a lack of awareness by any of the practitioners about contributing health problems or treatments, then this would influence higher anchor point scores for CHS2.

The transition of care for adolescents with health complexity from pediatricians and child mental health professionals to clinicians who will follow them through adulthood is a special contributor to persistence of complexity for youth. Difficulties with this transition process are assessed under the item labeled "Coordination of Care" (CHS2). As mentioned in the preceding general instructions, if the youth is experiencing good communication among child/youth-treating practitioners but is experiencing difficulty in identifying adult clinician counterparts to assume care responsibilities, then problematic transition may lead to anchor point scores of 2 or 3 based on the level of the barrier to improvement encountered.

HHS1	Access to care
0	Adequate access to care with insurance coverage stability
1	Some limitations in access to care due to financial/insurance problems, geographic reasons, family issues, language, or cultural barriers
2	Difficulties in accessing care due to financial/insurance problems, geographic reasons, family issues, language, or cultural barriers
3	No adequate access to care due to financial/insurance problems, geographic reasons, family issues, language, long waiting lists, or cultural barriers
HHS2	**Treatment experience**
0	No child/youth or parent/caregiver problems with health care professionals
1	Negative child/youth or parent/caregiver experience with health care professionals
2	Child/youth or parent/caregiver dissatisfaction with or distrust of doctors; multiple providers for the same health problem; trouble keeping consistent and/or preferred provider(s)
3	Repeated major child/youth or parent/caregiver conflicts with or distrust of doctors, frequent emergency room visits or involuntary admissions; forced to stay with undesirable provider because of cost, provider network options, or other reasons
CHS1	**Getting needed services**
0	Easily available treating practitioners and health care settings (general medical or mental health care); money for medications and medical equipment
1	Some difficulties in getting to appointments or needed services
2	Routine difficulties in coordinating and/or getting to appointments or needed services
3	Inability to coordinate and/or get to appointments or needed services

CHS2	Coordination of care
0	Complete practitioner communication with good coordination and transition of care
I	Limited practitioner communication and coordination of care; pediatrician coordinates medical and mental health services
2	Poor communication and coordination of care among practitioners; no routine pediatrician; difficulty in transitioning to age-appropriate care
3	No communication and coordination of care among practitioners; primary emergency room use to meet nonemergent health needs; systemic barriers to age-appropriate care transition
VHS	**Health system impediments**
0	No risk of impediments to coordinated physical and mental health care
I	Mild risk of impediments to care (e.g., insurance restrictions, distant service assess, limited provider communication and/ or care coordination/transition)
2	Moderate risk of impediments to care (e.g., potential insurance loss, inconsistent practitioners, communication barriers, poor care coordination/transition)
3	Severe risk of impediments to care (e.g., little or no insurance, resistance to communication and/or disruptive work processes that lead to poor coordination/transition among providers)

Activities Associated With IM-CAG Scores

Each of the INTERMED-Complexity Assessment Grid (IM-CAG) anchor points is designed to inform actions by case managers. The following is a list of actions that could be considered when a patient has a specific score on an item in the IM-CAG. *The actions listed in this appendix are not considered exhaustive but rather representative of the types of action that a case manager should consider on behalf of a patient.* Actions by case managers should be taken in an attempt to correct barriers to improvement, the primary goal of the IM-CAG and the central aim when working with patients suffering with health complexity.

In this appendix, actions are delineated for each score on each item in the IM-CAG. It should be noted that items within the grid are also often connected with each other. As a result, the case manager should not just consider the actions associated with an item score as he or she creates a care plan to assist a patient but should also consider how the item score relates to other items in the grid. For instance, a patient may change doctors often because of poor trust of doctors or the health industry (a score of 2 on HHS2). As a result, the patient may be nonadherent to treatment (a score of 3 on CP1). Since poor trust in such a patient is connected with nonadherence, actions on both items should be considered in tandem—for example, discuss barriers related to trust with the patient and his or her doctors (HHS2) and use education and motivational interviewing techniques to improve the patient's adherence (CP1).

Instructions to case managers:

1. The IM-CAG assesses complexity. Each item score (also called a "cell score") on the IM-CAG suggests actions by the case manager working on behalf of the patient or the patient on his or her own behalf within a time frame. A score of 1 (yellow) suggests the need for monitoring/prevention, 2 (orange) suggests the need to do something soon (i.e., intervention or develop a plan), and 3 (red) suggests the need for immediate intervention or plan implementation. To the extent possible, the actions taken by the case manager and the patient should be a part of a patient-manager developed care plan with goals and objectives. These care plans must then be communicated to the patient's practitioners with a request for their active participation.

2. *All care plans will include education of the patient and, when appropriate, significant others about the patient's illnesses, the interaction of illnesses, and treatments.* Often the case manager will provide information about diseases or help the patient formulate questions for his or her physicians. Physicians and other treating professionals should serve as the primary arbiter of information and treatment when possible. Thus, communication between the case manager and the patient's clinicians is also important.

3. Case managers do not treat patients; they support approaches to care that are likely to improve outcomes, break down barriers, and assist with health system navigation. They serve as health coaches to complex patients. Since the patient's clinicians are the focal point of effective treatment, it is important for case managers to form alliances with the patient's treatment team as they work with the patient. This can be facilitated by sending a flier and a letter to practitioners on case management and the role it plays in assisting with complex patient care (see Appendixes C and D, www.springer pub.com/kathol). Point out the intended limited duration of involvement by the case manager.

4. Many of the cells on the IM-CAG are associated with barriers to treatment adherence (Exhibit 7.1). Though active, patient-centered "Resistance to Treatment" (CP1) is one of the reasons, it is by no means the only, nor necessarily the main, reason. Other examples include, but are not limited to, insufficient funds to pay for treatment, religious objections, parental refusal, frequent family moves and practitioner changes, and so forth. Since nonadherence is clearly associated with worse clinical outcome, the case manager and patient should work together in all domains and in all cells to reverse barriers to treatment adherence.

5. No action is required for items in which a score of 0 is made.

TABLE A8.1	INTERMED—Complexity Assessment Grid Summary Form

ID Number _____ **Age** _____ **Gender** _____

Date	HEALTH RISKS AND HEALTH NEEDS					
Name	HISTORICAL		CURRENT STATE		VULNERABILITY	
Total score =	Complexity Item	Score	Complexity Item	Score	Complexity Item	Score
Biological Domain	Chronicity HB1		Symptom Severity/Impairment CB1		Complications and Life Threat VB	
	Diagnostic Dilemma HB2		Diagnostic/Therapeutic Challenge CB2			
Psychological Domain	Barriers to Coping HP1		Resistance to Treatment CP1		Mental Health Threat VP	
	Mental Health History HP2		Mental Health Symptoms CP2			
Social Domain	Job and Leisure HS1		Residential Stability CS1		Social Vulnerability VS	
	Relationships HS2		Social Support CS2			
Health System Domain	Access to Care HHS1		Getting Needed Services CHS1		Health System Impediments VHS	
	Treatment Experience HHS2		Coordination of Care CHS2			

Comments
(Enter pertinent information about the reason for the score of each complexity item here. For example, poor patient adherence, death in family with stress to patient, non-evidence-based treatment of migraine, etc.)

BIOLOGICAL DOMAIN

Actions related to items in the biological domain are intended to address barriers to improvement for physical conditions and their symptoms. In all situations, except anchor point 3 for item CB2, "Diagnostic/Therapeutic Challenge," these items refer specifically to taking action related to the physical health issues themselves. In fact, it is biomedical activity that forms the core of traditional case management, which focuses on correction of inconsistent adherence to evidence-based treatments for physical illness. Since the CB2 anchor point 3 includes nonphysical factors as a cause of physical symptoms, such as somatic preoccupation or somatic symptoms associated with a psychiatric illness, actions related to this item will also include assistance with cross-disciplinary (mental health) involvement and likely treatment.

In the current health care environment, few general practitioners are enthusiastic about addressing behavior-based issues without encouragement and assistance. Even in patient's with what would be considered subsyndromal mental health symptoms (CP2), treating minor mental health symptoms can be the tipping point between persistent biological symptoms with treatment nonresponse and health stabilization with reduced impairment. In patient's who score 3 on CB2, even when interacting CP2 or other nonbiological items are scored 1 or 2, clinicians should be encouraged to intervene related to the nonbiological items early in the integrated case management process as an indirect means of altering the 3 score on CB2.

HB1	Chronicity
1	**More than 3 months of physical dysfunction or several periods of less than 3 months**: review patient's understanding of persistent dysfunction; observe to see if condition turns chronic with physical limitations; ensure primary care or specialist follow-up

2	**A chronic disease**: review patient's understanding of the chronic illness and treatment; simplify and assist with a systematic approach to illness control; ensure active involvement and collaboration by primary care physician and medical specialists, if needed; assess and ensure treatment of co-occurring mental condition; confirm assessments of patient symptoms and/ or measure clinical outcomes over time (e.g., diabetic neuropathy, HbA1c, etc.); enable unfettered access to physical health and mental health records by all treating clinicians
3	**Several chronic diseases**: *immediately* perform actions under #2; include customized actions based on interview; review understanding of illnesses and treatments; confirm communication and coordination of care among practitioners
HB2	**Diagnostic dilemma**
1	**Easy diagnoses**: observe for changes in clinical status
2	**Diagnostic dilemma with single or multiple conditions**: review diagnoses, interventions, and treatments for fidelity with the patient's course and improvement with treatment; assess attitude of patient about diagnosis and workups; educate about process; bring in case management medical director to review if it is outside the case manager's level of expertise to get a big picture assessment of the accuracy of diagnoses and treatment; facilitate doctor-to-doctor communication, if needed; discuss ways that case management can assist the patient in improving outcomes; ensure assessment for concurrent mental conditions has been done and treatment is being given, if present; diplomatically communicate discordant understanding with patient and clinicians
3	**Diagnostic dilemma not solved despite considerable diagnostic efforts**: *immediately* perform actions under #2; include customized actions based on interview; seek patient's input about unresolved problems; case manager serves as link among clinicians caring for patient, the case management medical director, and the patient to maintain communication, collaboration, and outcome orientation
CB1	**Symptom severity/impairment**
1	**Mild symptoms; no functional impairment**: observe; review for less-invasive, less-expensive treatment options
2	**Moderate to severe symptoms; impairment present**: ensure treatment and follow-up provided is coordinated through efforts of primary care and specialty medical physicians; confirm active involvement of mental health team for patients with comorbid mental conditions; activate ongoing assessment of patient symptoms over time (e.g., labs, X-rays, complications, etc.); maximize adherence; enable unfettered access to physical health and mental condition records by all treating clinicians; evaluate patient's understanding of illness and impairment; educate if appropriate; delineate impairments and ensure rehabilitation and support measures
3	**Severe symptoms leading to inability to perform activities of daily living**: *immediately* perform actions under #1 and #2; include customized actions based on interview; find out what works best for the patient; assist with ongoing communication among practitioners; enlist family assistance when available; consider alternative treatment settings, living arrangements, rehabilitation services; augment home care availability; enlist case management medical director assistance and suggestions when needed
CB2	**Diagnostic/therapeutic challenge**
1	**Quick diagnoses expected with easy treatments**: ensure coordination of services
2	**Difficult to diagnose and treat, physical cause/origin and treatment expected**: scrupulously ensure that patient is following through on evaluations and treatments; make sure that clinicians know the outcomes of exams and tests done by colleagues; assist in measuring outcomes of interventions; maintain communications with and between patient and clinical team (e.g., using IM-CAG results); have case management medical director review case for additional ideas and talk to clinicians, if warranted; assist patient in getting answers to questions about health from practitioners; consider setting up a case conference among clinicians
3	**Difficult to diagnose and treat; psychological, social, economic issues cloud picture**: *immediately* perform actions under #2; include customized actions based on interview; make sure that clinicians know about mental conditions and/or social and health system factors that may be playing a role; confirm that the patient is being seen in a timely fashion by appropriate practitioners; have case management medical director talk with patient's clinician about expanded differential and potential treatments; facilitate mental health referral through primary care physicians if possible; include patient in discussions about roles of nonphysical factors in symptoms/treatment
VB	**Complications and life threat**
1	**Mild risk of premature physical complications or limitations in activities of daily living**: ensure adherence to treatment and troubleshoot barriers that crop up; consider transfer back to standard care
2	**Moderate risk of premature physical complications or permanent and/or substantial limitations in activities of daily living**: address issues causing nonadherence to treatment; establish continuity of physical and mental condition services; stabilize communication and collaboration among providers and patient; establish methodology to follow clinically relevant outcomes with patient and clinicians (e.g., HbA1c, visits to emergency room, missed work/disability, etc.); monitor with case management medical director through case conferences; consider intermittent long-term contact with patient
3	**Severe risk of physical complications and serious functional deficits and/or dying**: perform actions under #2; include customized actions based on interview; consider exploring alternative providers with patient after discussion with medical director; ensure physical health condition assessment and treatment follow through; intermittent long-term contact with patient until risks change; assist with hospice and long-term care, if appropriate

PSYCHOLOGICAL DOMAIN

Actions related to items in the psychological domain are intended to address barriers to improvement related to health behaviors, coping styles, prior mental conditions, and current psychiatric symptoms.

HP1	**Barriers to coping**
1	**Restricted coping skills**: provide active listening and patient education; ensure/encourage counseling on coping mechanisms; consider training in stress-reduction techniques (one to three sessions, often with a counselor)
2	**Impaired coping skills with frequent conflicts and/or substance abuse**: identify support for stressful situations; encourage counseling on coping mechanisms; enable training in stress-reduction and conflict-resolution techniques (one to five sessions, often with a counselor); involve employee assistance program (EAP) to address worksite-related stressors; suggest adjustments in living/work location/activities, if possible; endorse screening and brief intervention for alcohol abuse; consider talking with primary care physician about substance abuse counseling and/or mental health referral for assessment
3	**Minimal coping skills with dangerous behaviors**: *immediately* perform actions under #2; include customized actions based on interview; assist in support system or crisis management for patient through collaboration with providers; encourage providers to refer for mental health assessment and intervention (e.g. cognitive behavior therapy [CBT], dialectic behavior therapy [DBT], or medication; facilitate referral for substance abuse/dependence treatment
HP2	**Mental health history**
1	**Mental conditions resolved or without effect on life activities**: encourage regular primary care screenings for mental conditions with intervention, if appropriate; check for access to support from mental health professionals
2	**Mental conditions that interfered with life activities or required treatment**: ensure the patient's understanding of potential for recurrence of mental health conditions by using lay language; link potential for medical and physical condition interactions, if indicated; ensure potential for active involvement by psychiatrist and mental health team (psychologists, social workers, nurses, substance use disorder and other counselors, etc.) support when conditions destabilize; confirm maintenance and continuation treatment provided by primary care professionals (medical home) with mental health specialist assistance; facilitate ongoing monitoring of patient symptoms over time (e.g., PHQ-9, GAD-7, etc.); activate communication and unfettered access to physical and mental health records by all treating clinicians
3	**Psychiatric admissions and/or persistent effects on daily function**: *immediately* perform actions under #2; include customized actions based on interview; encourage primary involvement and treatment by a mental health team for mental conditions working in close collaboration with primary care physicians who care for concurrent physical illness; when possible, facilitate colocation of the patient's physical and mental health clinicians who actively interact in an integrated clinic setting
CP1	**Resistance to treatment**
1	**Ambivalence**: educate patient/family about illnesses; initiate discussions with patient about resistant behaviors using motivational interviewing and problem-solving techniques to reduce resistance; explore other barriers to treatment adherence (Exhibit 7.1); inform providers of adherence problems and work with them to consider alternative interventions, if needed
2	**Resistance, hostility, indifference**: perform actions under #1; review need for other health professional or clinic to provide care with case manager's medical director; actively explore and attempt to reverse other sources of resistance (e.g., family member's negativism, religious objections, cultural influences, relationships with treating physician)
3	**Active resistance**: *immediately* perform actions under #1 and #2; include customized actions based on interview; work with treating clinicians in considering and instituting alternative interventions; if needed, work with case management medical director to find second opinion practitioners; if irresolvable and pervasive, consider discontinuation of case management
CP2	**Mental health symptoms**
1	**Mild mental health symptoms**: ensure primary care treatment with access to support from mental health professionals; facilitate unfettered access to physical and mental health records by all treating clinicians
2	**Moderate mental health symptoms**: perform actions under #1; ensure that acute, maintenance, and continuation of treatment is being provided by primary care physicians with mental health support and backup; facilitate primary maintenance and continuation treatment provided by primary care physicians (medical home) with mental health specialist assistance—that is, a psychiatrist and mental health team (psychologists, social workers, nurses, substance abuse counselors, etc.)—when condition destabilizes, becomes complicated, or demonstrates treatment resistance; assist with instituting symptom documentation recording system, such as PHQ-9, GAD-7, and so forth; ensure crisis plan is available

3	**Severe psychiatric symptoms and/or behavioral disturbances**: *immediately* perform actions under #1 and #2; include customized actions based on interview; support active and aggressive treatment for mental conditions by a mental health team working in close collaboration with primary care physicians, who care for concurrent physical illness; when possible, encourage geographically collocated physical and mental health personnel to facilitate ease of coordinating treatment; confirm persistent symptom documentation recording system, such as PHQ-9, GAD-7, and so forth; ensure physical and mental health treatment adherence
VP	**Mental health threat**
1	**Mild risk of worsening mental health symptoms**: ensure access to support; ensure/encourage continuous follow-up care with intermittent mental health assessments, when appropriate; suggest booster sessions for coping and stress reduction, when needed; consider transfer back to standard care
2	**Moderate risk of worsening mental health symptoms**: perform actions under #1; set up maintenance and continuity program that involves the treating primary care physicians, clinical nurse specialists, and mental health specialists; assist in establishing a regular symptom documentation system, such as PHQ-9, GAD-7, and so forth; facilitate guideline development for mental health team involvement with patient in the primary care clinic to assist with treatment adjustments (best provided in an integrated primary care clinic); address adherence and patient-provider relationship issues; involve caregivers in all activities after informed consent obtained; institute verbal, paper, and electronic communication capabilities for all clinical professionals working with the patient
3	**Severe and persistent risk of psychiatric disorder with frequent health service use**: perform actions under #1 and #2; include customized actions based on interview; confirm care continuity with both general medical and mental health specialists; work with the patient's clinicians in establishing collaborative clinical goals with the patient; consider long-term involvement

SOCIAL DOMAIN

Actions related to items in the social domain are intended to address barriers to improvement related to difficulties in forming or maintaining relationships, establishing social connectedness and support, living arrangements; function in a community, or success in the job setting and with coworkers.

HS1	**Job and leisure**
1	**A job; few leisure activities**: explore interests/hobbies with the patient and encourage rekindling activity
2	**At least 6 months unemployed (but employable); leisure activities**: assist patient in getting disability assistance, exploring schooling opportunities, and so forth; educate patient on how to get public assistance for living and health care needs; set up with social service, job-finding services, vocational rehabilitation, or other community resources if a new job is a possibility; follow up; continue encouraging patient-initiated activities
3	**At least 6 months unemployed (but employable); few leisure activities**: *immediately* perform actions under #1 and #2; include customized actions based on interview; explore impact of no job and few activities on health access; explore community resources with patient
HS2	**Relationships**
1	**Mild social dysfunction; interpersonal problems**: observe interpersonal difficulties during patient interviews and adjust recommendations to accommodate for limitations (i.e., introversion, family discord, etc.)
2	**Moderate social dysfunction**: encourage social skills training (one to six sessions, often with a counselor); foster involvement of family, significant others, or social service; assess impact of social problems on patient's health issues, address if present; explore alternative socialization opportunities
3	**Severe social dysfunction**: *immediately* perform actions under #1 and #2; include customized actions based on interview; encourage mental health assessment and treatment if appropriate and/or needed through primary care physician
CS1	**Residential stability**
1	**Stable housing situation with support of others**: make sure vulnerability needs match support
2	**Unstable housing**: initiate contact with social service or other community resources to look into housing options; get assistance to help correct the cause of the residential instability, such as financial limitations, family conflict, natural disaster, and so forth; follow up on results of suggestions; use knowledge of community resources to push the system
3	**Unsafe or transient housing**: *immediately* connect the patient with social service to find a shelter, such as for battered women or other suitable housing; perform actions under #2; include customized actions based on interview

CS2	Social support
I	**Assistance generally available but possible delays**: initiate assistance mechanism, if needed
2	**Limited assistance readily available**: talk with patient's available personal contacts about what they can do along with the patient; set up with social services or other agency to assist patient in finding needed community resources; follow up on recommendation outcome; use knowledge of community resources to push the system; get ideas about options from other health professionals familiar with patient's social setting
3	**No assistance readily available**: *immediately* perform actions under #2; include customized actions based on interview; consider helping to transfer to a location with a higher level of care (e.g., group home, assisted living facility)
VS	**Social vulnerability**
I	**Some health assistance needs**: see if current location can accommodate potential need; consider transfer back to standard care
2	**Risk of need for alteration in social situation in the foreseeable future**: continue to work with family; assist, engage, and push social service to find resources and make ready the procedures for help and/or placement; follow outcomes of recommendations; use knowledge of community resources to push the system
3	**Risk of need for alteration in social situation now**: perform actions under #2; include customized actions based on interview; attempt to set up long-term living arrangements

HEALTH SYSTEM DOMAIN

Actions related to items in the health system domain are intended to address barriers to improvement caused by difficulties in accessing services, trusting and working with clinicians, getting to and coordinating appointments, or coordinating services due to noncommunication among the patient's providers and clinic settings.

There is a tendency for those working in different countries to think that the actions related to the following items do not fit their health system. For instance, in the U.S. system, lack of insurance coverage is a major barrier to care access but is much less of an issue in countries that have national health services with universal participation. Thus, those living in other countries with universal coverage feel that "Access to Care" (HHS1) is not a significant issue. Such knee-jerk reactions by case managers are to be discouraged, as has

become evident through discussions with the multinational professionals listed in the Acknowledgments.

For each item in the health system domain, case managers are instructed to systematically apply actions pertinent to their system. For instance, in several countries that use the IM-CAG, insurance coverage is not an issue; however, access problems do occur as a result of services distribution (e.g., rural care, language/cultural barriers such as treating immigrants, waiting lists, etc.). Similarly, communication among physical and mental health practitioners may be better in some countries than in others; however, there may remain major problems related to communication of hospital specialists with the patient's primary care physician and in transferring records from one location to another.

Health system domain actions should be customized to the health-related business practices used in each country so that barriers to care can be systematically corrected.

HHSI	Access to care
I	**Some limitation in accessing care:** assist in identifying culturally sensitive, willing providers, interpretation services, and ensure timely access to appointments
2	**Difficulties in accessing care:** work with patient in finding health insurance and in identifying willing providers; ensure timely culturally sensitive appointments and translation services (use conference calls or telephonic access if necessary); assist in flexing benefits (with health plan) when possible to get appropriate care (go up the supervisory ladder); push the system to shorten the wait list priority; connect physical and mental health financial/administrative support for services; assist with appeals of inappropriately denied care (use case management medical director, if necessary)
3	**No adequate access to care:** *immediately* perform actions under #2; include customized actions based on interview; enlist social service to assist with actions in #2 and in finding insurance product or general assistance clinic; assist with post-emergency room and posthospitalization follow-up locations; advocate for patient

HHS2	**Treatment experience**
1	**Negative experience with health care providers**: assess for adherence to assessment and treatment recommendations; periodically ask about current relationship with clinical practitioners; help patient to ask questions of or to challenge practitioners
2	**Changes doctors more than once because of dissatisfaction; multiple providers**: assess types of conflicts with practitioners; adjudicate conflict when possible (directly or indirectly); ensure treatment adherence; foster communication between patient and practitioner about conflicts; assist patient in getting to a different provider, if needed, where outcomes would be better; involve case management medical director for assistance
3	**Repeated major conflicts with doctors, frequent emergency room visits, or involuntary admissions**: *immediately* perform actions under #2; include customized actions based on interview; assist in finding someone to work with patient on conflict-resolution techniques; involve the case management medical director to talk with practitioners about relationship; consider assisting patient finding another professional or location of care; mental health consultation to assess for personality or chemical dependence issues contributing to conflict; look at insurance alternatives with patient
CHS1	**Getting needed services**
1	**Some difficulties in getting to appointments or needed services**: review correlation of disorders with treatment being given; check for barriers; assist with finding money for medications, equipment, and needed services
2	**Routine difficulties in coordinating and/or getting to appointments or needed services**: assess alternative care locations and practitioner availability; review options with the patient and ensure timely access; consider accessing services through telemedicine; assist with finding money for medications, equipment, and needed services; check for appointment flexibility in current clinic system; help patient find needed medical and/or mental health specialists and set up appointments (out of region/network if necessary); review difficulties with primary care physician (medical home)
3	**Inability to coordinate and/or get to appointments or needed services**: *immediately* perform actions under #2; include customized actions based on interview; establish medical home; work with primary care (or specialty) physician (medical home) to coordinate appointments (e.g., diabetologist and psychiatrist); assist with transportation for patient and coordination of assissments/follow-ups; enlist assistance of community agencies and social services
CHS2	**Coordination of care**
1	**Limited practitioner communication and coordination of care**: encourage record sharing and communication among clinicians, including mental health and complementary medicine; open links for important communication
2	**Poor communication and coordination of care among practitioners**: determine and augment communication links between physical and mental health practitioners; ensure note sharing, preferably common record system, among clinicians working with patient; assist in coordinating appointments and transportation; help patient get same-day appointments for different problems; investigate availability of integrated clinics; identify reasons for missed appointments to overcome barriers
3	**No communication and coordination of care among practitioners**: *immediately* perform actions under #1 and #2; include customized actions based on interview; serve as link for patient with various practitioners (i.e., with informed consent [see Appendix 3, if needed], obtain and fax notes for distribution to various clinic sites); talk with treating practitioners on behalf of patient but also educate patient on how to do so; create alternatives to emergency room use; enlist assistance from case management medical director to try to establish a medical home
VHS	**Health system impediments**
1	**Mild risk of impediments to care**: ensure insurance benefits cover health needs; assist in maintaining coverage; review practitioner communication procedures; consider transfer back to standard care
2	**Moderate risk of impediments to care**: work with patient, practitioner providing medical home, social services, and community agencies to establish the best health set-up possible in the region; assist in finding insurance products, needed providers, and communicating clinic systems; pay special attention to physical and mental health links
3	**Severe risk of impediments to care**: perform actions under #2; include customized actions based on interview; help patient find and establish a medical home that will persist over time; assist in overcoming barriers to practitioner involvement with patient; consider setting up a physical and mental health clinicians' case conference; attempt to enlist assistance of community-based case manager (public health); ensure insurance benefits cover health needs; assist in maintaining coverage; review and assist with practitioner communication procedures

Activities Associated With PIM-CAG Scores

Each of the Pediatric INTERMED-Complexity Assessment Grid (PIM-CAG) anchor points is designed to inform actions by case managers. The following is a list of actions that could be considered when a child/youth has a specific score on an item in the PIM-CAG. *The actions listed in this appendix are not considered exhaustive but rather representative of the types of action that a case manager could consider taking on behalf of a child/youth.* Actions by case managers should be taken in an attempt to correct barriers to improvement, the primary goal of the PIM-CAG and the central aim when working with children/youth suffering with health complexity.

In this appendix, actions are delineated for each score on each item in the PIM-CAG. It should be noted that items within the grid are also often connected with each other (i.e., they interact as barriers to improvement for children/youth). As a result, the case manager should not just consider the actions associated with the item score as he or she creates a care plan but should also consider how the item score relates to other item scores in the grid. For instance, the parents of a child/youth may change doctors often because of poor trust of doctors or the health industry (a score of 2 on HHS2). As a result, the child/youth is nonadherent to treatment (a score of 3 on CP1). Since poor trust by the parents (HHS2) is connected with nonadherence (CP1), actions on both items should be considered in tandem (e.g., discuss barriers related to trust with the parents and their doctors and use of education and motivational interviewing techniques to improve the parents' and child's/youth's adherence).

Working with children/youth creates an additional challenge for case managers since it is not just the child/youth but also the caregivers/parents who may be the objects of case managers' actions. It is important to remember that the child/youth is the primary target of the case management when the PIM-CAG is being used and the child/youth is considered to have health complexity. Having said this, in many situations, the caregivers/parents are just as complex or needy as the child/youth and thus require active participation in the child's/youth's intervention. In some situations, the actions that need to be directed at issues specifically for the caregiver/parent are in excess of time available to the case manager. When this occurs, the case manager will have to make a decision whether the caregivers/parents warrant referral to social service themselves, need assignment of their own case

manager, or whether child protective services should be considered. These are clinical questions that will require discussion with supervisors, medical directors, the child's/youth's clinicians, and perhaps others.

Instructions to case managers:

1. The PIM-CAG assesses complexity in children/youth. Each item score (also called a "cell score") on the PIM-CAG suggests the need for action by the case manager working, by the caregiver/parent, or the child/youth. A score of 1 (yellow) suggests the need for monitoring/prevention; 2 (orange) suggests the need to do something soon (i.e., intervention or develop a plan); and 3 (red) suggests the need for immediate intervention or plan implementation. To the extent possible, activities by the case manager, the child/youth, and the child/youth's caregivers/parents should be a part of a child/youth-parent-manager developed care plan with goals and objectives. These care plans must then be communicated to the child's/youth's practitioners with a request for their active participation.

2. *All care plans will include education of the child/youth and caregiver/parent about the child's/youth's illnesses, the interaction of illnesses, and treatments.* Often the case manager will provide information about diseases or help the child/youth and caregivers/parents formulate questions for their physicians. Physicians and other treating professionals should serve as the primary arbiter of information and treatment when possible. Thus, communication between the case manager and the child's/youth's clinicians is also important. Finally, when appropriate and with informed consent, school personnel who might be able to facilitate access to needed school resources or assist with maximizing educational and school experiences should also be informed of the health and health needs of the child/youth.

3. Pediatric case managers do not treat patients; they support approaches to care that are likely to improve outcomes, break down barriers, and assist with health system navigation. They serve as health coaches to complex children/youth and their caregivers/parents. Since clinicians are the focal point of effective treatment, it is important for case managers to form alliances with the child's/youth's treatment team as they work with the child/youth. This can be facilitated by sending a flier to practitioners on case management and

the role it can play in assisting with complex care (see Appendixes E and F, www.springerpub.com/kathol). Point out the intended limited duration of involvement by the case manager.

4. Many of the cells on the PIM-CAG are associated with barriers to treatment adherence (Exhibit 7.1). Though child/youth or caregiver/parent-based "Resistance to Treatment" (CP1) is one of the reasons, it is by no means the only, nor necessarily the main, reason. Other examples include, but are not limited to, insufficient funds to pay for treatment, cultural factors, language barriers, and religious objections. Since nonadherence is clearly associated with worse clinical outcome, the case manager, the child/youth, the caregiver/parent, and the child's/youth's care providers should work together in all domains and in all cells to reverse barriers to treatment adherence.

5. No action is required for items in which a score of 0 is made.

TABLE A9.1   **Pediatric INTERMED—Complexity Assessment Grid Summary Form**

ID Number _____ Age _____ Gender _____

Date	HEALTH RISKS AND HEALTH NEEDS					
Name	HISTORICAL		CURRENT STATE		VULNERABILITY	
Total score =	Complexity Item	Score	Complexity Item	Score	Complexity Item	Score
Biological Domain	Chronicity HB1		Symptom Severity/Impairment CB1		Complications and Life Threat VB	
	Diagnostic Dilemma HB2		Diagnostic/Therapeutic Challenge CB2			
Psychological Domain	Barriers to Coping HP1		Resistance to Treatment CP1		Learning and/or Mental Health Threat VP	
	Mental Health History HP2		Mental Health Symptoms CP2			
	Cognitive Development HP3					
	Adverse Developmental Events HP3					
Social Domain	School Functioning HS1		Residential Stability CS1		Family/School/Social System Vulnerability VS	
	Family and Social Relationships HS2		Child/Youth Support CS2			
	Caregiver/Parent Health and Function HS3		Caregiver/Family Support CS3			
			School and Community Participation CS4			
Health System Domain	Access to Care HHS1		Getting Needed Services CHS1		Health System Impediments VHS	
	Treatment Experience HHS2		Coordination of Care CHS2			
Comments						
(Enter pertinent information about the reason for the score of each complexity item here. For example, poor patient adherence, many recent homes and schools, no child psychiatrist available to see child/youth, etc.)						

BIOLOGICAL DOMAIN

Actions related to items in the biological domain are intended to address barriers to improvement for physical conditions and their symptoms. In all situations, except anchor point 3 for item CB2, "Diagnostic/ Therapeutic Challenge," these items refer specifically to taking action related to physical health issues themselves. In fact, it is biomedical activity that forms the core of traditional case management, which focuses on correction of inconsistent adherence to evidence-based treatments for physical illness. Since the CB2 anchor point 3 includes nonphysical factors as a cause of physical symptoms, such as poor family support, Munchausen's by proxy, or a psychiatric illness, actions related to this item diverge from traditional case management and include assistance with items in other domains with, perhaps, cross-disciplinary (mental health) involvement and likely treatment.

In the current health care environment, few pediatricians are enthusiastic about addressing behavior-based issues without encouragement and assistance. Even in children/youth with what would be considered subsyndromal mental health symptoms (CP2), treating minor mental health symptoms can be the tipping point between persistent biological symptoms with treatment nonresponse and health stabilization with reduced impairment. In children/youth who score 3 on CB2, even when interacting CP2 or other nonbiological items are scored 1 or 2, clinicians should be encouraged to intervene related to the nonbiological items early in the integrated case management process as an indirect means of altering the 3 score on CB2.

HB1	Chronicity
1	**Physical symptoms/dysfunction present for more than 3 months**: ensure child's/youth's/caregiver's understanding of the persistent dysfunction; observe to see if the condition turns chronic with physical limitations; ensure pediatric follow-up
2	**A chronic condition**: review child's/youth's/caregiver's understanding of illness and treatment; ensure active and collaborative involvement by pediatrician and medical specialists, if needed; assess and ensure treatment of co-occurring mental conditions; ongoing assessment of child/youth symptoms and/or measured outcomes over time (e.g., respiratory function, FEV1, etc.); unfettered access to physical health and mental health records by all treating clinicians
3	**Several chronic conditions**: *immediately* perform actions under #2; include customized actions based on interview; review child's/youth's/caregiver's understanding of illnesses and treatments; confirm communication and coordination of care among practitioners about all conditions
HB2	Diagnostic dilemma
1	**Easy diagnoses**: observe for changes in clinical status
2	**Diagnostic dilemma solved with diagnostic effort**: review diagnoses, interventions, and treatments for fidelity with the child's/youth's course and improvement with treatment; assess attitude of child/youth/caregiver about diagnosis and workups and educate about process; bring in case management medical director to review if it is outside the case manager's level of expertise to get a big picture assessment of accuracy of diagnoses and treatment; medical director to clinician communication if needed and appropriate to discuss ways that case management can assist the patient and practitioner in improving outcomes; ensure assessment for concurrent mental conditions has been done and treatment is being given, if present; communicate current understanding with child/youth/caregiver
3	**Diagnostic dilemma not solved despite considerable diagnostic efforts**: *immediately* perform actions under #2; include customized actions based on interview; case manager serves as communication link among physicians caring for patient, the case management medical director, and the child/youth/caregiver to maintain collaboration and outcome orientation; seek child/youth/caregiver input about their thoughts on the unresolved problem
CB1	Symptom severity/impairment
1	**Mild symptoms; no functional impairment**: observe; review for less invasive, less expensive treatment options
2	**Moderate symptoms; impairment present**: ensure treatment provided is coordinated through efforts of the pediatrician and other care professionals with active involvement of mental health team for children/youth with comorbid mental conditions when they destabilize; ongoing assessment of child/youth symptoms over time (e.g., labs, X-rays, complications, etc.); unfettered access to physical health and mental condition records by all treating clinicians; evaluate caregiver and child/youth understanding of illness and impairment; educate; assist with support and recovery from impairment; with permission, share summary of health situation with school
3	**Severe symptoms leading to inability to perform many functional activities**: *immediately* perform actions under #1 and #2; include customized actions based on interview; assist with ongoing communication among practitioners; maximize adherence; enlist caregiver assistance; consider alternative treatment settings, living arrangements, rehabilitation services; augment home care availability; enlist case management medical director assistance and suggestions when needed; find out what works best for the child/youth

CB2	Diagnostic/therapeutic challenge
1	**Quick diagnoses expected with easy treatments**: observe for change in status
2	**Difficult to diagnose and treat; physical cause/origin; invasive treatment expected**: scrupulously ensure that child/youth is following through on evaluations and treatments; involve caregiver; make sure that all clinicians know the outcomes of exams and tests done by colleagues; assist in measuring outcomes of interventions; maintain communications with patient and clinical team; have case management medical director review case for additional ideas and talk to clinicians, if warranted; assist child/youth/caregiver in getting answers to questions about health from practitioners; consider setting up a case conference among clinicians
3	**Difficult to diagnose with psychological, social, economic issues clouding picture; toxic and/or multidisciplinary treatments**: *immediately* perform actions under #2 and customized actions based on interview; make sure that clinicians know about mental conditions, social, and health system factors that may be playing a role and that child/youth is seen in a timely fashion; have case management medical director talk with child/youth's clinicians about expanded differential and potential treatment; facilitate mental health referral through pediatrician if possible; include child/youth/caregiver in discussions about the role of nonphysical factors in symptoms/treatment
VB	Complications and life threat
1	**Mild risk of premature physical complications or limitations in activities of daily living**: ensure adherence to treatment and troubleshoot barriers that crop up; consider transfer back to standard care
2	**Moderate risk of premature physical complications or permanent and/or substantial limitations in activities of daily living**: follow through on adherence to treatment and troubleshoot barriers that crop up; establish continuity of physical and mental condition services, including needed environmental aids, respite care, and palliative care; stabilize communication and collaboration among providers and with child/youth/caregivers; establish methodology to follow clinically relevant outcomes with child/youth and clinicians (e.g., HbA1c, visits to emergency room, missed school, etc.); monitor with case management medical director through case conferences; consider intermittent long-term contact with patient
3	**Severe risk of physical complications and serious permanent functional deficits and/or dying**: perform actions under #2; include customized actions based on interview; ensure follow-through; intermittent long-term contact with patient until risks change; assist with hospice or long-term care, if appropriate

PSYCHOLOGICAL DOMAIN

Actions related to items in the psychological domain are intended to address barriers to improvement related to health behaviors, coping styles, prior mental conditions, and current psychiatric symptoms. Children/youth exposed to early biological or psychological insults, which lead to altered emotions, behaviors, or cognitions, may also require action on the part of the case manager.

Among historical items, actions related to "Cognitive Development" (HP3) are separated from "Mental Health History" (HP2) since they require special attention to educational needs and participation of the school system. Among current items on the other hand, actions associated with active cognitive difficulties are included under "Mental Health Symptoms" (CP2) since they more likely require behavioral rather than system-level intervention.

While "Adverse Developmental Events" (HP4) can result from mental health (e.g., sexual abuse) and physical (e.g., fetal alcohol syndrome, lead exposure) causes, actions related to them are included in the psychological domain since they are typically associated with emotional, cognitive, or behavioral interventions, though additional physical testing may be warranted. When exposure to toxins leads to active physical symptoms or impairments, actions would be initiated under "Symptom Severity/Impairment" (CB1) in the biological domain.

"Barriers to Coping" (HP1) are to be differentiated from "Mental Health Symptoms" (CP2) since they relate more to the ability of the child/youth to react to life stresses than to the demonstration of psychologically abnormal behaviors. Coping issues are generally handled by assisting the child/youth with learning more adaptive coping skills and modifying the child's/youth's exposure to stressful situations, if possible. When problems with coping are associated with dangerous behaviors, such as substance dependence or self-damaging actions, mental health conditions often coexist that also require intervention. Providers involved in the child's/youth's care should be kept aware of a child's/youth's stress handling capacity.

HP1	**Barriers to coping**
1	**Restricted coping skills**: active listening and child/youth/caregiver education; ensure/encourage counseling for child/youth in coping skills consider training in stress-reduction techniques (one to three sessions, often with a child/youth through school counselor)
2	**Impaired coping skills with frequent conflicts and/or substance abuse**: identify support for stressful situations; counseling on coping mechanisms; training in stress-reduction and conflict-resolution techniques (one to five sessions, often with a child/youth through the school counselor); involvement by caregiver and educational system to address school-related issues/stressors; adjustments in living/school location/activities, if appropriate; consider talking with pediatrician about substance abuse and/or mental health referral for assessment
3	**Minimal coping skills with dangerous behaviors**: *immediately* perform actions under #2; include customized actions based on interview; activate support system or crisis management for child/youth in collaboration with providers; mental health assessment and intervention (e.g., psychotherapy or medication); encourage substance abuse/dependence treatment referral
HP2	**Mental health history**
1	**Mental conditions resolved or without effect on life activities**: regular pediatric screens for mental conditions with intervention if appropriate; check for access to support from child/youth mental health professionals
2	**Mental conditions that interfered with life activities or required treatment**: ensure understanding of conditions by child/youth/caregiver in lay language; link medical and physical conditions, if indicated; ensure active and appropriate involvement by child psychiatrist and mental health team (psychologists, social workers, nurses, substance use disorder and other counselors, etc.) when conditions destabilize; primary maintenance and continuation of treatment provided by pediatrician (medical home) with mental health specialist assistance; ongoing assessment of patient symptoms over time; communication and unfettered access to physical and mental health records by all treating clinicians
3	**Psychiatric admissions and/or persistent effects on daily function**: *immediately* perform actions under #2; include customized actions based on interview; primary involvement and treatment by a mental health team for mental conditions working in close collaboration with pediatrician who cares for concurrent physical illness; when possible, physical and mental health personnel should be located and actively interact in integrated clinic settings
HP3	**Cognitive development**
1	**Possible developmental delay or immaturity/low IQ**: assist in establishing level of impairment, including capacity of child to communicate physical needs and symptoms; discuss level of impairment and needs with caregivers, educator, and the pediatrician to ensure appropriate placement in school system; assess need for remedial educational assistance and home support; observe
2	**Delayed development; mild or moderate mental retardation**: perform actions under #1; assist caregiver/parent and pediatrician in identifying appropriate educational placement and support; review performance/adjustment issues with school facility; involve social services if needed; assess and assist with home support for child/youth based on functional capabilities and respite for caregivers/parents; assess and share child's/youth's ability to communicate
3	**Severe and pervasive developmental delays or profound mental retardation**: *immediately* perform actions under #1 and #2; include customized action based on interview; work with caregiver, pediatrician, and other clinicians to ensure appropriate support for child/youth special needs; consider and assist with placement options, if necessary
HP4	**Adverse developmental events**
1	**Traumatic prior experiences/injuries with no impact on child/youth**: observe for previously unrecognized symptoms; inform pediatrician of traumatic experiences/injuries
2	**Traumatic prior experiences/injuries with impairment in child/youth**: encourage referral to medical specialist for toxic exposure/brain injury assessment and/or mental health specialist for consideration of psychological intervention; confirm no further exposure to toxic cause; discuss insult and potential consequences with caregiver, pediatrician, and case management medical director
3	**Traumatic prior experiences with significant impairment in child/youth**: *immediately* perform actions under #2; include customized actions based on interview; ensure toxic event outcomes are being addressed (e.g., therapy or other mental health treatment, change in living situation, etc.); report any suspected abuse
CP1	**Resistance to treatment**
1	**Ambivalence**: educate child/youth/caregivers about illnesses/treatments; discussion between case manager and child/youth/caregivers about resistant behaviors using motivational interviewing and problem-solving techniques to reduce resistance (activity best performed sensitively by the case manager or the child's/youth's practitioner when he or she has been informed of the problem); inform providers of adherence problems and work with them to consider alternative interventions

2	**Resistance, hostility, indifference**: perform actions under #1; include customized actions based on interview; review need for other health professional or clinic to provide care with case manager's medical director; explore source of resistance (e.g., anxiety, home situation, family members, religion, complicated by school setting, culture, relationship with treating physician—try to correct)
3	**Active resistance**: *immediately* perform actions under #1 and #2; include customized actions based on interview; work with treating clinicians in considering and instituting alternative interventions; if needed, work with case management medical director to find second opinion practitioners; if irresolvable and pervasive, consider discontinuation of case management; report concerns about the safety and well-being of the child (e.g., parent treatment refusal for life-threatening but treatable medical illness in minor)
CP2	**Mental health symptoms**
I	**Mild mental health symptoms**: ensure pediatric treatment with access to support from mental health professionals; unfettered access to physical and mental health records by all treating clinicians
2	**Moderate mental health symptoms**: perform actions under #1; ensure that acute, maintenance, and continuation treatment is being provided by the pediatrician with mental health support and backup; facilitate primary maintenance and continuation treatment provided by pediatrician (medical home) with mental health specialist assistance—that is, a child psychiatrist and mental health team (psychologists, social workers, nurses, substance abuse counselors, etc.) when conditions destabilize, become complicated, and/or demonstrate treatment resistance; institute symptom documentation recording system; ensure crisis plan
3	**Severe psychiatric symptoms and/or cognitive disturbances**: *immediately* perform actions under #1 and #2; include customized actions based on interview; active and aggressive treatment for mental conditions by a mental health team working in close collaboration with the pediatrician, who cares for concurrent physical illness; when possible, geographic colocation of physical and mental health personnel to facilitate ease of coordinating treatment; confirm persistent symptom documentation recording system; ensure physical and mental health treatment adherence
VP	**Learning and/or mental health threat**
I	**Mild risk of worsening mental health or cognitive symptoms**: ensure access to support; ensure/encourage continuous follow-up care with intermittent mental health assessments when appropriate; booster sessions for coping and stress reduction when needed; educate caregiver about importance of mental health treatment; consider transfer back to standard care
2	**Moderate risk of mental health disorder or more impaired cognitive functioning**: perform actions under #1; set up maintenance and continuity program that involves the treating pediatrician, clinical nurse specialists, and mental health specialists in the pediatric clinic; establish a regular symptom documentation system; assist with guidelines for increased mental health team involvement in the pediatric clinic to assist with treatment adjustments (best provided in an integrated pediatric clinic); address adherence and patient-provider relationship issues; involve caregivers in all activities after informed consent obtained
3	**Severe risk of persistent psychiatric disorder or cognitive impairment with frequent health service use**: perform actions under #1 and #2; include customized actions based on interview; confirm care continuity; establish verbal, paper, and electronic communication capabilities for all clinical professionals working with the patient; work with the patient's clinicians in establishing clinical goals with the patient; consider long-term involvement

SOCIAL DOMAIN

Actions related to items in the family/social domain are intended to address barriers to improvement related to difficulties in forming relationships; establishing social connectedness and support; and functioning in a community, the school setting, and with peers. Actions in this domain also include those related to the child's/youth's primary caregivers'/parents' health and function and their support system. In these latter two content areas, actions are often directed specifically at helping to improve the situation of the caregiver, rather than the child/youth, since deficits in either can create barriers to optimal health for the child/youth.

The focus of the family/social domain is on ensuring the optimal health and well-being of the child/youth, though it includes the assessment of complexity issues related to the caregiver/parent. To the extent that the child/youth case manager can address caregiver/parent-related barriers to improvement within a reasonable time frame, they should be included in the actions of the case manager. There are, however, some situations in which the needs of the caregiver/parent are so severe that they are in excess of the time available for the case manager to effect change. In such situations, the caregiver/parent should be assigned his or her own case manager or should be connected with community resources in an effort to obtain needed assistance. Since this is not always possible, involvement of child protective services for the child/youth may be necessary.

In several family/social domain items—for example, "Family and Social Relationships" (HS2), "Caregiver/Parent Health and Function" (HS3), and "Residential Stability" (CS1)—the level of child/youth need may be due to dangerous caregiver/parent actions.

In these situations, the case manager may be required either by law or necessity to personally report or to work with the treating practitioners in reporting to oversight authorities situations that are dangerous to the child/youth. In these situations, it is important for case managers, who are health professionals with legal reporting obligations, to know when and how to take action when it is necessary.

HS1	School functioning
1	**Average to poor school performance and peer associations**: observe and initiate assistance mechanism if needed
2	**Disrupted school activity:** talk with child/youth, caregiver, and school officials to clarify cause of situation; consider assisting with care conference; assist in setting up help through school counselor; inform pediatrician of school-related activity
3	**Destructive school activity**: *immediately* perform actions under #2; include customized actions based on interview; assist pediatrician with referral for mental health assessment; assist in setting up conference with caregiver, school, pediatrician, and other health professionals about alternative schooling possibilities, corrective actions; involve case management medical director if needed
HS2	Family and social relationships
1	**Mild family problems; good social and peer relationships**: observe interpersonal difficulties during patient interviews and adjust recommendations to accommodate for limitations (e.g., introversion, family discord, etc.)
2	**Significant level of family problems; limited social and peer relationships**: encourage social skills training (one to six sessions, often with a counselor, include how to talk about health issues); family therapy; foster involvement with family, peers, school, social service, or legal system; assess impact of family problems on child/youth health issues (address if present); explore alternative socialization opportunities
3	**Severe family problems; no social or peer relationships**: *immediately* perform actions under #1 and #2; include customized actions based on interview; ensure social skills training; address bullying situation; consider school change, altered living situation; encourage mental health assessment and treatment if appropriate and/or needed through pediatrician; initiate family protective services and remediation if appropriate; report any suspected abuse
HS3	Caregiver/parent health and function
1	**Poor health and/or impairment in at least one caregiver with minimal impact on child's/youth's health**: document health and/or parental issue; share concern with case management medical director, school, and treating pediatrician as needed; observe child/youth and caregiver interactions to ensure minimal negative impact on child/youth; if appropriate provide suggestions and support to affected caregiver for deficits
2	**Poor health and/or impairment in at least one caregiver impacting child's/youth's health**: perform actions under #1 but also assist caregiver in obtaining services and/or intervention for deficits; include customized actions based on interview; consider working with pediatrician to involve social services, counseling, medical assistance, other medical providers, and so forth; review need for social skills training or conflict management
3	**Poor caregiver health and/or impairment with serious supervision deficits and/or danger for the child/youth**: *immediately* perform actions under #2; include customized actions based on interview; work with pediatrician and/or social service to determine need for corrective action; facilitate the initiation of child protective services; assist caregiver in obtaining services and/or intervention for deficits, including physical and/or mental health care; report any suspected abuse
CS1	Residential stability
1	**Inconsistent living situation**: make sure that child's/youth's safety, supervision, and nourishment needs are being met
2	**Unstable housing and/or living situation support**: in collaboration with the caregivers if possible, initiate contact with social service or other community resources to look into housing and food services options; get assistance to help correct the cause of the residential instability (e.g., financial limitations, family conflict, natural disaster, etc.); inquire about outcome; use knowledge of community resources to push the system
3	**Unsafe housing situation for child/youth**: *immediately* involve protective services to locate a safe living situation for the child/youth (e.g., foster home, youth facility); perform actions under #2; include customized actions based on interview; report concerns with the safety and well-being of the child

CS2	Child/youth support
1	**Supervision and/or assistance generally available but possible delays**: initiate assistance mechanism if needed
2	**Limited supervision and/or assistance readily available**: talk with child/youth's caregivers; consider talking with peer families for support; set up with social services or other agency to assist child/youth in finding needed community resources; assist caregiver/parent in correcting supervision disruption; follow up on outcome; use knowledge of community resources to push the system; involve pediatrician and other health professionals in remedying situation
3	**No supervision and/or assistance readily available**: *immediately* perform actions under #2; include customized actions based on interview; involve child protection to assist with placement in an alternative location (e.g., foster home, group home, friend's house, relative's house); report any suspected abuse
CS3	Caregiver/family support
1	**Assistance generally available but possible delays**: initiate assistance mechanism if needed
2	**Limited assistance readily available**: talk with needy caregiver's available personal contacts about what they can do to assist the caregiver; set up with social services or other agency to assist parent/caregiver find needed community resources, adjust work situation, and so forth; follow up on outcome; use knowledge of community resources to push the system; share situation with health professionals
3	**No assistance readily available**: *immediately* perform actions under #2; include customized actions based on interview; consider social services or individualized case management assistance for caregiver
CS4	School and community participation
1	**Missing up to one day of school/week and few extracurricular activities**: explore interests, hobbies with the child/youth and encourage initiation of activity; involve caregiver/parent in assisting child/youth to attend school more regularly and develop peer activities
2	**Missing average of 2 or more days of school/week with resistance to extracurricular activities**: assess reasons for resistance with child/youth, caregiver, and school; clarify school's understanding of child/youth health needs; assess reasons for peer activity nonparticipation, including health of child/youth; share information with pediatrician; collaborate with caregiver, educators, child/youth, and care providers in developing a remedial plan
3	**School nonattendance with no extracurricular activities or community connections**: *immediately* perform actions under #1 and #2; include customized actions based on interview; explore alternative ways to interact with peers; consider case management conference with caregivers, school personnel, pediatrician, mental health professionals, and others and work with them on potential solutions; follow through on initiated activities
VS	Family/school/social system vulnerability
1	**Some risk of housing, family, school, social needs**: see if current location can accommodate potential need; consider transfer back to standard care
2	**Risk of need for alteration in housing, family, school, social situation in the foreseeable future**: continue to work with family and pediatrician; assist, engage, and push social services and school to find resources and make ready the procedures for help and/or placement; follow up on outcome; use knowledge of community resources to push the system
3	**Risk of need for alteration in housing, family, school, social situation now and for the foreseeable future**: perform actions under #2; include customized actions based on interview; attempt to set up long-term social service assistance; consider long-term case management until situation stabilizes

HEALTH SYSTEM DOMAIN

Actions related to items in the health system domain are intended to correct barriers to care access at a system level, to repair child/youth- and/or caregiver/parent-doctor interactions, to help children/youth get needed health services, and to ensure that the clinicians treating the child/youth talk with each other and coordinate their care so that the child/youth returns to optimal health.

Health system domain actions should be customized to the health business practices used in each country so that barriers to care can be systematically corrected.

HHS1	**Access to care**
1	**Some limitation in accessing care**: assist in identifying culturally sensitive willing providers, interpretation of services, and ensuring timely appointments
2	**Difficulties in accessing care**: work with child/youth/caregiver in finding health insurance, in identifying culturally sensitive willing providers, and in ensuring timely appointments (use conference calls if necessary); assist in flexing benefits (with health plan) when possible to get appropriate care (go up the supervisory ladder); connect physical and mental health support for services; assist with appeals of inappropriately denied care (use case management medical director, if necessary)
3	**No adequate access to care**: *immediately* perform actions under #2; include customized actions based on interview; enlist social service to assist with actions in #2 and in finding insurance product or general assistance clinic; assist with post-emergency room and hospitalization follow-up locations; advocate for child/youth
HHS2	**Treatment experience**
1	**Negative child/youth or caregiver experience with health care providers**: assess for adherence to assessment and treatment recommendations; periodically ask about current relationship with clinical staff; help with asking questions of practitioners
2	**Child/youth and/or caregivers dissatisfaction with or distrust of doctors; multiple and/or inconsistent providers**: assess types of conflicts with practitioners; adjudicate conflict when possible (directly or indirectly); foster communication between child/youth/caregiver and practitioner about conflicts; assist in getting to a preferred provider if possible where outcomes would be better; involve case management medical director for assistance
3	**Repeated major child/youth or caregiver conflicts with or distrust of doctors, frequent emergency room visits, or involuntary admissions**: *immediately* perform actions under #2; include customized actions based on interview; assist in finding someone to work with child/youth or caregiver/parent on conflict-resolution techniques; involve the case management medical director to talk with practitioners about relationship; consider assisting child/youth and caregiver/parent in finding another professional or location of care; mental health consultation to assess for personality or chemical dependence issues contributing to conflict
CHS1	**Getting needed services**
1	**Some difficulties getting to appointments or needed services**: review correlation of disorders with treatment being given; check for barriers; assist with finding money for medications and needed services
2	**Routine difficulties in coordinating and/or getting to appointments or needed services**: assess alternative care locations and practitioner availability; review options with the child/youth/caregiver and ensure timely access; consider accessing services through telemedicine; assist with finding money for medications and needed services; help child/youth get same-day appointments for different problems; check for flexibility in current clinic system; help child/youth and caregiver find needed medical and mental health specialists and set up appointments (out of region if necessary); review difficulties with pediatrician (medical home)
3	**Inability to coordinate and/or get to appointments or needed services**: *immediately* perform actions under #2; include customized actions based on interview; establish pediatric medical home; work with pediatrician (or specialty physician) to coordinate services (e.g., diabetologist for brittle diabetic child/youth); assist with transportation for child/youth/caregiver and coordination of assessments/follow-ups; enlist assistance of community agencies and social services
CHS2	**Coordination of care**
1	**Limited practitioner communication and coordination of care**: encourage record sharing and communication among all clinicians, including mental health and complementary medicine; open links for important communication
2	**Poor communication and coordination of care among practitioners**: determine and augment communication links between physical and mental health practitioners; ensure note sharing among clinicians working with child/youth; assist in coordinating appointments and transportation; investigate availability of integrated clinics (medical home); assist with transition from pediatric care to adult practitioner care
3	**No communication and coordination of care among practitioners**: *immediately* perform actions under #1 and #2; include customized actions based on interview; serve as link for child/youth with various practitioners (i.e., fax accumulated clinical information to practitioners after release of information obtained); talk with treating practitioners on behalf of child/youth but also educate caregivers/parents on how to do so; consider setting up case conferences with treating providers; create alternatives to emergency room use; enlist assistance from case management medical director to try to establish a medical home
VHS	**Health system impediments**
1	**Mild risk of impediments to care**: ensure insurance benefits cover health needs; assist in maintaining coverage; review practitioner communication procedures; consider transfer back to standard care

2	**Moderate risk of impediments to care**: work with child/youth/caregiver, practitioner providing medical home, social services, and community agencies to establish the best health set-up possible in the region; assist in finding insurance products, needed providers, and communicating clinic systems; pay special attention to physical and mental health links
3	**Severe risk of impediments to care**: perform actions under #2; include customized actions based on interview; help child/youth and caregiver find and establish a medical home that will persist over time; assist in overcoming barriers to practitioner involvement with child/youth; consider setting up a physical and mental health clinicians case conference; attempt to enlist assistance of community-based case manager (public health); ensure insurance benefits cover health needs; assist in maintaining coverage; review and assist with practitioner communication procedures

Care Plan Development (CD)

BARRIERS	GOALS		ACTIONS
CAG items	*"Personal goals" followed by "health care goals"*		*Prioritized*
	Short-term		
	Ultimate		
	Short-term		
	Ultimate		
	Short-term		
	Ultimate		
	Short-term		
	Ultimate		
	Short-term		
	Ultimate		
	Short-term		
	Ultimate		
	Short-term		
	Ultimate		

Record of Outcome Measures (ROM)

OUTCOME MEASURES		BASELINE	FOLLOW-UP ASSESSMENTS		
	Time period recorded	Initial	2nd	3rd	4th
Clinical measure (personal goal)					
Functional measure (personal goal)					
Health-related quality of life					
Patient satisfaction					
CAG score					
Health care clinical measure (1)					
Health care clinical measure (2)					
Health care functional measure (1)					
Health care functional measure (2)					
Health care economic measure					

Measurement of Progress (MP3)

	GOAL	ACTION	OUTCOME
Barrier *CAG Item(s)* *#____*			
Barrier *CAG Item(s)* *#____*			
Barrier *CAG Item(s)* *#____*			
Barrier *CAG Item(s)* *#____*			
Barrier *CAG Item(s)* *#____*			

Abbreviations

AA:	Alcoholics Anonymous
ABI/TBI:	acute brain injury/traumatic brain injury
ACE:	angiotensin-converting enzyme
ACT:	assertive community treatment
CBT:	cognitive behavioral therapy
CAG:	Complexity Assessment Grid
CCM:	certified case manager
CHF:	congestive heart failure
CI:	confidence interval
CM:	case management
CMSA:	Case Management Society of America
CNS:	central nervous system
COPD:	chronic obstructive pulmonary disease
CPT:	current procedural terminology
CT:	computed tomography
CVD:	cardiovascular disease
DM:	disease management
DSM-IV-R:	*Diagnostic and Statistical Manual of Mental Disorders*-Revised, 4th edition
Dx:	diagnosis
EAP:	employee assistance program
EEG:	electroencephalogram
ER:	emergency room
FEV1:	forced expiratory volume at 1 second
GAD-7:	Generalized Anxiety Disorder Symptom Scale
GP:	general practitioner
HbA1c:	hemoglobin A1c
HIV:	human immunodeficiency virus
HM:	health (care) management
IBNR:	incurred but not reported
ICD-9:	*International Classification of Disease*, 9th edition
IM-CAG:	INTERMED-Complexity Assessment Grid

INF:	infection
INTERMED:	original name for the European version of the IM-CAG
IT:	information technology
LOS:	length of stay
MH:	mental health
MH/SUD:	mental health/substance use disorder
MI:	myocardial infarction
NIAAA:	National Institutes of Alcohol Abuse and Alcoholism
NIH:	National Institutes of Health
OR:	odds ratio
PC:	primary care
PCP:	primary care physician
PERFS:	peak expiratory flow rates
PH:	physical health
PHI:	personal health information
PHQ-2:	Patient Health Questionnaire-2
PHQ-9:	Patient Health Questionnaire-9
PIM-CAG:	Pediatric INTERMED Complexity Assessment Grid
PMPM:	per member, per month
PTSD:	posttraumatic stress disorder
RBRVS:	Resource-Based Relative Value Scale
RN:	registered nurse
ROI:	return on investment
RVU:	relative value units
Rx:	treatment
SMI:	serious mental illness
SPMI:	serious and persistent mental illness
SSRI:	selective serotonin reuptake inhibitor (class of antidepressant and antianxiety agents)
SUD:	substance use disorder
TTM:	transtheoretical model
UM:	utilization management

Definition of Terms

Acuity: related to the recentness with which an illness has shown presentation or increase in symptoms.

Age of consent: the minimum age at which a person is considered to be legally competent of consenting to sexual acts.

Age of majority: a legal definition that means that a person is legally an adult and responsible for the majority of his or her actions.

Allopathic medicine: the broad category of medical practice that is sometimes called Western medicine, which includes all medical disciplines represented in standard medical school curricula.

Care management: for purposes of this manual, this term is intended to encompass all forms of management activity, including health coaching (wellness), employee assistance, disability management and workers' compensation management, disease management, and case management. It is considered synonymous with "health management."

Child abuse and neglect: any type of cruelty inflicted on a child, including mental abuse, physical harm, neglect, and sexual abuse or exploitation.

Clinician: any clinical-based health care professional who assists the patient in receiving interventions that will lead to better clinical outcomes, such as nurse, social worker, counselor, pharmacist, doctor, and so forth in a clinical helper role, such as treating practitioner, case or disease manager, therapy provider, medication advisors, and so forth. Hospital or health plan administrators are not clinicians since they are not clinical-based health care professionals. Utilization managers, even though most often clinical-based health care professionals, are not clinicians since they are not functioning in a helper role.

Comorbidity: the occurrence of two or more illnesses or conditions in the same patient.

Complexity: the combination of biological, psychological, social, and health system circumstances that create barriers to improvement, making it difficult for a person with illness to regain or stabilize health.

Countertransference: a clinician's emotional reaction to a particular patient (psychiatric jargon).

Emancipated minor: a child who has been granted the status of adulthood by a court order or other formal arrangement.

Employee assistance program (EAP): employer-supported programs designed to assist employees with issues that lead to or perpetuate disability in an attempt to support health and reduce lost productivity.

Flex benefits: insurance contracts include specific language that describes the type of clinical services that are covered (i.e., the benefits in the plan). In most situations, there is no capability to adjust these benefits once the insurance contract has been signed during the contract period. The ability to flex benefits refers to permission given by the owner of the insurance contract—such as the health plan (fully insured) or employer (self insured)—to alter some components of the contract to meet the needs of a person covered under the contract. For instance, unused inpatient benefits could be used to extend the number of outpatient treatments or to support payment for case management services.

Generalized Anxiety Disorder-7 (GAD-7): standardized symptom scale for anxiety.

Health complexity: the interference with standard care by the interaction of biological, psychological, social, and health system factors. It includes two components, *case* and *care* complexity and requires a shift from standard (biomedical) care to individualized (integrated) care in order for patient outcomes to improve.

Hot transfer: the enrollment specialist keeps the patient on the line while the case manager who will be assuming responsibility for the case is brought on the line, personally introduced, and a short summary of the situation is given.

Individualized care: connecting a health professional with a general understanding of illnesses, treatments, the health system, and factors that create barriers to improvement, such as a case manager, to a patient/client with persistent health problems in an attempt to actively and personally assist him or her stabilize or return to health over a period of days to years. This form of care is patient-centered, focusing on all complexity domains, with an outcome orientation.

Insourced benefits: in the context of this manual, it refers to the process by which a medical health plan chooses to own (i.e., carve in) its behavioral health business for the people for whom it writes insurance rather than allowing an independent behavioral health insurer to manage and pay for behavioral health services used. This is a step toward integrating benefits, in which the medical health plan not only owns behavioral health management and payment (i.e. the adjudication of behavioral health claims) but actually makes mental health claims a part of the physical health benefits and adjudication process. Mental health and physical health claims are handled using the same rules and business procedures.

Integrated behavioral health benefits: in the context of this manual, it refers to the process by which a medical health plan not only owns behavioral health management and payment but also makes it a part of the physical health benefits and adjudication process.

Integrated care: for purposes of this manual, this term applies to the availability of coordinated health services from all complexity domains (biological, psychological, social, and health system) without hassle or impediment.

Likert scale: a question on a survey in which respondents answer by specifying their level of agreement to a statement with a fixed number of discrete, mutually exclusive options (e.g., a = strongly disagree; b = disagree; c = neutral; d = agree; e = strongly agree).

Long-term disability: generally employees with permanent conditions, requiring time away from work for more than 6 months and little likelihood of improvement; when long-term disability is supported by a documentable medical condition, (a) the disabled person is paid a percentage of his or her prior salary, (b) he or she must document persistence of disabling signs and symptoms over time, and (c) the employer has no obligation to take the person back to his or her prior position (unemployed—disabled).

Multimorbidity: the occurrence of multiple illnesses or conditions in the same patient.

Odds ratio: the likelihood of occurrence in relationship to a reference group (e.g., an odds ration of 2 for a heart attack in patients with high lipids means that those with high lipids are twice as likely to have a heart attack as those without).

Patient Health Questionnaire-9 (PHQ-9): standardized symptom scale for depression.

Prepopulate: a software capability in which data from an existing dataset automatically populates fields in a different but linked database (e.g., demographic information, laboratory results, diagnoses, admission dates, etc.) to prevent the need to spend time re-entering existing data.

Relative value unit (RVU) payment: This is payment based on the relative cost of doing the assessment and intervention, setting up the practice so that necessary components are available to support it, and the average cost of liability coverage associated with the services provided. (RVU work) + (RVU practice expense) + (RVU liability).

Severity: the seriousness of an illness; this is a component of complexity.

Short-term disability (STD): time-limited illness in an employee that prevents his or her ability to work (usually 6 months or less); during this time the employee retains his or her job, is paid during the time away from work, and cannot be fired or permanently replaced (employed—disabled).

Subthreshold symptoms: psychiatric symptoms reach threshold when they are sufficiently robust to allow a care professional to make a diagnosis of a psychiatric disorder, suggesting that specific treatments may be of value. When patients experience mental health symptoms (e.g., anxiety, sadness, obsessive behaviors, etc.) that influence thoughts and behavior but do not warrant a diagnosis, they are considered subthreshold.

Transference: the patient's emotional reaction to a clinician, which is hypothesized to emanate from relationships with others (psychiatric jargon).

Utilization management: the practice of approving or denying payment for services based on presence of covered benefit or medical necessity; this is *not* considered a form of care or health management.

European INTERMED in English: IM-CAG v6

BIOLOGICAL DOMAIN

Chronicity (History)
0. Less than 3 months of physical dysfunction
1. More than 3 months of physical dysfunction or several periods of less than 3 months
2. A chronic disease
3. Several chronic diseases

Diagnostic Dilemma (History)
0. No periods of diagnostic complexity
1. Diagnosis and etiology was clarified quickly
2. Diagnostic dilemma solved but only with considerable diagnostic effort
3. Diagnostic dilemma not solved despite considerable diagnostic efforts

Symptom Severity/Impairment (Current State)
0. No symptoms or symptoms reversible without intensive medical efforts
1. Mild but notable symptoms, which do not interfere with current functioning
2. Moderate to severe symptoms, which interfere with current functioning
3. Severe symptoms leading to inability to perform any functional activities

Diagnostic/Therapeutic Challenge (Current State)
0. Clear diagnoses and/or uncomplicated treatment
1. Clear differential diagnoses and/or diagnosis expected with clear treatments
2. Difficult to diagnose and treat, physical cause/origin and treatment expected
3. Difficult to diagnose or treat, other issues than physical causes interfering with the diagnostic and therapeutic process

Complications and Life Threat (Vulnerabilities)
0. No risk of limitations in activities of daily living
1. Mild risk of limitations in activities of daily living
2. Moderate risk of permanent or substantial limitations of activities in daily living
3. Severe risk of physical complications with serious permanent functional deficits or dying

PSYCHOLOGICAL DOMAIN

Barriers to Coping (History)
0. Ability to manage stress, such as through support seeking or hobbies
1. Restricted coping skills, such as need of control, illness denial, or irritability
2. Impaired coping skills, such as nonproductive complaining or substance abuse but without serious impact on medical condition, mental health, or social situation
3. Minimal coping skills, manifest by destructive behaviors, such as substance dependence, psychiatric illness, self-mutilation, or attempted suicide

Psychiatric Dysfunction (History)
0. No psychiatric dysfunction
1. Psychiatric dysfunction without clear effects on daily function
2. Psychiatric dysfunction with clear effects on daily function
3. Psychiatric admission(s) and/or permanent effects on daily function

Resistance to Treatment (Current State)
0. Interested in receiving treatment and willing to cooperate actively
1. Some ambivalence though willing to cooperate with treatment
2. Considerable resistance, such as nonadherence with hostility or indifference toward health care professionals or treatments
3. Active resistance to medical care

Psychiatric Symptoms (Current State)
0. No psychiatric symptoms
1. Mild psychiatric symptoms, such as problems with concentration or feeling tense
2. Moderate psychiatric symptoms, such as anxiety, depression or mild cognitive impairment
3. Severe psychiatric symptoms or behavioral disturbances, such as violence, self-inflicted harm, delirium, psychosis, or mania

Mental Health Threat (Vulnerabilities)
0. No risk of psychiatric disorder
1. Mild risk of psychiatric symptoms, such as stress, anxiety, feeling blue, substance abuse or cognitive disturbance; mild risk of treatment resistance (ambivalence)
2. Moderate risk of psychiatric disorder requiring psychiatric care; moderate risk of treatment resistance
3. Severe risk of psychiatric disorder requiring frequent emergency room visits or hospital admissions; risk of refusal of treatment for serious psychiatric disorder

SOCIAL DOMAIN

Job and Leisure Problems (History)
0. A job (including housekeeping, retirement, studying) and having leisure activities
1. A job (including housekeeping, retirement, studying) without leisure activities
2. Unemployed now and for at least 6 month with leisure activities
3. Unemployed now and for at least 6 month without leisure activities

Social Dysfunction (History)
0. No social disruption
1. Mild social dysfunction; interpersonal problems
2. Moderate social dysfunction, such as inability to initiate or maintain social relations
3. Severe social dysfunction, such as involvement in disruptive social relations or social isolation

Residential Instability (Current State)
0. Stable housing; fully capable of independent living
1. Stable housing with support of others (e.g., family, home care, or an institutional setting)
2. Unstable housing (e.g., no support at home or living in a shelter); change of current living situation is required
3. No current satisfactory housing (e.g., transient housing or dangerous environment); immediate change is necessary

Poor Social Support (Current State)
0. Assistance readily available from family, friends, or acquaintances, such as work colleagues, at all times
1. Assistance available from family, friends, or acquaintances, such as work colleagues, but possible delays
2. Limited assistance readily available from family, friends, or acquaintances, such as work colleagues
3. No assistance readily available from family, friends, or acquaintances, such as work colleagues, at all times

Social Vulnerability (Vulnerabilities)
0. No risk of changes in the living situation; adequate social support and integration
1. No risk of changes in the living situation but additional social support or increased integration is needed (e.g., home health care)
2. Risk of need for temporary or permanent admission to facility/institution in the foreseeable future
3. Risk of need for temporary or permanent admission to facility/institution now

HEALTH SYSTEM DOMAIN

Access to Care (History)
0. Adequate access to care
1. Some limitation in access to care due to insurance problems, geographical reasons, language, or cultural barriers
2. Difficulties in access to care due to insurance problems, geographical reasons, language, or cultural barriers
3. No adequate access to care due to insurance problems, geographical reasons, language, or cultural barriers

Treatment Experience (History)
0. No problems with healthcare professionals
1. Negative experience with healthcare professionals (self or relatives)
2. Requests for second opinions or changing doctors more than once; multiple providers; trouble keeping consistent or preferred provider(s)
3. Repeated conflicts with doctors, frequent emergency room visits, or involuntary admissions; forced to stay with undesirable provider because of cost, provider network options, or other reasons

Organization of Care (Current State)
0. Primary care/general practitioner only
1. Specialist services either in general health care or mental health/substance use disorder care
2. Both general health care and mental health/substance use disorder services
3. Hospitalization or transfer from a hospital of patients, who qualify in ambulatory care on Level 2

Coordination of Care (Current State)
0. Complete practitioner communication and good coordination of care
1. Limited practitioner communication and coordination of care; primary care physician coordinates medical and mental health/substance use disorder services
2. Poor communication and coordination of care among practitioners; no routine primary care physician
3. No communication and coordination of care among practitioners; primary emergency room use to meet non-emergent health needs

Health System Impediments (Vulnerabilities)
0. No risk of impediments to coordinated physical and mental health/substance use disorder care
1. Mild risk of impediments to care (e.g., insurance restrictions, distant service access, limited provider communication or care coordination)
2. Moderate risk of impediments to care (e.g., potential insurance loss, inconsistent practitioners, communication barriers)
3 Severe risk of impediments to care (e.g., little or no insurance, resistance to communication and coordination among providers)

Index